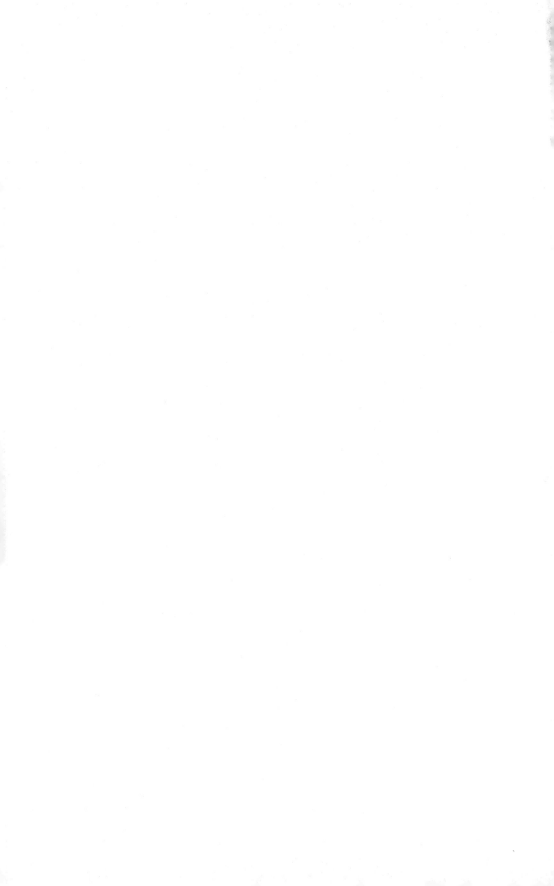

UPDATE IN INTENSIVE CARE MEDICINE

Series Editor: Jean-Louis Vincent

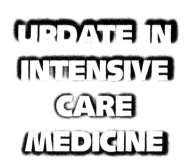

Springer Science+Business Media, LLC

MECHANICAL VENTILATION AND WEANING

Volume Editors:

Jordi Mancebo, MD
Associate Professor of Medicine
Hospital de la Sante Creu i Sant Pau
Servei de Medicina Intensiva
Barcelona, Spain

Alvar Net, MD
Professor of Medicine
Hospital de la Sante Creu i Sant Pau
Servei de Medicina Intensiva
Barcelona, Spain

Laurent Brochard, MD
Professor of Medicine
Hôpital Henri Mondor
Service Réanimation Médicale
Créteil, France

Series Editor:

Jean-Louis Vincent, MD, PhD, FCCM, FCCP
Head, Department of Intensive Care
Erasme University Hospital
Brussels, Belgium

With 85 Figures and 26 Tables

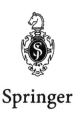

Springer

Jordi Mancebo, MD
Associate Professor of Medicine
Hospital de la Sante Creu i Sant Pau
Servei de Medicina Intensiva
Av. S.A. Maria Claret 167
08025 Barcelona, Spain

Alvar Net, MD
Professor of Medicine
Hospital de la Sante Creu i Sant Pau
Servei de Medicina Intensiva
Av. S.A. Maria Claret 167
08025 Barcelona, Spain

Laurent Brochard, MD
Professor of Medicine
Service Réanimation Médicale
Hôpital Henri Mondor
51, Av. Du M^{al} de Lattre de Tassigny
F-94010 Créteil cedex, France

Series Editor:
Jean-Louis Vincent, MD, PhD, FCCM, FCCP
Head, Department of Intensive Care
Erasme University Hospital
Route de Lennik 808
B-1070 Brussels, Belgium

Cataloging-in-Publication Data applied for

Die Deutsche Bibliothek - CIP-Einheitsaufnahme
Mechanical ventilation and weaning : with 26 tables / vol. ed.: Jordi Mancebo .... - New York ; Berlin ;
Heidelberg ; Hong Kong ; London ; Milan ; Paris ; Tokyo : Springer, 2003
(Update in intensive care medicine)
    ISBN 978-3-540-44181-6   ISBN 978-3-642-56112-2 (eBook)
    DOI 10.1007/978-3-642-56112-2

Printed on acid-free paper.

© 2003 Springer Science+Business Media New York
Originally published by Springer-Verlag New York, Inc. in 2003

Production managed by PRO EDIT GmbH, Heidelberg, Germany.
Typeset by TBS, Sandhausen, Germany.

9 8 7 6 5 4 3 2 1

Foreword

Do we really need a new book on mechanical ventilation? Initially, I thought: certainly not! This field of medicine is indeed moving rapidly, but clinicians have been given several excellent books in the recent past. However, when I went through this one, I was struck by a strong feeling of *jamais vu*. Indeed, it is focused mainly on new, difficult, practical issues such as complications of mechanical ventilation (Serrano, Esteban), patient-ventilator interaction, weaning, non-invasive ventilation, or artificial intelligence. Most of the members of the ventilator fan club are here, from Europe – a strong contributor – to North America, tracing an unexpected map where the capitals are St. Paul, Winnipeg, Barcelona, Créteil, Nashville, Boston and Pavia.

Subtleties of assisted modes are explained, including the still exotic PAV (Younes), from some very trivial but essential issues – what to do when the patient fights the ventilator (Tobin) – to the most sophisticated physiopathology (Sassoon). One major section is devoted to weaning. Weaning-induced cardiac failure is revisited (Jubran, Ferrer), as are all predictive tests (Mancebo, Epstein, Fernandez). Many of those who have recently contributed the most in this field are there: Ely and Epstein, who taught us that systematic and repetitive use of algorithms is better than plain medical judgement; Betbesé, who interpreted unplanned extubations; Tobin and Jubran, who did the same for shallow breathing. Another highlight is non-invasive ventilation, the new paradigm that is expanding so rapidly these days. The magic triangle here is clearly Créteil–Barcelona–Pavia. Finally, the opening to the future is represented by the fascinating knowledge-based system, recently implemented into a ventilator, which achieves the most ancient dream of ventilator users, an intelligent, auto-controlled machine....

Créteil   F. Lemaire

Contents

List of Contributors

Charles G. Alex
Associate Professor of Medicine, Division of Pulmonary and Critical Care Medicine, Loyola University of Chicago Stritch School of Medicine, Department of Veterans Affairs, Edward Hines Jr. Hospital, Hines, Illinois, USA

Inmaculada Alía Robledo
Assistant Physician, Intensive Care Unit, University Hospital of Getafe, Madrid, Spain

A.J. Betbesé
Servei de Medicina Intensiva, Hospital de la Santa Creu i Sant Pau, Av. S.A. Maria Claret 167, 08025 Barcelona, Spain

Lluis Blanch
Intensive Care Department, Hospital de Sabadell, Corporacio Parc Tauli, Parc Tauli s/n, 08208 Sabadell, Spain

Lucie Breton
Service de Réanimation Médicale, Hôpital Charles Nicolle, 1 rue de Germont, 76031 Rouen Cedex, France

Laurent Brochard
Hôpital Henri Mondor, Service Réanimation Médicale, 51 Avenue Du M^{al} de Lattre de Tassigny, 94010 Créteil, France

Kota G. Chetty
Department of Medicine, Veterans Affairs Medical Center, and the University of California, Irvine, California, USA

Christophe Delclaux
Servei de Medicina Intensiva, Hospital de Sant Pau, Universitat Autònoma de Barcelona, Av. S.A.M. Claret 167, 08025 Barcelona, Spain

Michel Dojat
Inserm U492, Hôpital Henri Moudor, 94010 Créteil, France

E. Wesley Ely
Division on Allergy, Pulmonary, and Critical Care Medicine, The Vanderbilt University Medical Center, 913 Oxford House, Nashville, TN 37232-4760, USA

Scott K. Epstein
New England Medical Center, Box 369, 750 Washington St., Boston, MA 02111, USA

Andrés Esteban de la Torre
Head of Department, Intensive Care Unit, University Hospital of Getafe,
Madrid, Spain

Patrick J. Fahey
Professor of Medicine, Chief, Department of Medicine,
Department of Veterans Affairs, Edward Hines, Jr. Hospital, Associate Chairman,
Department of Medicine, Loyola University of Chicago Stritch School of Medicine,
Hines, Illinois, USA

Rafael Fernández
Intensive Care Service, Hospital de Sabadell,
Parc Tauli s/n, 08208 Sabadell, Spain

Miquel Ferrer
UVIR. Servei de Pneumologia, Institut Clínic de Pneumologia i Cirurgia
Toràcica, Hospital Clínic, Villarroel 170, 08036 Barcelona, Spain

Fernando Frutos Vivar
Assistant Physician, Intensive Care Unit, University Hospital of Getafe,
Madrid, Spain

T. Scott Gallacher
Department of Medicine, Veterans Affairs Medical Center,
and the University of California, Irvine, California, USA

Isabel Illa
Neuromuscular Division, Department of Neurology,
Hospital de la Sta. Creu i St. Pau, C/Sant Antoni Mª Claret, 167,
08025 Barcelona, Spain

Amal Jubran
Division of Pulmonary and Critical Care Medicine, Edward Hines Jr.,
Veterans Affairs Hospital and Loyola University of Chicago Stritch School
of Medicine, Hines, IL 60141, USA

Sait Karakurt
Marmara University Hospital, Pulmonary and Critical Care Medicine,
81110 Istanbul, Turkey

Erwan L'Her
Réanimation et Urgences Médicales, CHU de la Cavale Blanche, Brest, France

Jordi Mancebo
Servei de Medicina Intensiva, Hospital de la Santa Creu i Sant Pau,
Av. S.A. Maria Claret 167, 08025 Barcelona, Spain

Albana Manka
Department of Medicine, Veterans Affairs Medical Center,
and the University of California, Irvine, California, USA

John J. Marini
Director of Pulmonary/Critical Care, St. Paul-Ramsey Medical Center,
640 Jackson Street, St. Paul, MN 55101-2595, USA

Elisa De Mattia
Respiratory Intensive Care Unit, Rehabilitation Center of Pavia,
S. Maugeri Foundation, Via Ferrata 8, 27100 Pavia, Italy

Gastón Murias
Intensive Care Service, Hospital de Sabadell, 08208 Sabadell, Spain

Stefano Nava
Respiratory Intensive Care Unit, Rehabilitation Center of Pavia,
S. Maugeri Foundation, Via Ferrata 8, 27100 Pavia, Italy

Avi Nahum
Pulmonary/Critical Care, St. Paul-Ramsey Medical Center,
640 Jackson St, St. Paul, MN 55101-2595, USA

Gian Carlo Piaggi
Respiratory Intensive Care Unit, Rehabilitation Center of Pavia,
S. Maugeri Foundation, Via Ferrata 8, 27100 Pavia, Italy

Jean-Christophe Richard
Service de Réanimation Médicale, Hôpital Charles Nicolle, 1 rue de Germont,
76031 Rouen Cedex, France

Josep Roca
Servei de Pneumologia i Allèrgia Respiratòria, Institut Clínic de Pneumologia i
Cirurgia Toràcica, Hospital Clínic, Barcelona, Spain

Robert Rodriguez-Roisin
Servei de Pneumologia i Allèrgia Respiratòria, Institut Clínic de Pneumologia i
Cirurgia Toràcica, Hospital Clínic, Barcelona, Spain

Pau V. Romero
Servei de Pneumologia, Hospital de Bellvitge,
Feixa Llarga s/n, 08907 L'Hospitalet, Spain

Catherine S.H. Sassoon
Pulmonary and Critical Care Section, VA Medical Center (111P),
5901 East Seventh Street, Long Beach, CA 90822, USA

Carmen Serrano-Munuera
Neuromuscular Division, Department of Neurology,
Hospital de la Sta. Creu i St. Pau, C/Sant Antoni Mª Claret, 167,
08025 Barcelona, Spain

Martin J. Tobin
Professor of Medicine, Chief, Division of Pulmonary and Critical Care Medicine,
Loyola University of Chicago Stritch School of Medicine,
Department of Veterans Affairs, Edward Hines, Jr. Hospital, Hines, Illinois, USA

Imma Vallverdú
Intensive Care Service, Hospital Universitari Sant Joan, Sant Joan s/n,
43201 Reus, Spain

Magdy Younes
RS 315, 810 Sherbrook Street, Winnipeg, Manitoba R3A 1R8, Canada

1 Mechanical Ventilation in Acute Respiratory Failure: What We Have Learnt and What We Still Need to Learn

J. Mancebo

Many advances have been seen over the past few years regarding supportive treatment (i.e., mechanical ventilation) of patients suffering acute respiratory failure (ARF) and needing clinical management in an ICU. This progress is the result of physiological studies specifically designed to answer relevant clinical questions or to more precisely understand physiopathological mechanisms of diseases. Such studies have usually been performed first with animals, on the bench, or with small series of selected patients under strict control. The data have then been transferred to the clinical arena and used to test a specific hypothesis in still small, open or controlled clinical trials. Finally, multicenter randomized clinical trials with large numbers of patients have been designed to ascertain the impact of certain ventilatory strategies on outcome variables. Very interestingly, some of the most important clinical trials in the field of mechanical ventilation published in recent years, for instance the impact of noninvasive positive-pressure ventilation (NPPV) in acute decompensation of chronic respiratory failure, the clinical relevance of different weaning strategies, and the impact of ventilating the lungs of acute respiratory distress syndrome (ARDS) patients with low tidal volumes, are nice examples of this commonly used, well thought-out approach. Even more important, such studies, based on robust experimental, physiological, and clinical data, have provided major improvements in patients' outcomes. In this chapter, I will comment on these seminal studies.

1.1 Noninvasive Positive-Pressure Ventilation

The technique of noninvasive positive-pressure ventilation consists of delivering mechanical ventilation without intubating the trachea. In this way, a ventilator delivers gas to the patient's lungs through an appropriate interface (a mask). In decompensated chronic obstructive pulmonary disease (COPD) the objectives are to improve gas exchange and to unload the respiratory muscles, these being the main physiopathological disturbances. The aim is to avoid endotracheal intubation and its short- and long-term sequelae, in particular, nosocomial infections. In the specific intensive care unit (ICU) setting this technique is quite new, and substantial knowledge appeared in the early 1990s. Since then, steady progress has been seen, not only in acutely decompensated COPD patients but also in patients with hypoxemic ARF, as a result of tantamount improvements in physiological and technical knowledge.

The first studies with COPD patients documented major benefits of pressure-support ventilation (PSV) delivered via a face mask. This technique induced considerable changes in the breathing pattern (decrease in respiratory rate and increase in tidal volume) and improvements in gas exchange (arterial PO_2 increases and hypercapnia decreases) and markedly unloaded the respiratory muscles (Brochard et al. 1990). It was later also well documented that these patients would also benefit from the addition of moderate external positive end-expiratory pressure (PEEP) levels, at least on a short-term basis and from a physiological point of view (Appendini et al. 1994; Nava et al. 1993). Nevertheless, of the two largest studies published to date, external PEEP was not used in one and was used in the other (Brochard et al. 1995; Plant et al. 2000). The results in terms of outcome, however, were identical: significant decreases in both intubation rate and mortality. The decreased incidence of nosocomial infections, attributable to the use of NPPV has recently been confirmed (Girou et al. 2000).

Important aspects related to NPPV are the interfaces, ventilatory modes and settings, and very probably humidification of the airways. With respect to the two former issues, much work has been done, and today we know that interfaces play a critical role in both tolerance and effects on gas exchange. In stable patients with chronic hypercapnic respiratory failure, the nasal mask provides the better tolerance, and the full-face mask provides for major decreases in $PaCO_2$ (Navalesi et al. 2000). Small-mask dead space is important to help reduce $PaCO_2$. Needless to say, CO_2 rebreathing should be avoided when a common inspiratory-expiratory line is used, to prevent persistent hypercapnia and subsequent clinical failures. Ventilatory mode is also important, and apart from providing highly sensitive trigger mechanisms, early high peak inspiratory flow, and minimal expiratory resistance, it is also crucial to avoid major leaks. When facing leaks at the patient-ventilator interface, it may be wise to switch from PSV (a flow-cycled form of ventilation) to pressure-controlled ventilation (a time-cycled form of ventilation). Patient-ventilator asynchrony due to leaks is thus prevented because machine-delivered positive pressure will end after a finite period of time, instead of after reaching a threshold flow value. When pressure-controlled ventilation is used, the inspiratory time is commonly adjusted to 0.8 s. It is conceivable that each one of these factors will improve tolerance of the technique, a fundamental issue that is directly associated with the success of NPPV. An additional cause of leaks may be glottic closure (Parreira et al. 1996). In normal volunteers the glottis tends to close when $PaCO_2$ decreases and also during sleep. Whether or not this is a relevant mechanism explaining leaks in patients receiving NPPV is not yet known.

Recent physiological studies (Jaber et al. 2000) have documented that gas mixtures containing helium and oxygen (instead of nitrogen and oxygen), can further reduce the inspiratory muscle effort developed by COPD patients and $PaCO_2$. Multicenter studies currently in progress are testing the hypothesis that NPPV with helium and oxygen is superior to NPPV with nitrogen and oxygen in terms of outcome. Quite recently acquired data (Richards et al. 1996) clearly indicate that nasal resistance dramatically increases when nasal continuous positive airway pressure is administered at different levels of humidity and different temperatures: This study documents that mucosal drying, rather than mucosal cooling, is the main factor explaining the increase in nasal resistance. Clearly, more work is needed in this area so as to further improve the comfort and tolerance of the technique, and hence its effects on outcome. Not all decompensated COPD patients will avoid intubation of the trachea and invasive mechanical ventilation. We have learnt that this is due to certain fundamental factors that clinicians should take into account: lack of tolerance to NPPV, severity of the underlying disease, and co-morbidity. For instance, it seems that patients with an arterial pH<7.30 at admission present a much higher rate of NPPV failures (Plant et al. 2000).

The usefulness of NPPV for hypoxemic ARF patients has also been tested in some studies. Among patients with acute hypoxemic ARF, Antonelli et al. (Antonelli et al. 1998) reported that intubation was avoided in 22 of 32 patients treated with NPPV using the PSV mode. The other ten patients needed intubation and mechanical ventilation and the ICU mortality in this subgroup was 90%, whereas the ICU mortality of the 32 patients who were initially intubated and treated with conventional mechanical ventilation was 47% (15/32). In another study the same group (Antonelli et al. 2000) compared NPPV (PSV) with supplemental oxygen in 40 solid organ transplant recipients. The rate of endotracheal intubation was significantly reduced in the NPPV group (20%, four of 20 patients) in comparison with the control group (70%, 14 of 20 patients), but in-hospital mortality did not differ. Another recent study (Delclaux et al. 2000) compared the usefulness of CPAP (n=62) versus supplemental oxygen (n=61) in patients with acute hypoxemic pulmonary edema, 83% of whom had an acute lung injury (ALI)/ARDS. No differences in intubation rate (34% CPAP and 39% oxygen), mortality (31% CPAP and 30% oxygen), or length of ICU stay (6.5 days CPAP and 6 days oxygen) were observed between the two groups. A significantly higher number of complications was observed in the CPAP group. Irrespective of whether NPPV was useful in hypoxemic respiratory failure, some fundamental issues remain unsolved: the physiological effects of NPPV in this patient population, and whether or not the effects of CPAP and NPPV (with PSV) may eventually differ, particularly in only-hypoxemic patients and in patients with a mixed hypoxemic and hypercapnic ARF. This may help us to understand the rationale (i.e., their respective effects on gas exchange and on respiratory muscle effort) for using these techniques in these patients.

1.2 Ventilatory Strategies in Patients with ARDS

An overwhelming number of data have been published in the past 15 years indicating that, in certain circumstances, some combinations of mechanical ventilator settings do more harm than good. This is not only because these could induce barotrauma, but also, more importantly, because ventilatory strategies allowing repetitive opening and collapse of alveolar units, or those using high teleinspiratory volumes, clearly generated increased permeability pulmonary edema in experimental animals (Dreyfuss and Saumon 1998). More recently, it has become clear that the use of these injurious ventilatory patterns, through mechanisms of cellular mechanotransduction, is also accompanied by a significant release of proinflammatory cytokines from the lungs to the bloodstream, in animals as well as in human beings (Ranieri et al. 1999; Slutsky and Tremblay 1998). Additionally, experimental studies have demonstrated that ventilatory strategies using high tidal volumes and low PEEP are able to induce bacterial translocation within the lungs (Nahum et al. 1997; Verbrugge et al. 1998).

In 1990, Hickling and co-workers (Hickling et al. 1990) reported that a ventilatory strategy entailing low tidal volumes and low driving pressures and leading to hypercapnia was associated with reduced mortality in ARDS patients. In these past few years, several large multicenter trials have compared ventilatory strategies using high and low tidal volumes. The first of these studies was published by Amato and colleagues (Amato et al. 1998), who randomized a group of 53 ARDS patients to treatment either with a conventional strategy (high tidal volume, 12 ml/kg, to allow normocapnia, and the lowest PEEP to keep acceptable arterial oxygenation) or with a protective strategy (PEEP titrated according to the inspiratory shape of pressure-volume (P/V) curves, and low tidal volumes, below 6 ml/kg, thus leading to hypercapnia, and frequent use of recruitment maneuvers). Mortality after 28 days was significantly higher in the control group (71%, 17 of 24 patients) than in the "protected" group (38%, 11 of 29 patients). Another study, by Stewart and co-workers (Stewart et al. 1998), randomized a group of 120 patients considered at high risk for ARDS. Sixty patients were assigned to a pressure-volume limitation (peak inspiratory pressure maintained at 30 cmH_2O or less and tidal volume of 8 ml/kg or less), and 60 were treated with conventional tidal volumes (between 10 and 15 ml/kg) allowing peak inspiratory pressure to reach 50 cmH_2O. Mortality was 50% in the limited ventilation group and 47% in the control group. However, in the limited-ventilation group a significantly higher requirement for paralytic agents and dialysis for renal failure was observed. A randomized multicenter study by Brochard and co-workers (Brochard et al. 1998), analyzing 126 patients with ARDS, showed no benefits of a strategy limiting end-inspiratory plateau pressure and tidal volume below 10 ml/kg when compared with a strategy using a tidal volume of 10 ml/kg or above. At 60 days, mortality was 47% in the low tidal volume group and 38% in the control group. The ARDS network recently published the largest study carried out in ARDS patients (The Adult Respiratory Distress Syndrome Network 2000). In this investigation including a total of 861 patients, the authors compared traditional treatment, 12 ml/kg (predicted body wt.) and plateau pressures up to 50 cmH_2O, with a low tidal volume strategy, 6 ml/kg (predicted body wt.) and plateau pressures up to 30 cmH_2O. After 28 days of randomization, the mortality and ventilator-free days were significantly worse in the control group (40% and 10 days, respectively) in comparison with the low tidal volume group (31% and 12 days, respectively).

Where have these studies led us? In the study by Amato et al., the control group reached average end-inspiratory plateau pressures of 37 cmH_2O, whereas the protective ventilation group reached an average plateau pressure of 30 cmH_2O in the first 36 h. PEEP was 9 cmH_2O in the former and 16 cmH_2O in the latter group. The incidence of barotrauma was also significantly higher in the control group (42% versus 7%). In the study by Stewart et al., plateau pressures were 27 and 22 cmH_2O and PEEP levels 7 and 9 cmH_2O in the control and intervention groups, respectively. In Brochard's study, PEEP levels were about 11 cmH$_2$O in both groups, but plateau pressure was 32 cmH$_2$O in the control group and 26 cmH$_2$O in the low tidal volume group. In the ARDS Network study, PEEP levels were about 9 cmH$_2$O in both groups, and mean plateau pressures were 25 cmH$_2$O in the low tidal volume group and 33 cmH$_2$O in the control group. Taken together, these data indicate that high end-inspiratory plateau pressures, i.e., above 30–35 cmH$_2$O, are harmful and high swings in driving pressures are also probably harmful (the association of a high mortality with high tidal volumes and a relatively low PEEP level in the control group of Amato's study suggests this). Also, the impressive results of the ARDS Network study can be explained by the fact that, apart from the large number of patients, the two arms of the study did not have major overlaps in tidal volumes. In other words, the tidal volume was really low in the intervention group and the tidal volume was indeed high in the control group. The lower mortality in the low tidal volume group suggests this approach was better.

There are still some interesting questions to answer with regard the ventilatory strategy to be followed in ARDS patients. For instance, although the above-mentioned studies have shown that hypercapnia is remarkably well tolerated, patients in the ARDS -Network study had relatively normal PaCO$_2$ and pH values. Whether or not this can be an added benefit is not known. Also, patients in the low tidal volume group had a respiratory rate almost twofold higher than the respiratory rate in the control group (29 breaths/min vs 16 breaths/min). High respiratory rates, especially when associated with high peak pulmonary artery pressures, have been reported to magnify lung edema formation in isolated rabbit lungs (Hotchkiss et al. 2000). Recruitment maneuvers have recently been claimed as an important adjunct to the common ventilatory strategies. Nevertheless, experimental data have showed that not all lungs are susceptible to be recruited (Van der Kloot et al. 2000). This seems to depend on what predominates, whether it is edema/collapse or consolidation, and also on the previous ventilatory strategy. For instance, a sustained improvement in oxygenation after a recruitment maneuver was observed in a model of ALI induced by lavage, but when relatively high PEEP and tidal volumes were used, the effects of recruitment maneuvers on lung volume were almost nil. The physiological data concerning recruitment in human ARDS lungs are very scarce. Although it is physiologically sound, we still do not know how recruitment should be evaluated (i.e., in terms of lung volume, arterial oxygenation, or both), how much recruitment pressure should be applied, what type of ventilatory settings should be used to recruit the lungs, or for how long and how often these maneuvers have to be applied. Neither do we know what type of risks such maneuvers can entail.

A useful tool for evaluating respiratory system mechanics and the influence of ventilatory settings on the lungs is the pressure-volume curve. Indeed, this technique has been used for many years to help adjust ventilatory parameters and to evaluate PEEP-induced alveolar recruitment and overdistension, according to the shape of the inflation limb of the pressure-volume relationship. The lack of a simple, safe, and reproducible measurement technique at the bedside has limited its use. It is conceivable, however, that new technical developments implemented in modern ventilators will make this tool widely available at the bedside quite soon.

More importantly, if this technique is made clinically available, it will enable us to study the mechanical characteristics of the respiratory system (during inspiration and expiration as well) on an ongoing basis, and hence to modify and tailor the ventilatory settings according to the different evolutive phases of the ARDS and according to each patient's need. Of course, the importance of imaging should not be neglected. Indeed, thoracic computed tomographic scan studies have recently provided new clues to understanding the relationships between lung morphology and lung mechanics (Puybasset et al. 2000a,b; Rouby et al. 2000). It is conceivable that this technique will provide new physiological data to further improve mechanical ventilation delivery to ARDS patients.

Finally, another strategy worthy of discussion is prone position. In the clinical setting, prone positioning (PP) has repeatedly been associated with significant improvements in arterial oxygenation and a lack of clinically relevant untoward effects in short-term studies (Blanch et al. 1997; Chatte et al. 1997; Jolliet et al. 1998; Nakos et al. 2000; Servillo et al. 1997). From a physiological standpoint, during PP the vertical gravitational gradient in pleural pressure is more evenly distributed than in the supine position (Mutoh et al. 1992). This implies a better distribution of ventilation in the dorsal areas of the lung during PP. Because regional lung perfusion is almost unaffected by the turn, this strategy results in a decrease in both intrapulmonary shunting of blood and in the heterogeneity of the ventilation/perfusion relationships when compared with the supine position (Lamm et al. 1994). Besides, it has been demonstrated in the experimental setting that the severity of lung lesions induced by high tidal volumes and low PEEP is considerably reduced in PP in comparison with supine position (Broccard et al. 1997). This strategy could theoretically minimize the cyclic alveolar opening and closing phenomena, thus decreasing shear stress. Better oxygenation could also be useful to decrease the FiO_2 and help diminish the possibility of oxygen toxicity. The effects of PP on outcome are currently being, or have just been, tested in ALI/ARDS patients in large randomized multicenter trials. One of these trials, carried out in Italy and yet not published, has not shown differences in mortality between the control group (supine position) and the intervention group (prone position). At least two more trials are underway, one in France and another in Spain, and the results are not yet known.

1.3 Weaning from Mechanical Ventilation

Unnecessary prolongation of mechanical ventilation increases the risk of complications, including, among others, bronchopulmonary infections, cardiovascular compromise, laryngotracheal injuries, and skeletal muscle deconditioning. At the same time, premature discontinuation of mechanical ventilation leading to reintubation may also increase morbidity, mortality, and duration of ICU stay. About 25% of patients who require intubation and mechanical ventilation for longer than 24 h cannot tolerate initial attempts to breathe without the mechanical ventilator. Typically, patients who present with weaning failure develop a rapid shallow-breathing pattern shortly after disconnection from the mechanical ventilator, and this is accompanied by a progressive worsening in respiratory system mechanics, an increase in inspiratory muscle effort, and CO_2 retention (Jubran and Tobin 1997; Tobin et al. 1986). The presence of cardiovascular dysfunction can be a non-negligible contributor to weaning failure in a number of patients. Jubran et al. (Jubran et al. 1998) examined hemodynamic data in patients during weaning trials. Successfully weaned patients demonstrated increases in cardiac index and oxygen transport compared with values during mechanical ventilation. Patients who failed weaning also failed to increase O_2 delivery, due, in part, to elevated right- and left-ventricular afterloads. Patients who failed also experienced increased peripheral oxygen extraction, which, combined with relative decreases in O_2 delivery, resulted in reduced mixed oxygen saturations.

Several techniques can be used to withdraw the ventilator in those patients who fail initial weaning attempts. In one randomized multicenter study (Brochard et al. 1994), PSV weaning was superior to weaning by T-piece trials or decremental synchronized intermittent mandatory ventilation (SIMV) in patients who failed initial spontaneous breathing trials. These results, however, were not reproduced in another similar multicenter randomized trial (Esteban et al. 1995). In this latter study, once-daily T-piece trials shortened the period of weaning compared with PSV or SIMV. The contradictory results of these studies could be explained by methodological differences. In actual fact, the algorithms for reducing PSV and the criteria for extubation were different. In other words, the way the techniques were used differed and probably influenced the final results. Interestingly, both studies agreed that SIMV weaning prolonged the duration of mechanical ventilation. Indeed, the use of SIMV has been very disappointing. This is a typical example of how a new ventilatory mode was launched and widely used in the clinical scenario without appropriate studies having been done to analyze its physiological effects on inspiratory muscle effort and gas exchange. We know now that whereas PSV provides a progressive unloading of inspiratory muscles, SIMV does not. In other words, SIMV reloads very early because the respiratory centers are probably unable to instantaneously adapt to machine-assisted intermittent breaths (Imsand et al. 1994; Leung et al. 1997; Marini et al. 1988; Viale et al. 1998). What we do not know is whether SIMV can do so better if used in a different way; for instance, pressure-controlled mandatory breaths interspersed with spontaneous pressure-supported breaths.

Another technique that can be used to hasten weaning from mechanical ventilation is early extubation followed by PSV applied noninvasively via a face mask. A prospective randomized trial (Nava et al. 1998) studied a group of patients with COPD who failed an initial SBT and who were extubated to noninvasive PSV. These patients were liberated from ventilators more quickly (10.2 vs 16.6 days), spent less time in the ICU (15.1 vs 24 days), and were more likely to survive (92% vs 72%) than patients conventionally weaned with PSV. In another investigation, Girault et al. (Girault et al. 1999) prospectively studied 33 COPD patients who failed a 2-h T-piece trial. Although weaning with noninvasive PSV significantly reduced the total duration of invasive mechanical ventilation and the probability of remaining intubated compared with conventional PSV (delivered via an endotracheal tube), the total duration of ventilatory support related to weaning was greater in the noninvasive PSV group. The lengths of ICU and hospital stay and mortality at 3 months were similar in both groups as well.

There are also important data, apart from those on ventilatory modalities, suggesting that other major factors influence the outcome of mechanically ventilated patients. It appears that a protocol-directed weaning strategy (Ely et al. 1996) leads not only to a significant reduction in the duration of mechanical ventilation but also to a significant decrease in the number of complications and costs. However, even following a protocol-directed weaning strategy, it is possible that weaning duration can be further reduced. This is confirmed by several studies dealing with unplanned extubation (Betbesé et al. 1998; Boulain et al. 1998; Chevron et al. 1998; Epstein et al. 2000). Taken together, these data suggest that there are still some patients (about 20%) who remain intubated and mechanically ventilated for a longer period of time than necessary, simply because when unplanned extubation occurs they do not need to be reintubated. In other words, from a clinical point of view, it is crucial to realize that every effort should be made, at least once a day, to ascertain whether or not a patient can be successfully liberated from the ventilator. Indeed, there are data to reinforce the notion that the way we implement our clinical practice is critical with respect to the total duration of mechanical ventilation and other outcomes. A significant number of patients (about 15%) who are deemed clinically ready to be extubated will need subsequent reintubation in the following 48 h (Epstein et al. 1997; Epstein and Ciubotaru 1998; Vallverdú et al. 1998). Very importantly, this patient group will have a high mortality, about 30%, and physiological data are badly needed to fully understand why these patients fail and how this can eventually be prevented. Some data indicate that this is quite frequent in patients who require intubation and mechanical ventilation because of neurological disturbances (Vallverdú et al. 1998), although this was not confirmed in a subsequent study using different clinical criteria to evaluate extubation readiness (Coplin et al. 2000). Strategies that could be envisaged as theoretically useful in this particular setting (failed extubation) are the use of NPPV to avoid reintubation or to perform early tracheostomies in neurological patients. Unfortunately, we do not have data regarding the impact of these interventions. Finally, recently published data (Kress et al. 2000) clearly indicate that one of the pharmacological treatments most widely used for intubated ICU patients, i.e., the administration of sedatives, is a fundamental intervention that influences outcome. In a randomized controlled trial the authors analyzed whether daily interruption of sedative infusions might accelerate withdrawal of mechanical ventilation. They found that daily interruption, as compared with continuous sedative infusions, significantly decreased the duration of mechanical ventilation and the length of stay in the ICU, without increasing the number of complications.

1.4 Other Recent Advances in Mechanical Ventilation

Other recent advances are explained in detail in the chapters that follow. In particular, I would like to draw your attention to the chapters dealing with the knowledge-based expert systems to hasten the process of weaning from mechanical ventilation (by L. Brochard), the physiopathological determinants of patient-ventilator interaction (by C.S.H. Sassoon), and the new and fascinating ventilatory mode called proportional assist ventilation (by M. Younes). Finally, a new technology, with direct clinical applications for patients with an intact neural pathway to the diaphragm, the neural adjusted ventilatory assist (i.e., the electrical activity of the diaphragm is used to trigger the ventilator), has recently been described by Sinderby and co-workers (Sinderby et al. 1999). All these areas will probably constitute a phenomenal avenue of physiological and clinical research in the next few years and, I hope, will bring our patients new opportunities for improved outcomes.

1.5 Corollary

We have learned much in the past decade about the effects of mechanical ventilation in diseased lungs and how we can improve the beneficial effects of this life-saving technique, applied either invasively or noninvasively. In terms of clinical outcomes, major benefits have arisen from the investigation of physiologically relevant issues. The information gathered in this way has then been applied to a large number of patients in well-designed, randomized clinical and usually multicenter trials. Close cooperation between clinicians, physiologists, and engineers has been essential to the success of this endeavor. Astonishing results have been seen from two perspectives: Our ignorance is clearly a source of problems for our patients, but at the same time all the strenuous efforts that investigators have made to date have produced enormous benefits. Indeed, it seems that adapting our approach to a more scientifically oriented clinical practice provides major benefits to our patients in terms of outcome. To conclude, a recent editorial by M.J. Tobin (Tobin 2000) emphasized the following: *"For 30 years, investigators have bemoaned the fact that increased oxygen delivery or treatment with glucocorticoids, surfactant, prostacyclin, or nitric oxide does not decrease mortality among patients with the ARDS....But this research has not resulted in any identifiable improvement in the outcome."* We have realized that a clinical intervention in ARDS as simple as turning the tidal volume knob down significantly decreased mortality. We have to keep up this pace so as to improve the clinical care of our critically ill patients. There are many problems yet to be solved and they will keep us very busy for life. Although we have made much progress, we are still not good enough and can do even better.

1.6 References

Amato MBP, Barbas CSV, Medeiros DM, Magaldi RB, Schettino GPP, Lorenzi-Filho G, Kairalla RA, Deheinzelin D, Munoz C, Oliveira R, et al (1998) Effect of a protective-ventilation strategy on mortality in the acute respiratory distress syndrome. N Engl J Med 338:347–354
Antonelli M, Conti G, Rocco M, Bufi M, De Blasi RA, Vivino G, Gasparetto A, Meduri GU (1998) A comparison of noninvasive positive-pressure ventilation and conventional mechanical ventilation in patients with acute respiratory failure. N Engl J Med 339:429–435
Antonelli M, Conti G, Bufi M, Costa M, Lappa A, Rocco M, Gasparetto A, Meduri G (2000) Noninvasive ventilation for treatment of acute respiratory failure in patients undergoing solid organ transplantation: a randomized trial. JAMA 283:235–241
Appendini L, Patessio A, Zanaboni S, Carone M, Gukov B, Donner CF, Rossi A (1994) Physiologic effects of positive end-expiratory pressure and mask pressure support during exacerbations of chronic obstructive pulmonary disease. Am J Respir Crit Care Med 149:1069–1076

Betbesé AJ, Perez M, Bak E, Rialp G, Mancebo J (1998) A prospective study of unplanned endotracheal extubation in intensive care unit patients. Crit Care Med 26:1180–1186

Blanch L, Mancebo J, Perez M, Martinez M, Mas A, Betbese A, Joseph D, Ballus J, Lucangelo U, Bak E (1997) Short-term effects of prone position in critically ill patients with acute respiratory distress syndrome. Intensive Care Med 23:1033–1039

Boulain T and the Association des Réanimateurs du Centre-Ouest (1998) Unplanned extubations in the adult intensive care unit. A prospective multicenter study. Am J Respir Crit Care Med 157:1131–1137

Broccard AF, Shapiro RS, Schmitz LL, Ravenscraft SA, Marini JJ (1997) Influence of prone position on the extent and distribution of lung injury in a high tidal volume oleic acid model of acute respiratory distress syndrome. Crit Care Med 25:16–27

Brochard L, Isabey D, Piquet J, Amaro P, Mancebo J, Messadi AA, Brun-Buisson C, Rauss A, Lemaire F, Harf A (1990) Reversal of acute exacerbations of chronic obstructive lung disease by inspiratory assistance with a face mask. N Engl J Med 323:1523–1530

Brochard L, Rauss A, Benito S, Conti G, Mancebo J, Rekik N, Gasparetto A, Lemaire F (1994) Comparison of three methods of gradual withdrawal from ventilatory support during weaning from mechanical ventilation. Am J Respir Crit Care Med 150:896–903

Brochard L, Mancebo J, Wysocki M, Lofaso F, Conti G, Rauss A, Simonneau G, Benito S, Gasparetto A, Lemaire F, et al (1995) Noninvasive ventilation for acute exacerbations of chronic obstructive pulmonary disease. N Engl J Med 333:817–822

Brochard L, Roudot-Thoraval F, Roupie E, Delclaux C, Chastre J, Fernandez-Mondéjar E, Clémenti E, Mancebo J, Factor P, Matamis D, et al (1998) Tidal volume reduction for prevention of ventilator-induced lung injury in the acute respiratory distress syndrome. Am J Respir Crit Care Med 158:1831–1838

Chatte G, Sab JM, Dubois JM, Sirodot M, Gaussorgues P, Robert D (1997) Prone position in mechanically ventilated patient with severe acute respiratory failure. Am J Respir Crit Care Med 155:473–478

Chevron V, Ménard J-F, Richard J-C, Girault C, Leroy J, Bonmarchand G (1998) Unplanned extubation: risk factors of development and predictive criteria for reintubation. Crit Care Med 26:1049–1053

Coplin W, Pierson D, Cooley K, Newell D, Rubenfeld G (2000) Implications of extubation delay in brain-injured patients meeting standard weaning criteria. Am J Respir Crit Care Med 161:1530–1536

Delclaux C, L'Her E, Alberti C, Mancebo J, Abroug F, Conti G, Guérin C, Schortgen F, Lefort Y, Antonelli M, et al (2000) Treatment of acute hypoxemic nonhypercapnic respiratory insufficiency with continuous positive airway pressure delivered by a face mask. A randomized controlled trial. JAMA 284:2352–2360

Dreyfuss D, Saumon G (1998) Ventilator-induced lung injury: lessons from experimental studies. Am J Respir Crit Care Med 157:294–323

Ely EW, Baker AM, Dunagan DP, Burke HL, Smith AC, Kelly PT, Johnson MM, Browder RW, Bowton DL, Haponik EF (1996) Effect on the duration of mechanical ventilation of identifying patients capable of breathing spontaneously. N Engl J Med 335:1864–1869

Epstein S, Nevins M, Chung J (2000) Effect of unplanned extubation on outcome of mechanical ventilation. Am J Respir Crit Care Med 161:1912–1916

Epstein SK, Ciubotaru RL (1998) Independent effects of etiology of failure and time to reintubation on outcome for patients failing extubation. Am J Respir Crit Care Med 158:489–493

Epstein SK, Ciubotaru RL, Wong JB (1997) Effect of failed extubation on the outcome of mechanical ventilation. Chest 112:186–192

Esteban A, Frutos F, Tobin MJ, Alia I, Solsona JF, Valverdu I, Fernandez R, De la Cal MA, Benito S, Tomas R, et al (1995) A comparison of four methods of weaning patients from mechanical ventilation. N Engl J Med 332:345–350

Girault C, Daudenthun I, Chevron V, Tamion F, Leroy J, Bonmarchand G (1999) Noninvasive ventilation as a systematic extubation and weaning technique in acute or chronic respiratory failure. A prospective, randomized controlled study. Am J Respir Crit Care Med 160:86–92

Girou E, Schortgen F, Delclaux C, Brun-Buisson C, Blot F, Lefort Y, Lemaire F, Brochard L (2000) Association of noninvasive ventilation with nosocomial infections and survival in critically ill patients. JAMA 284:2361–2367

Hickling KG, Henderson SJ, Jackson R (1990) Low mortality associated with low-volume pressure-limited ventilation with permissive hypercapnia in severe adult respiratory distress syndrome. Intensive Care Med 16:372–377

Hotchkiss J, Blanch L, Murias G, Adams A, Olson D, Wangensteen O, Leo P, Marini J (2000) Effects of decreased respiratory frequency on ventilator-induced lung injury. Am J Respir Crit Care Med 161:463–468

Imsand C, Feihl F, Perret C, Fitting JW (1994) Regulation of inspiratory neuromuscular output during synchronized intermittent mechanical ventilation. Anesthesiology 80:13–22

Jaber S, Fodil R, Carlucci A, Boussarsar M, Pigeot J, Lemaire F, Harf A, Lofaso F, Isabey D, Brochard L (2000) Noninvasive ventilation with helium-oxygen in acute exacerbations of chronic obstructive pulmonary disease. Am J Respir Crit Care Med 161:1191–1200

Jolliet P, Bulpa P, Chevrolet J (1998) Effects of the prone position on gas exchange and hemodynamics in severe acute respiratory distress syndrome. Crit Care Med 26:1977–1985

Jubran A, Tobin MJ (1997) Pathophysiologic basis of acute respiratory distress in patients who fail a trial of weaning from mechanical ventilation. Am J Respir Crit Care Med 155:906–915

Jubran A, Mathru M, Dries D, Tobin M (1998) Continuous recordings of mixed venous oxygen saturation during weaning from mechanical ventilation and the ramifications thereof. Am J Respir Crit Care Med 158:1763–1769

Kress J, Pohlman A, O'Connor M, Hall J (2000) Daily interruption of sedative infusions in critically ill patients undergoing mechanical ventilation. N Engl J Med 342:1471–1477

Lamm W, Graham M, Albert R (1994) Mechanism by which the prone position improves oxygenation in acute lung injury. Am J Respir Crit Care Med 150:184–193

Leung P, Jubran A, Tobin M (1997) Comparison of assisted ventilator modes on triggering, patient effort and dyspnea. Am J Respir Crit Care Med 155:1940–1948

Marini JJ, Smith TC, Lamb VT (1988) External work output and force generation during synchronized intermittent mechanical ventilation. Am Rev Respir Dis 138:1169–1179

Mutoh T, Guest R, Lamm W, Albert R (1992) Prone position alters the effect of volume overload on regional pleural pressures and improves hypoxemia in pigs in vivo. Am Rev Respir Dis 146:300–306

Nahum A, Hoyt J, Schmitz L, Moody J, Shapiro R, Marini JJ (1997) Effect of mechanical ventilation strategy on dissemination of intratracheally instilled *Escherichia coli* in dogs. Crit Care Med 25:1733–1743

Nakos G, Tsangaris I, Kostanti E, Nathanail C, Lachana A, Koulouras V, Kastani D (2000) Effect of the prone position on patients with hydrostatic pulmonary edema compared with patients with acute respiratory distress syndrome and pulmonary fibrosis. Am J Respir Crit Care Med 161:360–368

Nava S, Ambrosino N, Rubini F, Fracchia C, Rampulla C, Torri G, Calderini E (1993) Effect of nasal pressure support ventilation and external PEEP on diaphragmatic activity in patients with severe stable COPD. Chest 103:143–150

Nava S, Ambrosino N, Clini E, Prato M, Orlando G, Vitacca M, Brigada P, Fracchia C, Rubini F (1998) Noninvasive mechanical ventilation in the weaning of patients with respiratory failure due to chronic obstructive pulmonary disease. A randomized, controlled trial. Ann Intern Med 128:721–728

Navalesi P, Fanfulla F, Frigerio P, Gregoretti C, Nava S (2000) Physiologic evaluation of noninvasive mechanical ventilation delivered with three types of masks in patients with chronic hypercapnic respiratory failure. Crit Care Med 28:1785–1790

Parreira V, Jounieaux V, Aubert G, Dury M, Delguste P, Rodenstein D (1996) Nasal two-level positive pressure ventilation in normal subjects. Am J Respir Crit Care Med 153:1616–1623

Plant P, Owen J, Elliott M (2000) Early use of non-invasive ventilation for acute exacerbations of chronic obstructive pulmonary disease on general respiratory wards: a multicentre randomised controlled trial. Lancet 355:1931–1935

Puybasset L, Cluzel P, Gusman P, Grenier P, Preteux F, Rouby J (2000a) Regional distribution of gas and tissue in ARDS. I. Consequences for lung morphology. Intensive Care Med 26:857–869

Puybasset L, Gusman P, Muller J, Cluzel P, Coriat P, Rouby J (2000b) Regional distribution of gas and tissue in ARDS. III. Consequences for the effects of positive end-expiratory pressure. Intensive Care Med 26:1215–1227

Ranieri V, Suter P, Tortorella C, De Tullio R, Dayer J, Brienza A, Bruno F, Slutsky A (1999) Effect of mechanical ventilation on inflammatory mediators in patients with acute respiratory distress syndrome: a randomized controlled trial. JAMA 282:54–61

Richards G, Cistulli P, Ungar R, Berthon-Jones M, Sullivan C (1996) Mouth leak with nasal continuous positive airway pressure increases nasal airway resistance. Am J Respir Crit Care Med 154:182–186

Rouby J, Puybasset L, Cluzel P, Richecoeur J, Lu Q, Coriat P (2000) Regional distribution of gas and tissue in ARDS. II. Physiological correlations and definition of an ARDS severity score. Intensive Care Med 26:1046–1056

Servillo G, Roupie E, De Robertis E, Rossano F, Brochard L, Lemaire F, Tufano R (1997) Effects of ventilation in ventral decubitus position on respiratory mechanics in adult respiratory distress syndrome. Intensive Care Med 23:1219–1224

Sinderby C, Navalesi P, Beck J, Skrobik J, Comtois N, Friberg S, Gottfried S, Lindström L (1999) Neural control of mechanical ventilation in respiratory failure. Nat Med 5:1433–1436

Slutsky AS, Tremblay LN (1998) Multiple system organ failure. Is mechanical ventilation a contributing factor? Am J Respir Crit Care Med 157:1721–1725

Stewart TE, Meade MO, Cook DJ, Granton JT, Meade MO, Hodder RV, Lapinsky S, Mazer CD, McLean RF, Rogovein TS, et al (1998) Evaluation of a ventilation strategy to prevent barotrauma in patients at high risk for acute respiratory distress syndrome. N Engl J Med 338:355–361

The Adult Respiratory Distress Syndrome Network (2000) Ventilation with lower tidal volumes as compared with traditional tidal volumes for acute lung injury and the acute respiratory distress syndrome. N Engl J Med 342:1301–1308

Tobin M (2000) Culmination of an era in research on the acute respiratory distress syndrome. N Engl J Med 342:1360–1361

Tobin MJ, Perez W, Guenther SM, Semmens BJ, Mader MJ, Allen SJ, Lodato RF, Dantzker D (1986) The pattern of breathing during successful and unsuccessful trials of weaning from mechanical ventilation. Am Rev Respir Dis 134:1111–1118

Vallverdú I, Calaf N, Subirana M, Net A, Benito S, Mancebo J (1998) Clinical characteristics, respiratory functional parameters and outcome of a 2-hour T-piece trial in patients weaning from mechanical ventilation. Am J Respir Crit Care Med 158:1855–62

Van der Kloot T, Blanch L, Youngblood A, Weinert C, Adams A, Marini J, Shapiro R, Nahum A (2000) Recruitment maneuvers in three experimental models of acute lung injury. Effects on lung volume and gas exchange. Am J Respir Crit Care Med 161:1485–1494

Verbrugge SJC, Sorm V, Van't Veen A, Mouton JW, Gommers D, Lachmann B (1998) Lung overinflation without positive end-expiratory pressure promotes bacteremia after experimental *Klebsiella pneumoniae* inoculation. Intensive Care Med 24:172–177

Viale JP, Duperret S, Mahul P, Delafosse BX, Delpuech C, Weismann D, Annat GJ (1998) Time course evolution of ventilatory responses to inspiratory unloading in patients. Am J Respir Crit Care Med 157:428–434

2 Controlled Mechanical Ventilation

J.J. Marini

2.1 Definition of Controlled Ventilation

Although any form of pressure-*assisted* breathing (such as assist/control, synchronized mandatory ventilation, or pressure support) can provide the power required to accomplish the breathing workload, effort during these cycles may be highly variable [1, 2]. The term "controlled ventilation" (CMV) implies that all ventilatory support is provided mechanically and that the patient's efforts to breathe have been effectively silenced. Accordingly, the pressure applied at the airway opening accounts for the entire inspiratory transpulmonary pressure gradient.

2.2 Indications for Controlled Ventilation

Virtually all indications for establishing controlled ventilation can be classified as needs to manipulate the ventilatory pattern, to reduce agitation and the oxygen cost of breathing, to facilitate nonventilatory medical treatment, or to prevent exposure of the lungs to excessive pressure. Perhaps the most common indication for CMV, however, is to provide maximal support to a patient with such marginal reserve that the work of breathing compromises comfort, gas exchange, or cardiac function. Reducing the amount of oxygen consumed by a patient with critical coronary ischemia, for example, may prove lifesaving, especially in the setting of circulatory shock or acute pulmonary edema.

Silencing ventilatory effort can also improve arterial oxygenation in agitated patients with acute lung injury (ARDS) [3]. The precise explanation for improved oxygenation after paralysis may well vary among different patients and involve several mechanisms. Almost invariably, cardiac output falls in parallel with declining oxygen consumption as ventilatory control is established. Because venous admixture tends to respond in the same direction as cardiac output, reducing pulmonary blood flow diminishes the shunt fraction [4]. A second possibility is that the decline in oxygen consumption occurs out of proportion to the reduction in cardiac output, thereby restoring an appropriate balance between O_2 supply and O_2 delivery [5]. The resultant increase in mixed venous O_2 saturation could account, in part, for the apparently improved oxygen exchange across the lung. A third possibility is that the distribution of ventilation might improve as the respiratory muscles relax. Finally, most patients who experience improved gas exchange after the institution of controlled ventilation vigorously use their expiratory muscles prior to paralysis in an attempt to avoid hyperinflation or minimize inspiratory effort through "work sharing" [3, 6, 7] (Fig. 2.1). Preventing expiratory activity may allow positive end-expiratory pressure (PEEP) to recruit significantly more lung volume, especially from basilar regions.

Apart from its influence on oxygen consumption and cardiac output and its value in keeping patient effort from interfering with intended patterns of conventional ventilation, establishing ventilatory control greatly facilitates the application of therapeutic but "nonphysiological" breathing patterns. Such interventions as inverse ratio ventilation [8–10], independent lung ventilation [11], low-frequency positive-pressure ventilation [12], and enforced CO_2 retention ("permissive hypercapnia") [13–18] usually require silencing or attenuating breathing effort. Intentional hyperventilation may be the appropriate therapeutic strategy when reduction of cerebral blood volume and intracranial pressure are urgent priorities, as after cranial surgery or closed head injury.

Although a continuing need to evaluate the respiratory system is seldom sufficient reason in itself to undertake deep sedation or paralysis, the need to monitor respiratory system mechanics is greatly facilitated by controlling ventilation [19]. Unless controlled conditions are assured, airway pressure alone does not provide sufficient information to enable the clinician or investigator to directly assess any aspect of respiratory mechanics with precision or confidence. When passive conditions are achieved, however, respiratory system impedance and its subcomponents (resistance, compliance, and auto-PEEP), as well as estimates of the mechanical work of spontaneous breathing (and the pressure time product) are readily measured or calculated from airway pressure and flow signals [19]. The same information can be obtained for the lungs when an esophageal balloon catheter is inserted, whether or not ventilatory control has been established. The mechanical properties of the chest wall can be determined with an estimate of pleural pressure, but only under passive conditions.

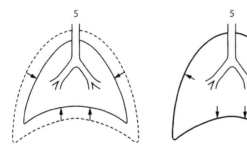

Fig. 2.1. Relationship of PEEP, lung volume, and expiratory muscle activity. By forcing the chest to a volume below the equilibrium position appropriate to the applied level of end-expiratory pressure (5 cmH₂O), the mechanical advantage of the inspiratory muscles is improved ("inspiratory work sharing"). Furthermore, the potential energy stored in the chest wall during expiration (*left*) can be released to aid inflation (*right*). (From [132] with permission)

2.3 Requirements for Establishing Ventilatory Control

The rhythm controller of the respiratory system is strongly influenced by non-chemical factors, especially in the nonhypercapnic subject. Consequently, the apneic threshold of a normal awake individual lies well below the usual CO_2 set point of 40 mmHg [20, 21]. Typically, this value approximates 30 mmHg, but there is wide individual variation. Although not well characterized for critically ill patients, these thresholds for apnea induction are likely to be even lower in those with increased ventilatory drive [21]. Moreover, the apneic threshold might be expected to vary with the rapidly changing levels of metabolism and alertness that characterize this setting. Sedation, often supplemented by protracted skeletal muscle relaxation (paralysis), is almost routinely required to establish ventilatory control in the conscious and critically ill patient.

Muscle relaxants must be employed with careful regard for their potential to produce psychological distress and physical injury [22]. These agents must not be used in the conscious or lightly sedated patient. Therefore, concomitant and continuous suppression of consciousness with a benzodiazepine (often supplemented by an opioid) is standard practice in most North American intensive care units. Although short-term suppression of neuromuscular tone seldom results in lasting impairment, protracted therapeutic paralysis is often accompanied by undesirable or even catastrophic sequelae:

- Accelerated wasting of skeletal muscle
- Electrolyte imbalance/H_2O retention
- Reduced tissue turgor and vascular tone
- Sustained paralytic syndrome
- Dependent infiltration and atelectasis
- Cardiovascular effects
- Obstipation

Accelerated wasting of skeletal protein, electrolyte depletion, water retention, deterioration of tissue turgor, and diminished vascular tone are to be anticipated when paralysis is maintained for longer than 3 days [23, 24]. It may be important to insure that some neural traffic to the muscle continues during the period over which muscle relaxants are employed. To achieve this end, many practitioners use a percutaneous nerve stimulator to guide the infusion rate of the blocking agent. Others prefer to use drug boluses that are administered only as needed to suppress movement. With either technique, the muscle fibers should not be totally isolated from neural stimulation. A paralytic agent must not be administered at an unchanging rate without its impact on the therapeutic target, as well as the need for its continued use, being frequently reassessed. Relaxants and sedatives should be withdrawn expeditiously when no longer necessary.

The choice of agents used in sedation and paralysis should be individualized. It is generally understood that morphine has unparalleled anxiolytic, analgesic, and ventilatory drive-suppressing properties. However, its venodilating action, while highly desirable in certain settings (e.g., cardiogenic pulmonary edema), may prove detrimental when a high level of vascular tone is needed to preserve adequate venous return (e.g., right heart failure, high levels of positive end-expiratory alveolar pressure). The benzodiazepines generally have less vascular and gut-immobilizing effects but vary in their duration of action. Because of long-acting metabolites, it is not uncommon for sedation to persist for days following attempted reversal.

Many reports documenting protracted weakness after therapeutic paralysis concern treatment of patients with status asthma who were simultaneously given corticosteroids [22, 25–29]. Myonecrosis with systemic release of muscle enzymes into the blood can be detected in a high percentage of patients given both medications [25]. Although the precise mechanism for the phenomenon and the specific role of muscle relaxants are not currently known, adverse effects have been suggested to occur more frequently with agents having a "steroid" nucleus (e.g., vecuronium). Other types of muscle relaxants (e.g., atracurium) are not free of this complication [28, 29]. Paralytic agents vary in their metabolic and excretion pathways, as well as in the activity and cumulation rates of their metabolites. Pancuronium and vecuronium, if not operationally adjusted using a nerve stimulator, should be given in doses that reflect the status of their primary route of excretion (renal and hepatic, respectively). Atracurium appears to be degraded primarily by tissue metabolism.

Dependent atelectasis and infiltration undoubtedly contribute to veno-arterial shunting in the patient receiving CMV, especially in supine postures. In the early phase of acute lung injury, infiltrates are usually distributed in a gravity-dependent fashion in the supine position [30–34]. This gravitational dependence may help to explain the striking improvement in gas exchange that often accompanies a shift to the prone position, which evens the distribution of pleural pressure [35]. Muscle relaxation entails monotonous breathing and impaired coughing. Moreover, failure to change position encourages the accumulation of airway secretions in these same dependent regions. The lateral decubitus position is associated with a higher average FRC than the supine position [36]. The nondependent lung assumes a resting volume greater than in the sitting position, while it drains airway secretions more effectively. For these reasons, special effort should be made to vary posture and to maintain the airways bronchodilated and free of retained secretions whenever deep sedation and muscle relaxants are used.

2.4 Appropriate Therapeutic Targets

Given the injurious potential of positive-pressure ventilation, it seems prudent to question the therapeutic end points which drive current ventilatory strategy. Apart from relieving the work of breathing, most clinicians focus on achieving acceptable gas exchange with the lowest levels of applied pressure and inspired oxygen that accomplish this therapeutic objective. Two major questions immediately arise: What is adequate gas exchange? What are dangerous levels of applied pressure?

The intensive care unit is populated by patients whose reserves, tolerance, compensatory potential, and diseases span a wide spectrum. Even among patients of similar age and illness severity, the pace at which the problem evolves can differ strikingly, allowing either ample or insufficient time for physiological adaptation. Two primary goals of ventilation are to eliminate metabolic CO_2 at an appropriate rate and to assure adequate transpulmonary transfer of oxygen. Because both objectives are tightly linked to the airway pressure requirement, it is essential to identify the minimum levels of PaO_2, $PaCO_2$, and pH needed for satisfactory vital organ function. Although a substantial body of scientific data addresses these crucial points in normal healthy subjects, until recently, surprisingly little was known about the tolerance limits and adaptability of critically ill patients to abnormalities of arterial blood gases. Whereas extensive experience with permissive hypercapnia has been gathered rapidly, there still is no consensus as to whether subacute hypoxemia can be tolerated. Supraphysiological levels of O_2 delivery do not appear to benefit patients with diseases such as sepsis or ARDS [37].

2.4.1 Oxygen Tension

High concentrations of inspired oxygen and elevated airway pressures are both potentially injurious. Debate continues as to the highest safe inspired oxygen fraction (FiO_2), but it appears likely that an FiO_2 >0.65 will eventually harm the normally aerated and functional lung parenchyma or impede healing. Many patients with ARDS have half or more of all lung units collapsed, flooded, or infiltrated. These diseased alveoli may be shielded from long-term O_2 toxicity. Unfortunately, the least injurious combination of applied pressure and FiO_2 to achieve a targeted PaO_2 is not known with certainty.

Normal values for PaO_2 in a healthy patient living at sea level generally fall within a narrow, well-defined range. Although PaO_2 declines somewhat with advancing age [38], arterial hemoglobin remains almost entirely saturated with oxygen throughout life.

At a normal pH, blood O_2 saturation and content remain nearly normal until PaO_2 declines to less than 60 mmHg. Several important physiological responses are evoked when this saturation threshold has been crossed. These include increased (hypoxic) ventilation, pulmonary arterial vasoconstriction, and erythropoietin release. Although the physiological significance of desaturation cannot be denied, it is apparent that brief episodes of modest desaturation evoke little dysfunction of vital organs and produce no lasting effect in healthy subjects, provided that O_2 delivery can be maintained by cardiovascular compensation. In an otherwise healthy individual with ample cardiovascular reserves, overt cerebral dysfunction requires arterial oxygen tension to fall below 40 mmHg, and consciousness is lost only at levels lower than 30 mmHg [39]. Without concomitant ischemia, permanent cerebral damage is unlikely if PaO_2 exceeds 20 mmHg.

Given a few days to accommodate to hypoxemia, vigorous work can be accomplished by healthy individuals in hypoxic environments (e.g., high altitude) [40, 41]. The extent and pace at which different critically ill patients "acclimatize" to hypoxemia remains an important but unresolved question. Therefore, although achieving full O_2 saturation seems an appropriate clinical objective for a patient with multisystem organ failure [42], it is not entirely clear that high ventilating pressures or toxic O_2 concentrations should be applied in pursuit of this goal when managing a patient with isolated lung failure, normal hemoglobin concentration, and a healthy heart.

Until recently, it has generally been assumed that hypoxemia plays a central role in the generation of multiple-system organ failure. Such thinking has been reinforced by reports that O_2 delivery correlates with survival in sepsis [43] and that supernormal O_2 delivery improves survival in postoperative patients [44]. This presumption, however, has been challenged by work demonstrating that accelerated glycolysis, rather than delivery dependence of oxygen consumption, best explains the lactic acidosis of sepsis [45]. Targeting mixed venous oxygen saturation and oxygen delivery to higher values does not appear to confer a survival advantage to patients with acute respiratory failure [37].

2.4.2 Carbon Dioxide

Concerning patients without concomitant metabolic acidosis, severe hypoxemia, beta-adrenergic blockade, or acute cerebral injury, a compelling argument can be made in favor of abandoning the traditionally targeted range for carbon dioxide tension (~35–45 mmHg) when insistence on those values requires hazardous treatment. Although CO_2 is the major end-product of cellular metabolism, carbon dioxide itself is remarkably free of noxious effects [14–16]. Most problems associated with CO_2 retention either do not apply to the patient receiving controlled ventilation or are associated with concomitant plasma or cellular acidosis [46]. The great majority of adverse effects related to hypercapnia are produced by the rapid, unbuffered retention of CO_2. These include cerebral vascular congestion, central nervous system dysfunction, skeletal muscle weakness, bronchoconstriction, heightened adrenergic activity, pulmonary hypertension, and cardiovascular impairment. Because the cellular membrane is more permeable to carbon dioxide than to $[HCO_3]^-$, important disparities can develop between plasma and intracellular pH during rapid accumulation or elimination of CO_2. Conversely, paradoxical intracellular acidosis can result from overzealous administration of bicarbonate [47, 48].

Few important physiological effects ensue when CO_2 accumulates slowly enough to permit intracellular pH adjustment and compensatory renal retention of $[HCO_3]^-$ [14, 16, 49]. Such adjustments of intracellular pH may be largely completed within a few hours of initiating the $PaCO_2$ elevation, depending on its magnitude. Although sensitivity of the respiratory drive center to changes in ventilation is blunted by compensatory elevations in tissue $[HCO3]^-$ concentration, any resulting acidosis tends to be well buffered [47]. Furthermore, such considerations have little import for the patient receiving controlled ventilation. For the spontaneously breathing patient with a chronically elevated breathing workload, deliberately resetting the "homeostatic set point" for CO_2 appears to be an appropriate strategy for reducing breathing effort without adverse sequelae. With well-functioning kidneys, sufficient bicarbonate ion is retained to keep pH within normal limits until $PaCO_2$ exceeds ≈ 65 mmHg [50]. Consequently, there is some reason to believe that the patient with seriously compromised ventilatory function might naturally seek or tolerate a higher $PaCO_2$ than that set by the well-meaning clinician.

In acute respiratory failure, using permissive hypercapnia to control airway pressure often presents an attractive therapeutic option. Allowing carbon dioxide retention decreases the work of breathing because fewer breaths and less ventilatory effort are required to maintain hypercapnia. The feasibility of this approach has been clearly demonstrated in asthmatics receiving mechanical ventilation, all of whom survived without barotrauma or ventilator-induced lung injury [13]. Such encouraging results suggest that in this reversible condition with uniorgan failure, the traditional therapeutic paradigm (which uses high ventilating pressure in an attempt to maintain eucapnia) may itself present the greatest threat to full recovery.

The need to keep $PaCO_2$ targeted at the normal level must also be questioned in forms of lung disease not usually characterized by CO_2 retention [51, 52]. The therapeutic approach to the adult respiratory distress syndrome (ARDS) has been under intense recent scrutiny, with interest piqued by the experimental observations that high transpulmonary pressures applied in the setting of tissue edema and atelectasis may disrupt delicate alveolar-capillary membranes [53–56]. Strikingly improved survival has been reported when care is taken to maintain a certain critical end-expiratory volume and to prevent exposure to excessively high or low tidal pressures [17, 18, 57–59].

Such observations seem consistent with the idea that the pathology of ARDS is heterogeneous, and that lung tissue capable of effectively participating in gas exchange is fragile and susceptible to injury. It seems reasonable, therefore, that the lung should not be subjected to stresses beyond those encountered during health. Adherence to this principle often requires that $PaCO_2$ be allowed to rise, buffering CO_2 accumulation and/or utilizing dialysis, when necessary, to avert serious acidemia.

2.4.3 Hydrogen Ion Concentration and pH

For most patients, pH is more significant as a *marker* of the underlying disease process than for its inherent physiological actions. Diabetic ketoacidosis, for example, may produce extremely low pH values without notable cardiovascular problems, assuming that circulating volume has been adequately restored and adrenergic reflexes are intact [60, 61]. Severe acidosis is not always well tolerated, however, and sedation and paralysis are frequently required. Even mild acidosis (7.20<pH<7.40) accentuates the drive to breathe, alters the O_2 binding affinity of hemoglobin, and acts synergistically with alveolar hypoxia to cause pulmonary vasoconstriction [62]. The strength of this effect varies widely among individuals [60–62]. Mild acidemia may be well tolerated physiologically by the great majority of patients, only to prove problematic for the patient with pulmonary hypertension. Conversely, even though pH values lower than 7.20 tend to impair normal cardiovascular function, intact adrenergic tone may mask all cardiodepressant effects of failing pH until acidemia is extreme.

Acidosis may be well tolerated when pH falls slowly. On the other hand, the pressure cost of maintaining a normal pH may be unacceptably high. Increased ventilatory dead-space fractions and the pre-existence of auto-PEEP predispose to a high pressure cost of additional alveolar ventilation. A patient with severe airflow obstruction, or one being supported with inverse ratio ventilation, may experience greatly accentuated air trapping with comparatively minor increases in the minute ventilation requirement. As already noted, a strategy of permissive hypercapnia may not be feasible in the setting of concomitant metabolic acidosis.

2.5 Adverse Consequences of Airway Pressure

2.5.1 Consequences of High Pressure

Neonatologists have long been aware that survival in the infant respiratory distress syndrome often hinges on avoiding barotrauma [63]. Until recently, comparatively little attention had been paid to pressure-related injury in adults, since clinicians lacked evidence that adult patients are susceptible to the same types of injury encountered by their younger counterparts. It is now recognized, however, that the spectrum of injury is virtually identical even though the susceptibility and frequency of certain types of barotrauma undoubtedly differ with age.

Over the past two decades, interstitial emphysema [64], tension cyst formation [65], and systemic gas embolism [66] have been demonstrated in patients with ARDS – problems unreported and unsuspected only a short time ago. Moreover, damage to the small airways can be identified on pathological specimens of adult lungs ventilated for long periods by high pressure [67–69].

Pressure-related damage is not confined to extravasation of alveolar gas. As already noted, acute lung injury is heterogeneously distributed. Aerated portions participating in gas exchange constitute approximately one third of the total volume occupied by these wet, partially collapsed, and cell-infiltrated lungs [70]. Overall lung and chest wall volumes remain approximately normal. Heterogeneous ventilation/perfusion distributions documented by inert gas analysis are accompanied by disproportional radiographic infiltrates in dependent areas, a finding best explained by the topography of pulmonary and pleural pressures and by hydrostatic compression of dependent airways [71]. The sum of available information suggests, therefore, that the aeratable, functioning lung in ARDS is less stiff than it is undersized [72].

Given the high dead-space fraction and increased CO_2 production associated with ARDS, insistence on maintaining normal arterial $PaCO_2$ may expose residual lung tissues to high pressure and to wide excursions of tidal volume. In a normal subject, exposure to a transmural alveolar (transalveolar) pressure of 30–35 cmH$_2$O will achieve the alveolar size associated with total lung capacity. It may not be surprising, therefore, that transmural alveolar pressures exceeding this value render normal alveolar membranes permeable to water and protein [53–56]. As little as 20–25 cmH$_2$O plateau pressure may be sufficient to overdistend some lung units in ARDS [73]. Following membrane injury, even lower pressures may increase the rate of edema formation. Furthermore, wide tidal excursions of transpulmonary pressure overventilate patent lung units, a process which may cause regional alkalosis, deplete surfactant, produce damaging shear stresses, or otherwise accentuate tissue injury. According to current understanding, therefore, high tidal pressures and wide tidal excursions of pressure and volume are deleterious in the setting of lung edema [74–76] (Fig. 2.2). Nonetheless, the lung may need periodic inflation to total lung capacity in order to open and maintain patency of all recruitable units.

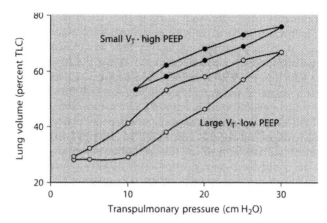

Fig. 2.2. Lung volume as a function of transpulmonary pressure for two patterns of ventilation in dogs with acute lung injury. Both patterns maintained peak airway pressure <30 cmH$_2$O. However, the large V$_T$-low PEEP group experienced worse gas exchange and edema. (From [74] with permission)

2.5.2 Consequences of Low Pressure

Recognizing that excessive pressures must be avoided, there are equally convincing data showing that tidal *alveolar* pressures must not be allowed to fall too far in the acutely injured lung. Simply ventilating the surfactant-depleted small animal lung at modest peak pressures but low levels of PEEP causes evidence of lung injury [77]. The appropriate level of PEEP varies with tidal volume. In the earliest stages of acute lung injury, a certain minimal pressure – typically in the range of 10–15 cmH$_2$O for moderate tidal volumes – seems needed to prevent tidal end-expiratory collapse of edematous lung tissue [78, 79]. Stresses applied at the junctions of inflating and collapsed tissues may greatly exceed those within inflated units imbedded in well-aerated regions. It has been estimated that alveolar wall tensions at such boundaries may be five to tenfold higher than the inflating pressure suggests [80]. Over time, the process of tidal recruitment and collapse may promote a sequence of edema and consolidation, thereby creating an even smaller (and apparently stiffer) lung [75, 79, 81]. Elimination of "tidally phasic" atelectasis, therefore, may be a key to minimizing injury. In fact, persistent collapse may itself be deleterious; even high-frequency oscillation can produce barotrauma unless enough PEEP is applied [79].

Early in the course of ARDS, failure to provide adequate end-expiratory alveolar pressure is often manifested by low compliance and a static pressure-volume curve characterized by hysteresis and distinct upper and lower zones of inflection [78]. These features are blurred or obliterated by adding sufficient end-expiratory alveolar pressure [74, 78]. Raising end-expiratory alveolar pressure (total PEEP or P$_{ex}$) can be accomplished either by directly applying end-expiratory airway pressure (PEEP) or by encouraging the development of dynamic hyperinflation and "auto-PEEP". Thus, P$_{ex}$=PEEP+auto-PEEP.

These arguments do not generally apply to the patient mechanically ventilated for severe airflow obstruction. In such patients peak airway pressures are high, but maximum *alveolar* pressures are usually held within acceptable limits. More importantly, air trapping – not atelectasis – presents the primary problem. Thus, whereas the addition of PEEP or CPAP can often help the spontaneously breathing or machine-assisted patient cope with the work of breathing [82, 83], there currently is no compelling evidence that PEEP has any other therapeutic benefit. Adding PEEP usually accentuates hyperinflation, particularly when PEEP exceeds the original level of auto-PEEP [82, 84]. The distribution of ventilation may improve if PEEP replaces auto-PEEP [85]. Although some have suggested that this hyperinflation could have therapeutic benefit, PEEP-induced hyperinflation is likely to be hazardous and poorly tolerated hemodynamically by the heavily sedated or paralyzed patient receiving controlled ventilation.

2.5.3 Influence of Transvascular Pressure on Lung Injury

Recent work has demonstrated that high transvascular pressures can cause capillary stress failure [86, 87]. Such evidence provides a good rationale for limiting the amount of fluid administered to patients with lung injury. Moreover, transvascular forces are increased at high lung volumes, especially at the boundaries of collapsed and inflated lung tissue [80, 86]. Therefore, to minimize ventilator-induced lung injury and speed healing of tissues already damaged, it seems prudent to avoid both widespread atelectasis and high end-inspiratory lung volumes. This goal can be accomplished with a ventilation strategy that simultaneously provides a certain minimum end-expiratory pressure and constrains both end-inspiratory alveolar pressure and tidal volume.

2.6 Importance of Mean Airway Pressure

The preceding discussion has argued that neither should tidal alveolar pressures be driven too high (at end-inspiration), nor in certain settings – exemplified by ARDS – should end-expiratory alveolar pressure dip too low. Whether the objectives of controlled ventilation are achieved within these guidelines depends upon the objectives for ventilation (adequate gas exchange, tolerable adverse effects), the ventilatory pattern, and (under passive conditions) the mean airway pressure.

2.6.1 Relationship of Mean Airway to Mean Alveolar Pressure

Although the terms "mean *airway* pressure" (mP_{aw}) and "mean *alveolar* pressure" (mP_{alv}) are used almost interchangeably in the medical literature, they are not synonymous. A minority of clinicians fully understand the exact basis for the relationship between them. At any instant, the pressure applied across the passive respiratory system, (i.e., pressure at the airway opening) must be entirely accounted for by its conserved (elastic) and dissipated (nonelastic) components [88, 89]. During passive exhalation, alveolar pressure conserved during inflation drives expiratory flow, so that the tidal component of elastic pressure must dissipate before exhalation stops. Equivalence between mean airway and mean alveolar pressures depends upon the identity of frictional ("resistive") pressure losses that occur during the inspiratory and expiratory periods. The relevant expression is:

$$mP_{alv}=mP_{aw}+[V_E (R_x-R_i)]/60,$$

where mP_{alv} and mP_{aw} are mean alveolar and mean airway pressures, V_E is minute ventilation (l/min), and R_i and R_x are volume-averaged values for inspiratory and expiratory "resistance" (the quotient of driving pressure to flow, expressed in $cmH_2O/l/s$) [90]. Since R_x normally exceeds R_i by only a small amount, mean airway pressure tends to provide a good first approximation of mP_{alv}, especially when V_E is modest. Equivalence between these two mean pressures is *not* preserved, however, in the setting of severe airflow obstruction, where R_x may be several-fold higher than R_i [82, 91]. As the above equation predicts, increases in the delivered minute ventilation accentuate differences between mP_{alv} and mP_{aw}.

2.6.2 Physiological Significance of Mean Airway Pressure

The concept of mP_{aw}, or more precisely, mean alveolar pressure, is central to understanding the benefits and hazards of controlled mechanical ventilation. Under the *passive* conditions of controlled ventilation, mean alveolar pressure (mP_{alv}) is linked to five key outcomes of ventilatory support. In a sense, mP_{aw} can be considered associated with two beneficial actions (ventilation, oxygenation) and three potentially noxious ones (hemodynamic compromise, fluid retention, and barotrauma).

Ventilation is driven by pressure differences developed between the airway opening and the alveolus. The average pressure required to inflate the respiratory system during a single tidal cycle (P_{avg}) can be expressed in terms of its modified "equation of motion" [89]:

$$P_{avg}=R_i [Vt/ti]+V_{avg}/C+auto\text{-}PEEP$$

where R_i is inspiratory resistance, t_i is inspiratory flow duration, and V_{avg} is average volume above FRC. Here, the first term is the flow-resistive pressure, the second is the average inspiratory tidal elastic pressure. When rewritten in terms of minute ventilation, the expression becomes:

$$P_{avg}=R_i [Ve/60D]+V_{avg}/C+Ve/\{fC[e^{60(1-D)/(fR_xC)}-1]\}$$

where D is inspiratory duty cycle, t_i/t_{tot}, R_x is expiratory resistance, and f is frequency. This equation emphasizes the fact that mean airway pressure ($mP_{aw}=P_{avg} \times D+PEEP$) is strongly influenced by the minute ventilation requirement.

Mean alveolar pressure, closely indexed by mP_{aw}, relates directly to mean alveolar volume, and therefore to oxygen exchange across the lung. Once a certain minimum level of end-expiratory volume has been ensured, further increases of PEEP or extensions of inspiratory time fraction (e.g., inverse ratio ventilation) may enhance arterial oxygenation primarily by increasing average lung volume and mP_{alv}. Redistribution of alveolar liquid may also occur.

The place of mP_{alv} in the generation of – or protection from – barotrauma is less clear. Although mean airway pressure correlates reasonably well with the incidence of alveolar rupture, it is not certain that mP_{alv} itself (separated from concomitant increases of peak alveolar pressure) poses an independent risk for barotrauma [92]. It seems reasonable to assume that peak transalveolar pressure, an indicator of the maximal stretching forces applied to distensible alveoli, is more important in *causing* the injury. Once rupture has occurred, however, a high level of mean alveolar pressure may be instrumental in *exacerbating* the damage or *accentuating* gas leakage through rents in the alveolar tissues, i.e., in bringing alveolar rupture to clinical attention. The role of mP_{aw} in ventilator-induced lung injury may vary with its potential to recruit lung units.

2.6.3 Hemodynamic Consequences of Controlled Ventilation

Vigorous spontaneous breathing increases cardiac output requirements and causes mean intrathoracic pressure to fall in proportion to the intensity of the ventilatory workload. Phasic and tonic muscle activity during expiration helps drive venous return. In patients with limited reserve, this fall of intrapleural pressure may congest the central vasculature and afterload the left ventricle excessively. In this setting, passive inflation is often accompanied by the opposite problem; when controlled ventilation is first initiated, cardiac output and blood pressure almost routinely fall as oxygen demands lessen, vascular tone relaxes, and the normal pressure gradient for venous return is reduced.

During *controlled* ventilation mean airway pressure is a close and easily measurable correlate of these adverse hemodynamic sequelae [93]. Raising mP_{alv} during passive ventilation increases both lung and chest volume by similar amounts. Lung expansion tends to increase right ventricular afterload – which poses a life-threatening problem for many patients in the latter phases of acute respiratory failure. More importantly, the increase of intrapleural pressure boosts right atrial pressure, thereby impeding venous return [94]. Rising backpressure is made even more significant by the impaired systemic venous tone and tissue turgor consequent to sedation/paralysis.

The retention of sodium and water were among the earliest recognized complications of positive-pressure ventilation [95]. Fluid retention correlates with the magnitude of average airway (and therefore alveolar and intrapleural) pressure and can be reliably elicited by PEEP [96]. The mechanism remains uncertain, but it could involve reflex-mediated corticomedullary shunting within the kidney, globally reduced renal perfusion, or interference with the humoral control of renal adjustment of fluid balance [97].

2.7 A Strategy for Implementing Controlled Ventilation

In formulating a rational strategy for implementing *controlled* ventilation, the clinician should apply only those pressure levels absolutely required to meet unequivocally important clinical objectives. The minute ventilation requirement should be reduced by treating fever, sepsis, metabolic acidosis, agitation, and the breathing workload, while avoiding excessive calorie and carbohydrate loading. Apart from applying sufficient end-expiratory pressure to maximize compliance, aeration of potentially recruitable lung units should be ensured by maintaining appropriate fluid status and secretion clearance, and by changing position frequently. Upright and prone positioning may be especially helpful in this regard.

For patients in the first stages of acute lung injury, a minimum of 8–10 cmH$_2$O of end-expiratory alveolar pressure (and sometimes as much as 15–20 cmH$_2$O) is usually required to maintain patency of recruited units; for patients with acute airflow obstruction, no added PEEP may be needed or desirable during controlled ventilation. PEEP should not be added beyond levels which cause compliance to deteriorate or peak transpulmonary pressure to exceed safe limits. Judging from the characteristics of normal parenchyma and from limited clinical data, this upper target for *transalveolar* pressure should not exceed 30–35 cmH$_2$O, a value that corresponds to a maximal static airway pressure ("plateau pressure") of 35–40 cmH$_2$O, depending on the stiffness or flexibility of the chest wall. The most appropriate ceiling for alveolar pressure has not yet been determined for patients with acute lung injury and may well be lower than such guidelines suggest [73]; regional alveolar dimensions vary throughout the lung. Moreover, patients who require extended ventilatory support and those with pre-existing lung injury or edema may be more susceptible to damage by mechanical stresses. On the other hand, strong counterarguments can also be mounted for the opposite conclusion; the answer is not currently available to settle the question.

With these requirements satisfied, mPalv should be raised just enough to keep the lung fully inflated and to assure adequate O$_2$ exchange across the lung at safe concentrations of inspired oxygen. In making a judgment regarding adequacy of perfusion and oxygenation, standard methods for assessing vital organ function (e.g., mental status and urine flow) are supplemented by metabolic indicators, such as the serum anion gap and the arterial lactate concentration.

For patients with single organ (lung) failure – whether acute lung injury, asthma, or decompensated COPD – the threshold for increasing ventilator pressures to support gas exchange should be considerably higher than for cardiac dysfunction, shock, or multisystem organ failure. (In the latter cases, reserves and compensatory mechanisms that ensure adequate oxygen extraction cannot be assumed.) The appropriate lower limit for pH is undefined and is almost certain to vary with the nature and severity of the underlying problem. Nonetheless, pH generally can be allowed to fall to 7.25 or less, provided that acidemia is primarily or exclusively respiratory in origin, that pH falls gradually to its nadir and thereafter remains stable, and that acidemia does not develop in the setting of overt pulmonary hypertension or vital organ compromise. Bicarbonate infusion is a rational adjunct to this strategy when the salt and water loads can be easily dealt with. Dialysis or hemofiltration may be required when they cannot. Permissive hypercapnia is of limited effectiveness when there is an important underlying component of metabolic acidosis.

It is widely recognized that a PaCO$_2$ of 40 mmHg should not be the therapeutic goal for an acutely ill patient with airflow obstruction or neuromuscular weakness who normally maintains hypercapnia. In fact, under the worsened conditions of an acute exacerbation, accepting a PaCO$_2$ value somewhat *higher* than the chronically elevated baseline may accelerate machine withdrawal.

2.8 Mode and Machine Settings for Controlled Ventilation

Within the general framework of the strategy just outlined, the clinician must choose the tidal volume and cycling frequency, the inspiratory flow waveform, the end-inflation pause length, the duration of the inspiratory duty cycle, and the mode of machine cycling (the inspiratory "off switch").

2.8.1 Tidal Volume and Cycling Frequency

Reducing the need for ventilatory support is an essential component of a rational strategy for controlled ventilation, whatever the disease being treated. The traditional guideline for tidal volume of 10–15 ml/kg lean body wt. is often too high for safety in patients with severe lung injury or profound air trapping; a selection of 6–8 ml/kg is usually more consistent with the pressure constraints mentioned earlier. In the early phase of ventilatory support, periodic sighs of increased duration may be needed to prevent progressive derecruitment and hypoxemia. With V$_T$ selected, frequency is adjusted to keep PaCO$_2$ at the desired level (dictated by pH and the need to keep peak and mean cycling pressures within acceptable bounds).

2.8.2 Inspiratory Flow Rate and Waveform

In the setting of exacerbated chronic airflow obstruction, where the principal objective is to improve alveolar ventilation and reduce air trapping, rapid inspiratory flows (60–100 l/min) lengthen expiratory time, tending to reduce dynamic hyperinflation and improve gas exchange [98]. Although the shape of the inspiratory flow waveform has little impact on oxygen exchange once mean airway pressure and duty cycle length are taken into account, a decelerating flow profile may improve the ventilation homogeneity achieved by a constant flow profile of similar duration. Slowing end-inspiratory flow improves the distribution of ventilation and reduces the dead-space fraction, enhancing the efficiency of ventilation [99, 100]. Deceleration of end-inspiratory flow can be achieved with pressure-controlled ventilation, by adding a brief end-inspiratory pause to a constant-flow, volume-cycled pattern [100] or by using a linearly decelerating flow profile as an option for volume-cycled ventilation [101].

2.8.3 Duty Cycle and Extended (Inverse) Ratio Ventilation

Inverse ratio ventilation (IRV), a form of controlled ventilatory support introduced more than 25 years ago in the care of neonates with the infant respiratory distress syndrome, has been a subject of recent interest among clinicians treating adult patients as well [8–10]. Extending the duty cycle (inspiratory time fraction) appears to improve oxygenation, primarily by increasing the mean airway and alveolar pressures [90, 101, 102, 103]. Prolonged traction may also facilitate recruitment of lung units that would otherwise remain collapsed. Consistent with this notion, the tidal compliance of the respiratory system tends to improve after starting IRV, and oxygen exchange efficiency may demonstrate time dependence [8, 104]. Improved ventilatory efficiency would be expected for a waveform that inherently decelerates flow and automatically provides an end-inspiratory pause. In fact, on the basis of meager comparative data it appears that IRV may be somewhat more effective in achieving CO_2 elimination than conventional ventilation using PEEP to provide an identical mean airway pressure [99, 105].

Extending the duty cycle is a logical means of raising mean airway pressure once the lower and upper bounds of the tidal cycle have been adjusted to their safe limits. A further rise in end-expiratory pressure causes peak alveolar pressure to encroach on the upper pressure boundary, forcing a reduction in tidal volume. Lengthening the duty cycle may achieve the desired mP_{aw} with less interference with ventilation. Having justified its rationale, existing clinical data are insufficient to prove its superiority [9, 10, 106–109]. Inversion of the inspiratory/expiratory ratio would appear hazardous and counterproductive for the patient with severe airflow obstruction. Here, where unnecessary elevations of mean airway pressure often present serious clinical problems, ratio inversion would appear to have little rationale.

2.8.4 Selection of "Controlled" Parameter During Controlled Ventilation

The clinician has the option of controlling flow and tidal volume or applied pressure and tidal volume, but not all three at once. Traditionally, flow-controlled, volume-cycled modes have been employed, an option which guarantees minute ventilation but allows airway and alveolar pressures to rise when impedance deteriorates.

Volume-Cycled, Flow-Controlled Ventilation
Under conditions of passive inflation, selecting the flow waveform allows the physician to specify delivered tidal volume and minute ventilation. The airway and alveolar pressures developed are then a function of inflation impedance (resistance and elastance) of the respiratory system. As already discussed, increas-

es of alveolar pressure may result in lung injury, and under passive conditions, raising mean airway pressure increases lung and chest wall volumes, impeding venous return. When leakage of gas occurs in the endotracheal tube or external circuitry, airway pressure falls, and only a portion of the machine-generated tidal volume is effective. To avert microcollapse, relatively large tidal volumes (10–15 ml/kg) have traditionally been selected. Although generally a rational practice, insistence on such large tidal volumes may cause alveolar pressures to rise excessively. When tidal volumes fall to <7 ml/kg, many clinicians add one or more recruiting "sigh" breaths of extended duration 2–12 times per hour so as maintain optimal recruitment.

Pressure-Controlled Ventilation

With better understanding of pressure-related tissue injury interest has refocused on the pressure-controlled, time-cycled modes of ventilation. The primary variants of pressure-preset ventilation are pressure-controlled ventilation (PCV), PC-IRV, airway pressure-release ventilation (APRV), and Bi-Phasic airway pressure (Bi-PAP), a mode in which CPAP is varied about two levels [108]. This should not be confused with the mode for noninvasive ventilation known commercially as Bi-PAP, which is essentially pressure support. Although APRV and Bi-PAP combine patient efforts and machine cycles, both revert to pressure-controlled ventilation when ventilatory efforts cease.

Unlike volume-cycled ventilation, pressure-controlled ventilation applied by a machine with high flow capacity automatically compensates for minor circuit leaks and augments flow as necessary to maintain the targeted circuit pressure. However, fixing the upper and lower limits for applied pressure restricts the ventilating pressure gradient. Consequently, even though pressure control effectively regulates peak and mean airway pressures, the relationship between ventilation and the clinician-set variables (frequency, applied pressure, and duty cycle) is not intuitive or straightforward [110–112]. Ventilation during PCV is the result of the interaction between the applied pattern and the impedance to ventilation. The latter is characterized by inspiratory (R_i) and expiratory (R_x) resistance and compliance (C). Decreases of compliance will reduce the tidal volume, and increases of resistance may do so unless sufficient inspiratory and expiratory times are allowed. Thus, tidal volume tends to vary with changes of position, bronchial tone, and central airway secretions. The ventilatory parameters selected by the clinician include the set pressure target, PEEP, frequency, and duty cycle.

Qualitatively similar curves relating ventilation to cycling frequency can be drawn for restrictive and obstructive disease. For both, a fixed upper limit for total ventilation can be determined mathematically for any given set of impedance parameters and P_{set}. However, the *shape* of the curves and, specifically, the rate at which the plateau of each is approached, differ considerably (Fig. 2.3). As frequency increases, tidal volume decreases. Consequently, as frequency increases, peak alveolar pressure and ventilation both reach maximum values and then decline. Moreover, for a fixed frequency, variations in duty cycle demonstrate an optimum value which is more distinct for obstructive than for restrictive disease (Fig. 2.4).

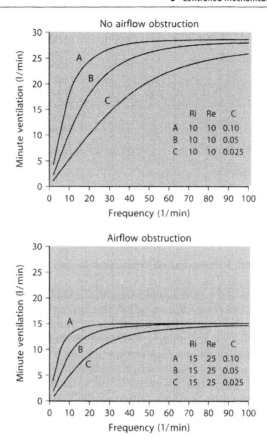

Fig. 2.3. *Top panel*: Minute ventilation (V_E) as a function of frequency for three values of respiratory system compliance, with $R_i = R_e$ and no major degree of airflow obstruction ($P_{set}=20$, $D=0.4$). Whatever the compliance value, V_E rises toward a final plateau determined only by inspiratory time fraction and resistance. However, compliance determines rate of rise of these curves and, over the clinically relevant frequency range, exerts a profound influence on V_E. *Bottom panel*: During simulated airflow obstruction (moderately severe), the maximum V_E achievable with the same P_{set} and D is sharply lower and closely approached at frequencies well within the clinically observable range. *C*, compliance; R_i, inspiratory resistance; R_e, expiratory resistance; *D*, duty cycle (t_i/t_{tot}). (From [110] with permission)

Because auto-PEEP is defined as a positive difference between alveolar and airway pressures at end-expiration, auto-PEEP represents a counterpressure detracting from the ventilatory effectiveness of the applied P_{set}. To the extent that dynamic airway compression and flow limitation accompany auto-PEEP, the addition of PEEP will minimally affect the ventilation resulting from a given peak pressure. Conversely, if auto-PEEP develops without tidal limitation of airflow, the addition of PEEP while maintaining the same value for P_{set} will diminish its ventilatory effectiveness. For PCV, therefore, close volume monitoring is essential.

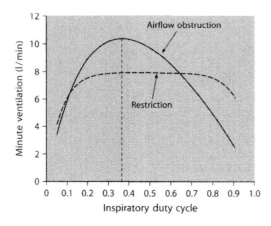

Fig. 2.4. Relationship of minute ventilation to inspiratory duty cycle length during pressure-control ventilation. Unlike severe restrictive disease, obstructive disease is characterized by a distinctly optimal inspiratory duty cycle length. (From [110] with permission)

2.8.5 Converting from Volume-Cycled Ventilation to Pressure Control

Many critically ill patients have limited tolerance for changes in machine settings. Therefore, it is important to accomplish transitions between volume-cycled and pressure-controlled ventilation smoothly, matching inspired tidal volume and mean airway pressure and holding PEEP and cycling frequency unchanged. Because PCV inherently applies a decelerating flow waveform, the simplest lateral conversion is generally made from volume-cycled decelerating flow [112]. The procedure begins by first noting the exhaled tidal volume, the mean airway pressure, and the I:E ratio. The pressure setting for PCV (including PEEP) should approximate the end-inspiratory plateau pressure. (Note that on some machines the excursion of pressure *above* PEEP is the set variable). Next, the inspiratory time fraction should be adjusted so as to match volume cycled ventilation. The resulting values should be similar to those existing prior to the conversion. However, if the V_T that results is somewhat smaller than desired, auto-PEEP may be an explanation. P_{set} can be adjusted to compensate. If the transition from volume-cycled ventilation is made from *constant* (rather than from linearly decelerating) flow, a small ($\approx$2–3 cmH$_2$O) decline in mean airway pressure should be anticipated. Mean airway pressure can be altered, as indicated, by extending or contracting T_i/T_{TOT}.

2.9 Future Directions in Controlled Mechanical Ventilation

Experimental and clinical evidence strongly suggests that a spectrum of innovative techniques ranging in invasiveness from extracorporeal oxygenation and CO$_2$ removal to retargeting of the fundamental goals of mechanical ventilation themselves may allow controlled ventilation to achieve its full potential as a life-support technique.

2.9.1 Controlled Ventilation and Permissive Hypercapnia

As already noted, CO_2 retention may be an inevitable consequence of a lung-protective strategy that tightly restricts applied pressure and maintains a certain minimum lung volume [75, 110, 111]. Although gradual elevations of $PaCO_2$ are often tolerated remarkably well, hypercapnia may not be advisable for all patients (e.g., those with coexisting head injury, recent cerebral vascular accident, significant cardiovascular dysfunction, severe hypoxemia, or β-blockade) [14]. Acute elevations in $PaCO_2$ increase sympathetic activity, increase cardiac output, increase the pulmonary vascular resistance, alter bronchomotor tone, dilate cerebral vessels, and disturb functions of the central nervous system [16]. The consequences of CO_2 retention are related to changes of intracellular pH and therefore dissipate with the passage of time.

2.9.2 Decreasing Series Dead Space by Tracheal Gas Insufflation (TGI)

A possible alternative to allowing extreme or rapidly developing hypercapnia in ALI would be to enhance the efficiency of CO_2 elimination at low tidal volumes and cycling pressures. Techniques to improve the efficiency of cyclical ventilatory pressure would be desirable when hypercapnia must be minimized or when the pace at which hypercapnia develops must be slowed. One recent approach is to insufflate fresh gas into the trachea (TGI) in order to reduce the concentration of CO_2 in the series (anatomic) dead space.

The idea of bypassing the anatomic dead space has been applied to *spontaneously* breathing patients for many years. A variant of this technique, for example, was employed in the early 1960s, when tracheostomy was used to treat patients with severe emphysema and ventilatory failure [113]. In 1968, Stresemann demonstrated the potential utility of flushing the proximal anatomic dead space in normal subjects and in two patients with obstructive lung disease [114, 115]. More recently, forms of TGI have been shown to be effective in spontaneously breathing hypercapnic animals and patients [116–124].

TGI-aided ventilation should be particularly effective in a lung-protective ventilatory strategy for two important reasons: (a) small tidal volumes are associated with a relatively high percentage of series dead space; (b) when $PaCO_2$ is very elevated, small reductions of V_D/V_T are associated with large decreases of $PaCO_2$ [120]. During TGI-aided ventilation, fresh gas delivery occurs either throughout the respiratory cycle (continuous catheter flow) or only during a segment of it (phasic catheter flow) [120, 123]. During expiration, low-to-moderate continuous flows of fresh gas introduced near the carina dilute the proximal anatomic dead space (dead space flushing) (Fig. 2.5). During inspiration, catheter flow contributes to the total inspired V_T but also bypasses the anatomic dead space mouthward (proximal) of the gas jet. At high catheter flow rates, turbulence generated at the catheter tip can also enhance gas mixing in regions beyond its orifice, thereby contributing to CO_2 elimination [125–127]. Selective expiratory TGI retains the gas exchange efficiency of continuous TGI with several distinct benefits: (a) alveolar pressures do not rise when inspirato-

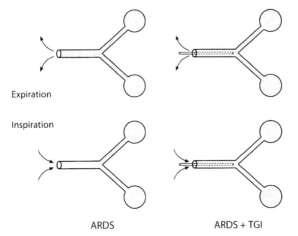

Fig. 2.5. Concept of tracheal gas insufflation. The removal of CO_2 from the central airway at end expiration improves the ventilatory efficiency of small tidal volume breaths. (From [133] with permission)

ry time is extended; (b) higher flows can be utilized without increasing either tidal volume or peak alveolar pressure; (c) unlike continuous TGI, plateau pressure can be effectively monitored. The efficiency of expiratory TGI appears to parallel the volume of fresh gas injected per exhalation, and not the TGI flow rate itself [128].

The ventilatory benefit which occurs from TGI is often modest in lungs with large alveolar dead space. However, its benefit should be substantial in the settings of hypercapnia and small tidal volumes – two features of the modern strategy for controlled ventilation. Optimal usage and long-term safety are yet to be fully defined. Moreover, its potential for causing mucosal damage, secretion retention, and barotrauma remains to be determined. Nonetheless, the experience of workers using transtracheal oxygen in patients with COPD and other stable conditions [116–119], as well as that of our group and others using TGI in critically ill patients [122, 129–131], indicates that it may eventually prove helpful in a variety of acute and chronic settings. Because of its potential to moderate the rate and extent of CO_2 retention, TGI would appear well-suited as an adjunct to a pressure-targeted, lung-protective ventilatory support.

2.10 References

1. Marini JJ, Rodriguez RM, Lamb VJ (1986) The inspiratory workload of patient-initiated mechanical ventilation. Am Rev Respir Dis 134:902–909
2. Marini JJ, Smith TC, Lamb VJ (1988) External work output and force generation during synchronized intermittent mechanical ventilation. Effect of machine assistance an breathing effort. Am Rev Respir Dis 138:1169–1179
3. Coggeshall JW, Marini JJ, Newman JH (1985) Improved oxygenation after muscle relaxation in the adult respiratory distress syndrome. Arch Intern Med 145:1718–1720

4. Lynch JP, Mhyre JG, Dantzker DR (1979) The influence of cardiac output on intrapulmonary shunt. J Appl Physiol 46:315-321
5. Schumacker PT, Cain SM (1987) The concept of critical oxygen delivery. Intensive Care Med 13:223-229
6. Chandra A, Coggeshall JW, Ravenscraft SA, Marini JJ (1994) Hyperpnea limits the volume recruited by positive end-expiratory pressure. Am J Respir Crit Care Med 150:911-917
7. Lessard MR, Lofaso F, Brochard L (1995) Expiratory muscle activity increases intrinsic positive end-expiratory pressure independently of dynamic hyperinflation in mechanically ventilated patients. Am J Respir Crit Care Med 151:562-569
8. Gurevitch MJ, Van Dyke J, Young ES, Jackson K (1986) Improved oxygenation and lower peak airway pressure in severe adult respiratory distress syndrome: treatment with inverse ratio ventilation. Chest 89:211-213
9. Lessard MR, Guerot E, Lorino H, et al (1994) Effects of pressure-controlled with different I:E ratios versus volume-controlled ventilation on respiratory mechanics, gas exchange, and hemodynamics in patients with adult respiratory distress syndrome. Anesthesiology 80:983-991
10. Marcy TW, Marini JJ (1991) Inverse ratio ventilation: rationale and implementation. Chest 100:495-504
11. Westenskow DR, Pace NL (1982) Differential lung ventilation. In: Prakash O (ed) Applied physiology in clinical respiratory care. Martinus Nijhoff, Boston, pp 313-324
12. Gattinoni L, Pesenti A. Mascheroni D, et al (1986) Low frequency positive pressure ventilation with extracorporeal CO_2 removal in severe acute respiriratory failure. JAMA 256:881-886
13. Darioli R, Perret C (1984) Mechanical controlled hypoventilation in status asthmaticus. Am Rev Respir Dis 129:385-387
14. Feihl F, Perret C (1994) Permissive hypercapnia. How permissive should we be? Am J Respir Crit Care Med 150: 1722-1737
15. Tuxen DV (1994) Permissive hypercapnic ventilation. Am J Respir Crit Care Med 150:870-874
16. Hickling KG, Joyce C (1995) Permissive hypercapnia in ARDS and its effect on tissue oxygenation. Acta Anaesthesiol Scand 107:201-208
17. Hickling KG, Henderson SJ, Jackson R Low mortality associated with low volume pressure limited ventilation with permissive hypercapnia in severe adult respiratory distress syndrome. Int Care Med 1990 16:372-377
18. Hickling KG, Walsh J, Henderson S, et al (1994) Low mortality rate in adult respiratory distress syndrome using low-volume, pressure-limited ventilation with permissive hypercapnia: a prospective study. Crit Care Med 22:1568-1578
19. Truwit JD, Marini JJ (1988) Evaluation of thoracic mechanics in. the ventilated patient. 1: Primary measurements. 2: Applied mechanics. J Crit Care 3:133-150, 199-213
20. Cunningham DJC, Robbins PA, Wolff CB (1986) Integration of respiratory responses to changes in alveolar partial pressures of CO_2 and O_2 and in arterial pH. In: Geiger SR (ed) Handbook of physiology, sect 3: The respiratory system, vol 2. American Physiology Society, Bethesda, pp 475-528
21. Prechter GC, Nelson SB, Hubmayr RD (1990) The ventilatory threshold for carbon dioxide. Am Rev Respir Dis 141:758-764
22. Hansen-Flaschen J, Cowe J, Raps EC (1993) Neuromuscular blockade in the intensive care unit - more than we bargained for. Am Rev Respir Dis 147:234-236
23. Greenleaf JE, Kozlowski S (1982) Physiological consequences of reduced physical activity during bed rest. Exerc Sport Sci Rev 10:84-119
24. Bolton CF (1996) Sepsis and the systemic inflammatory response syndrome: neuromuscular manifestations. Crit Care Med 24:1408-1416
25. Douglass JA, Tuxen DV, Horne M, et al (1992) Myopathy in severe asthma. Am Rev respir Dis 146:517-519
26. Brun-Buisson C, Gherardi R (1988) Hydrocortisone and pancuronium bromide: acute myopathy during status asthmaticus (letter). Crit Care Med 16:732

27. Segredo V, Caldwell JE, Matthay MA, Sharma ML, Gruenke LD, Miller RD (1992) Persistent paralysis in critically ill patients after long-term administration of vecuronium. N Engl J Med 327:524–528
28. Leatherman JW, Fluegel WL, David WS, et al (1996) Muscle weakness in mechanically ventilated patients with severe asthma. Am J Respir Crit Care Med 153:1686–1690
29. Hoey LL, Joslin SM, Nahum A, et al (1995) Prolonged neuromuscular blockade in two critically ill patients treated with atracurium. Pharmacotherapy 15:254
30. Gattinoni L, Pelosi P, Crotti S, et al (1995) Effects of positive end-expiratory pressure on regional distribution of tidal volume and recruitment in adult respiratory distress syndrome. Am J Respir Crit Care Med 151:1807–1814
31. Gattinoni L, Bombino M, Pelosi P, et al (1994) Lung structure and function in different states,of severe adult respiratory distress syndrome. JAMA 271:1772–1779
32. Pelosi P, D'Andrea L, Vitale G, et al (1994) Vertical gradient of regional lung inflation in adult respiratory distress syndrome. Am J Respir Crit Care Med 149:8–13
33. Gattinoni L, Pesenti A, Avalli L, Rossi F, Bombino M (1987) Pressure-volume curve of total respiratory system in acute respiratory failure. Computed tomographic scan study. Am Rev Respir Dis 136:730–736
34. Maunder RJ, Shuman WP, McHugh JW, Marglin SI, Butler J (1986) Preservation of normal lung regions in the adult respiratory distress syndrome. Analysis by computed tomography. JAMA 255:2463–2465
35. Lamm WJ, Graham MM, Albert RK (1994) Mechanism by which the prone position improves oxygenation in acute lung injury. Am J Respir Crit Care Med 150:184–193
36. Marini JJ, Tyler ML, Hudson LD, Davis BS, Huseby JS (1984) Influence of head-dependent positions on lung volume and oxygen saturation in chronic airflow obstruction. Am Rev Respir Dis 129:101–105
37. Gattinoni L, Brazzi L, Pelosi P, et al (1995) A trial of goal–oriented hemodynamic therapy in critically ill patients. S_VO_2 Collaborative Group. N Engl J Med 333:1025–1032
38. Raine JM, Bishop JM (1963) A-a difference in O_2 tension and physiological dead space in normal man. J Appl Physiol 18:284–288
39. Refsum HE (1963) Relationship between state of consciousness and arterial hypoxemia and hypercapnia in patients with pulmonary insufficiency breathing own. Clin Sci 25:361–367
40. Schoene RB, Horbein TF (1988) High altitude adaptation. In: Murray JF, Nadel JA (eds) Textbook of respiratory medicine. Saunders, Philadelphia, pp 196–220
41. Hochachka PW (1996) Metabolic defense adaptations to hypobaric hypoxia in man. In: Fregly MJ, Blatteis CM (eds) Environmental physiology, vol II, chap 48. Handbook of physiology, sect 4. Oxford University Press, New York, pp 1115–1124
42. Schumacker PT, Samsel RW (1990) Oxygen supply consumption in ARDS. Clin Chest Med 11:715–722
43. Tuchschmidt J, Fried J, Astiz M, Rackow E (1992) Elevation of cardiac output and oxygen delivery improves outcome in septic shock. Chest 102:216–222
44. Shoemaker WC, Appel PL, Kram KB, Waxman K, Lee TS (1988) Protective trial of supranormal values of survivors as therapeutic goals in high risk surgical patients. Chest 94:1176–1186
45. Hotchkiss RS, Karl IE (1992) Re-evaluation of the role of cellular hypoxic and bioenergetic failure in sepsis. JAMA 267:1503–1510
46. Nunn JF (1977) Applied respiratory physiology, 2nd edn. Butterworths, Boston, pp 460–470
47. Narins RG (1985) Alkali therapy of metabolic acidosis due to organic acids: the case for the judicious use of sodium bicarbonate. AKF Nephrol Lett 2:13
48. Arieff AI, Leach W, Park R, Lazarowitz VC (1982) Systemic effects of $NaHCO_3$ in experimental lactic acidosis in dogs. Am J Physiol 242:F586–591
49. Kacmarek R, Hickling KG (1993) Permissive hypercapnia. Respir Care 38:373–387
50. Kilburn KH, Dowell AR (1971) Renal function in respiratory failure. Arch Int Med 127:754–762
51. Pesenti A (1990) Target blood gases during ARDS ventilatory management. Int Care Med 16:349–351

52. Marini JJ (1991) Controlled ventilation: targets, hazards and options. In: Marini JJ, Roussos C (eds) Ventilatory failure. Springer, Berlin Heidelberg New York, pp 269–292
53. Dreyfuss D, Basset G, Soler P, Saumon G (1985) Intermittent positive pressure hyperventilation with high inflation pressures produces pulmonary microvascular injury in rats. Am Rev Respir Dis 132:880–884
54. Kolobow T, Moretti MP, Furmagalli R, et al (1987) Severe impairment in lung function induced by high peak airway pressure during mechanical ventilation. Am Rev Respir Dis 135:312–315
55. Dreyfuss D, Saumon G (1994) Should the lung be rested or recruited? The Charybdis and Scylla of ventilatory management. Am J Respir Crit Care Med 149:1066–1067
56. Dreyfuss D, Saumon G (1993) Role of tidal volume, FRC, and end-inspiratory volume in the development of pulmonary edema following mechanical ventilation. Am Rev Respir Dis 148:1194–1203
57. Morris AH, Wallace CJ, Menlove RL, Clemmer TP, Orme JF Jr, Weaver LK, Dean NC, Thomas F, East TD, Pace NL, et al (1994) Randomized clinical trial of pressure-controlled inverse ratio ventilation and extracorporeal CO_2 removal for adult respiratory distress syndrome. Am J Respir Crit Care Med 149: 295–305
58. Amato MBP, Barbas CSV, Medeiros DM, Schettino GDP, Filho GL, et al (1995) Beneficial effects of the "open lung" approach with low distending pressures in acute respiratory distress syndrome. Am J Respir Crit Care Med 152: 1835–1846
59. Amato MBP, Barbas CSV, Medeiros D, et al (1996) Improved survival in ARDS: beneficial effects of a lung protective strategy. Am J Respir Crit Care Med 153:A531
60. Narins RG, Bastl CP, Rudnick MR, et al (1982) Acid-base metabolism. In: Golnick HC (ed) Current nephrology. Wiley, New York, pp 7–9
61. Mitchell JH, Wildenthal K, Johnson RL Jr (1972) The effects of acid base disturbances on cardiovascular and pulmonary function. Kidney Int 1:375
62. Housley E, Clarke SW, Hedworth-Whitty RB, Bishop JW (1970) Effect of acute and chronic acidemia and associated hypoxemia on the pulmonary circulation of patients with chronic bronchitis. Cardiovasc Res 4:482–489
63. Reynolds EOR (1975) Management of hyaline membrane disease. Br Med Bull 31:18–24
64. Woodring JH (1985) Pulmonary interstitial emphysema in the adult respiratory distress syndrome. Crit Care Med 13:786–791
65. Albelda SM, Gefter WB, Kelley MA, et al (1983) Ventilator-induced subpleural air cysts: clinical, radiographic, and pathologic significance. Am Rev Respir Dis 127:360–365
66. Marini JJ, Culver BH (1989) Systemic air embolism consequent to mechanical ventilation in ARDS. Ann Intern Med 110:699–703
67. Churg A, Golden J, Fligiel S, Hogg JC (1983) Bronchopulmonary dysplasia in the adult. Am Rev Respir Dis 127:117–120
68. Slavin G, Nunn JF, Crow J, Core C (1982) Bronchiolectasis – a complication of artificial ventilation. Br Med J 285:931–934
69. Rouby JJ, Lherm T, de Lasale E, et al (1993) Histologic aspects of pulmonary barotrauma in critically ill patients with acute respiratory failure. Intensive Care Med 19:383–389
70. Pesenti A, Pelosi P, Gattinoni L (1990) Lung mechanics in ARDS. In: Vincent JL (ed) Update in intensive care and emergency medicine. Springer, Berlin Heidelberg New York, pp 231–238
71. Gattinoni L, D'Andrea L, Pelosi P, Vitale G, Pesenti A, Fumagalli R (1993) Regional effects and mechanism of positive end-expiratory pressure in early adult respiratory distress syndrome. JAMA 269:2122–2127
72. Gattinoni L, Mascheroni D, Basilco E, Foti G, Pesenti A, Avalli L (1987) Volume/pressure curve of total respiratory system in paralyzed patients: artefacts and correction factors. Intensive Care Med 13:19–25
73. Roupie E, Dambrosio M, Servillo G, et al (1995) Titration of tidal volume and induced hypercapnia in acute respiratory distress syndrome. Am J Respir Crit Care Med 152:121–128
74. Corbridge TC, Wood LDH, Crawford GP, Chudoba MJ, Yanos J, Sznajder JI (1990) Adverse effects of large tidal volume and low PEEP in canine acid aspiration. Am Rev Respir Dis 142:311–315

75. Marini JJ (1996) Evolving concepts in the ventilatory management of ARDS. Clin Chest Med 17: 555–575
76. Marini JJ (1994) Ventilation of the acute respiratory distress syndrome. Looking for Mr. Goodmode. Anesthesiology 80: 972–975
77. Muscedere JG, Mullen JB, Gan K, et al (1994) Tidal ventilation at low airway pressures can augment lung injury. Am J Respir Crit Care Med 149:1327–1334
78. Matamis D, LeMaire F, Harf A, et al (1984) Total respiratory pressure volume curves in the adult respiratory distress syndrome. Chest 86:58–66
79. Bryan AC, Froese AB (1991) Reflections on the HIFI trial. Pediatrics 87:565
80. Mead J, Takishima T, Leith D (1970) Stress distribution in lungs: a model of pulmonary elasticity. J Appl Physiol 28:596–608
81. Koltan M, Cattran CB, Kent G (1982) Oxygenation during high-frequency ventilation in two models of lung injury. Anesth Analg 61:323–327
82. Smith TC, Marini JJ (1988) Impact of PEEP on lung mechanics and work of breathing in severe airflow obstruction. The effect of PEEP on auto-PEEP. J Appl Physiol 65:1488–1499
83. Petrof BJ, Legare M, Goldberg P, Milic-Emili J, Gottfried SB (1990) Continuous positive airway pressure reduces work of breathing and dyspnea during weaning from mechanical ventilation in severe chronic obstructive pulmonary disease. Am Rev Respir Dis 141:281–289
84. Tuxen D (1989) Detrimental effects of positive end expiratory pressure during controlled mechanical ventilation of patients with severe airflow obstruction. Am Rev Respir Dis 140:5–9
85. Hotchkiss JR, Crooke PS, Adams AB, Marini JJ (1993) Implications of a biphasic two-compartment model of constant flow ventilation for the clinical setting. J Crit Lit Care 2:114–123
86. Fu Z, Costello ML, Tsukimoto K, et al (1992) High lung volume increases stress failure in pulmonary capillaries. J Appl Physiol 73:123–133
87. Mathieu-Costello O, Willford DC, Fu Z, et al (1995) Pulmonary capillaries are more resistant to stress failure in dogs than in rabbits. J Appl Physiol 79:908
88. Otis AB, Fenn WO, Rahn H (1950) Mechanics of breathing in man. J Appl Physiol 2:592–607
89. Marini JJ (1990) Lung mechanics in ARDS: recent conceptual advances and implications for management. Clin Chest Med 11:673–690
90. Marini JJ, Ravenscraft SA (1992) Mean airway pressure: physiological determinants and clinical importance. 2: Clinical implications. Crit Care Med 20:1604–1616
91. Hyatt RE (1983) Expiratory flow limitation. J Appl Physiol: Respirat Environ Exercise Physiol 55:1–8
92. Gammon BR, Shin MS, Buchalter SE (1992) Pulmonary barotrauma in mechanical ventilation: patterns and risk factors. Chest 102:568–572
93. Cournand A, Motley HL, Werko L, Richards DW (1948) Physiologic studies of the effects of intermittent positive pressure breathing on cardiac output in man. Am J Physiol 152:162–174
94. Guyton AC, Jones CE, Coleman TC (1973) Circulatory physiology. In: Cardiac output and its regulation. W.B. Saunders, Philadelphia, p 193
95. Sladen A, Laver MB, Pontoppidan H (1968) Pulmonary complications and water retention in prolonged mechanical ventilation. N Engl J Med 279:448–453
96. Kumar A, Falke K, Geffin B, Aldredge CF, Laver MB, Lowenstein E, Pontoppidan H (1970) Continuous positive pressure ventilation in acute respiratory failure. N Engl J Med 283:1430–1436
97. Manquez JM, Douglas ME, Downs JB, et al (1979) Renal function and cardiovascular responses during positive airway pressure. Anesthesiology 50:393–398
98. Connors AF, McCaffree DR, Gray BA (1981) Effect of inspiratory flow rate on gas exchange during mechanical ventilation. Am Rev Respir Dis 124:537–543
99. Cole AGH, Weller SF, Sykes MK (1984) Inverse ratio ventilation compared with PEEP in adult respiratory failure. Intensive Care Med 10:227–232
100. Fuleihan SF, Wilson RS, Pontoppidan H (1976) Effect of mechanical ventilation with end-inspiratory pause on blood-gas exchange. Anesth Analg 55:122–130

101. Ravenscraft SA, Burke WC, Marini JJ (1992) Volume-cycled decelerating flow: an alternative form of mechanical ventilation. Chest 101:1342–1351
102. Toben BP, Lewandowski V (1988) Nontraditional and new ventilatory techniques. Crit Care Nurs Q 11:12–28
103. Kacmarek RM, Hess D (1990) Pressure controlled inverse ratio ventilation. Panacea or auto-PEEP? Respir Care 35:945–948
104. Tharatt RS, Allen RP, Albertson TE (1988) Pressure controlled inverse ratio ventilation in severe adult respiratory failure. Chest 94:755–762
105. Pesenti A, Marcolin R, Prato P, Borelli M, Riboni A, Gattinoni L (1985) Mean airway pressure vs. positive end-expiratory pressure during mechanical ventilation. Crit Care Med 13:34–37
106. Marini JJ (1995) Inverse ratio ventilation – simply an alternative, or something more? Crit Care Med 23: 224–228
107. Armstrong BW Jr, MacIntyre NR (1995) Pressure-controlled, inverse ratio ventilation that avoids air trapping in the adult respiratory distress syndrome. Crit Care Med 23:279–285
108. Sydow M, Burchardi H, Ephraim E, et al (1994) Long-term effects of two different ventilatory modes an oxygenation in acute lung injury. Comparison of airway pressure release ventilation and volume-controlled inverse ratio ventilation. Am J Respir Crit Care Med 149:1550–1556
109. Shanholtz C, Brower R (1994) Should inverse ratio ventilation be used in adult respiratory distress syndrome? Am J Respir Crit Care Med 149:1354
110. Marini JJ, Crooke PS, Truwit JD (1989) Determinants and limits of pressure preset ventilation: a mathematical model of pressure control. J Appl Physiol 67:1081–1092
111. Marini J.J, Crooke PS (1993) A general mathematical model for Respiriratory dynamics relevant to the clinical setting. Am Rev Respir Dis 147:14–24
112. McKibben AW, Ravenscraft SA (1996) Pressure controlled and volume-cycled ventilation. Clin Chest Med 17 395–410
113. Cullen JH (1963) An evaluation of tracheostomy in pulmonary emphysema. Ann Intern Med 58:953–960
114. Stresemann E (1968) Washout of anatomical dead space. Design of a method and experimental study using an external dead space. Respiration 25:281
115. Stresemann E, Votteri BA, Sattler FP (1969) Washout of anatomical dead space for alveolar hypoventilation. Respiration 26:425–434
116. Hurewitz A, Bergofsky E, Vomero E (1991) Airway insufflation: Increasing flow rates progressively reduce dead space in respiratory failure. Am Rev Respir Dis 144:1229–1233
117. Bergofsky EH, Hurewitz AN (1989) Airway insufflation: physiologic effects on acute and chronic gas exchange in humans. Am Rev Respir Dis 140:885–890
118. Long SE, Menon AS, Kato H, Goldstein RS, Slutsky AS (1988) Constant oxygen insufflation (COI) in a ventilatory failure model. Am Rev Respir Dis 138:630–635
119. Benditt J, Pollock M, Roa J, Celli B (1993) Transtracheal delivery of gas decreases the oxygen cost of breathing. Am Rev Respir Dis 147:1207–1210
120. Nahum A, Burke WC, Ravenscraft SA, Marcy TW, Adams AB, Crooke PS, Marini JJ (1992) Lung mechanics and gas exchange during pressure controlled ventilation in dogs: augmentation of CO_2 elimination by an intratracheal catheter. Am Rev Respir Dis 146:965–973
121. Nahum A, Ravenscraft SA, Adams AB, et al (1995) Inspiratory tidal volume sparing effects of tracheal gas insufflation in dogs with oleic acid-induced lung injury. J Crit Care 10:115–121
122. Belghith M, Fierobe L, Brunet F, et al (1995) Is tracheal gas insufflation an alternative to extrapulmonary gas exchangers in severe ARDS? Chest 107:1416
123. Burke WC, Nahum A, Ravenscraft SA, Nakos G, Adams AB, Marcy TW, Marini JJ (1993) Modes of tracheal gas insufflation: comparison of continuous and phase specific gas injection in normal dogs. Am Rev Respir Dis 148:562–568
124. Nahum A, Ravenscraft, SA, Nakos G, Burke WC, Adams AB, Marcy TW, Marini JJ (1992) Tracheal gas insufflation during pressure controlled ventilation: effect of catheter position, diameter, and flow rate. Am Rev Respir Dis 146:1411–1418
125. Slutsky AS, Watson J, Leith DE, Brown R (1985) Tracheal insufflation O_2 (TRIO) at low flow rates sustains life for several hours. Anesthesiology 63:278–286

126. Isabey D, Boussignac G, Harf A (1989) Effect of air entrainment on airway pressure during endotracheal gas injection. J Appl Physiol 67:771–779
127. Slutsky AS, Menon AS (1987) Catheter position and blood gases during constantflow ventilation. J Appl Physiol 62:513–519
128. Ravenscraft SA, Shapiro RS, Nahum A, Burke WC, Adams AB, Nakos G, Marini JJ (1996) Tracheal gas insufflation: catheter effectiveness is determined by expiratory flush volume, Am J Respir Crit Care Med 153:1817–1824
129. Gilbert J, Larsson A, Smith RB, Bunegin L (1991) Intermittent-flow expiratory ventilation (IFEV): delivery technique and principles of action – a preliminary communication. Biomed Instrum Technol 25:451–456
130. Jonson B, Similowski T, Levy P, Vires N, Pariente R (1990) Expiratory flushing of airways: a method to reduce dead space ventilation. Eur Respir J 3:1202
131. Ravenscraft SA, Burke WC, Nahum A, Adams AB, Nakos G, Marcy TW, Marini JJ (1993) Tracheal gas insufflation augments CO_2 clearance during mechanical ventilation. Am Rev Respir Dis 148:345–351
132. Marini JJ (1990) Ventilatory management of chronic obstructive pulmonary disease. In: Cherniack NS (ed) Chronic obstructive pulmonary disease. W.B. Saunders, Philadelphia, pp 495–506
133. Marini JJ, Wheeler AW (1997) Critical care medicine – the essentials, 2nd edn. Williams and Wilkins, Baltimore

3 Proportional Assist Ventilation

M. Younes

Supported by the Respiratory Health Network of Centres of Excellence (INSPIRAPLEX) and by the Medical Research Council of Canada Proportional Assist Ventilation and PAV are trademarks of the University of Manitoba

3.1 Definition

Proportional assist ventilation (PAV) is a form of synchronized partial ventilatory support in which the ventilator generates pressure in *proportion to the patient's instantaneous effort,* and this proportionality applies from breath to breath as well as continuously throughout each inspiration [1]. In effect, patient effort is amplified, as if the patient has acquired additional inspiratory muscles that remain under the control of the patient's own respiratory control system (Fig. 3.1).

Unlike other modes of partial support, there is no target flow, tidal volume, ventilation or airway pressure. Rather, the objective of PAV is to allow the patient to comfortably attain whatever ventilation and breathing pattern his or

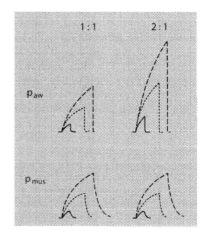

Fig. 3.1. Idealized representation of ventilator response during PAV. Ventilator output (P_{aw}) tracks patient's inspiratory muscle output (P_{mus}). What is adjusted is proportionality between P_{aw} and P_{mus}. Two examples are represented where the proportionalities are 1:1 and 2:1. Clearly, other ratios are possible

her control system sees fit. The responsibility for determining level and pattern of breathing is shifted entirely from the caregiver to the patient.

3.2 How to Get the Ventilator to Respond to the Patient's Instantaneous Inspiratory Effort

The objectives of PAV can, theoretically, be accomplished by recording the activity from a respiratory muscle (EMG) or nerve (ENG) and using the signal to drive the ventilator. Systems of this kind have been developed and used to produce a "normal" breathing pattern in experimental animals subjected to thoracotomy or paralysis [2, 3].

Alternatively, the pressure output of an inspiratory muscle, for example the diaphragm (P_{di}), may be used as the command signal to the ventilator. Although this would theoretically accomplish the same objectives, there are practical difficulties, including the need for invasive monitoring (esophageal and gastric catheters) and the substantial artifacts produced in this signal by the heart beat and by swallowing.*

The method proposed to accomplish the objectives of PAV [1], and which is suitable for clinical application, is to provide pressure assist in proportion to ongoing inspiratory flow (flow assist, FA) and volume (volume assist, VA). For FA and VA to result in airway pressure (P_{aw}) being proportional to instantaneous effort (i.e. PAV) the following two conditions must be met:

1. Both FA and VA need to be used.
2. FA (which is expressed in $cmH_2O/l/s$) and VA (expressed in cmH_2O/l) must be *less than the patient's resistance (R_{rs}) and elastance (E_{rs})*, respectively, and the fractions (i.e. FA/R_{rs} and VA/E_{rs} should, ideally, be similar.

Figure 3.2 illustrates how applying these two principles can result in proportionality between P_{aw} and patient's inspiratory effort (P_{mus}). Assume a flow pattern of the form shown in the first column (nearly sinusoidal, as is most often the case during normal breathing). Volume, which is the integral of flow, rises in a completely different pattern and reaches its peak at the end of inspiration. The total pressure used to generate flow (P_{res}) is a function of $\dot{V}$ and resistance (R_{rs}). If R_{rs} is constant (i.e. not flow dependent) the time course of P_{res} will resemble the time course of flow ($P_{res} = \dot{V} \cdot R_{rs}$), as shown by the outer envelope of the P_{res} waveform. The total pressure used to overcome elastic recoil (P_{el}) is a function of volume above FRC and respiratory system elastance (E_{rs}, E_{rs} = l/compliance). In the case where E_{rs} is constant in the V_T range, the time course of P_{el} resembles the time

---

* Pleural (esophageal) pressure (P_{pl}) alone is not a suitable signal. Apart from being subject to the same difficulties of P_{pl} (invasiveness and artifacts), P_{pl} during mechanical ventilation does not bear a fixed relation to the pressure generated by respiratory muscles (P_{mus}), since P_{pl} represents P_{mus} after subtracting the pressure dissipated in moving the chest wall [4]. In fact, P_{pl} can be increasing (i.e. becoming more positive) in the course of inspiration even as inspiratory P_{mus} is increasing (which should reduce P_{pl}). (See [4] for details).

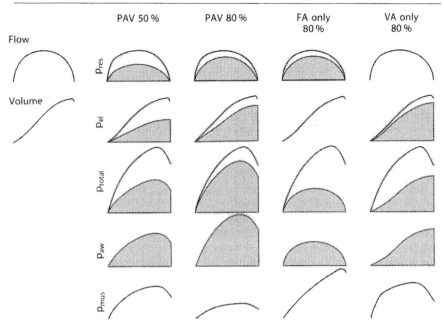

Fig. 3.2. Schematic representation of how using both flow assist (*FA*) and volume assist (*VA*) in the same fraction of resistance (R) and elastance (E) results in ventilator pressure (P_{aw}) becoming a function of respiratory muscle pressure (P_{mus}). Hypothetical flow and volume waveforms are used, but the results are similar regardless of waveform shape. P_{res} is the pressure used to overcome resistance and equals $\dot{V}_R$. P_{el} is the pressure used to overcome elastic recoil and equals V_E. P_{total} is the sum of P_{res} and P_{el}. In this example elastic and resistive losses are approximately equal. The *shaded area* represents the pressure provided by the ventilator. At 50% assist the ventilator provides half P_{el} and P_{res} at all times. Note that total ventilator output (*shaded area*, P_{total}) is, necessarily, half P_{total} at all times. P_{mus} is patient's contribution and is the difference between P_{total} and P_{aw}. Note that P_{aw} and P_{mus} resemble each other, and the proportionality is 1:1. A similar analysis, but with FA and VA representing 80% of R and E, results in P_{aw} again resembling P_{mus}, but the proportionality is 4:1. When FA is given alone, the shapes of P_{aw} and P_{mus} differ substantially and there is minimal assist near the end of inspiration where inspiratory effort is maximal. With VA, the assist lags behind P_{mus}. There is little assist at the beginning of inspiration. Furthermore, at the end of neural inspiration P_{aw} is rising as the patient reduces his effort in order to terminate flow

course of volume ($P_{el} = V \cdot E_{rs}$), as shown in the outer envelope of the P_{el} waveform. During mechanical ventilation the pressure used to generate flow and to offset elastic recoil is provided jointly by the ventilator (P_{aw}) and the patient (P_{mus}). At any instant during inspiration the combined pressure (P_{tot}) is used to offset resistive and elastic losses. The time course of P_{tot} is therefore the sum of the P_{res} and P_{el} outer envelopes, as shown by the outer envelope of the P_{tot} waveform (Fig. 3.2).

Consider the case where the ventilator is set to deliver FA (in cmH$_2$O/l/s) that is 50% of the patient's resistance and VA (in cmH$_2$O/l) that is 50% of the patient's elastance (2nd column, Fig. 3.2). The ventilator will thus deliver 50% of total P_{res}

and 50% of total P_{el} at all times during inspiration. Thus, if at a given instant $\dot{V} = 1$ l/s and resistance is 10 cmH$_2$O/l/s, total P_{res} at this moment is 10 cmH$_2$O. If FA is set at 50% (or 5 cmH$_2$O/l/s in this case), the ventilator provides 5 cmH$_2$O in relation to this flow. The patient is providing the balance. The same can be said for other flow rates occurring at different times and also for volume and its related P_{el}. With 50% assist the ventilator's contribution is 50% of P_{res} and P_{el} throughout inspiration (shaded areas in P_{res} and P_{el} waveforms, Fig. 3.2, 50% column). The shaded area in the P_{tot} waveform is the sum of the ventilator's contribution towards P_{res} and P_{el}. It should be evident that the height of this shaded area should equal 50% of the height of the outer P_{tot} envelope at all times. Since the balance must be derived from the patient, the patient's contribution must also be 50% at all times. At the 50% setting, therefore, P_{aw} and P_{mus} must equal each other throughout inspiration. Their shapes will accordingly be similar, and the proportionality is 1:1. P_{mus} has been amplified by a factor of two.

It should be emphasized that the flow pattern need not be sinusoidal to accomplish this result. Regardless of the flow and volume patterns, as long as the ventilator provides 50% of P_{res} and P_{el}, it is providing 50% of total pressure throughout inspiration. The patient is providing the other 50%; the shapes of P_{aw} and P_{mus} will be similar and the proportionality will be 1:1.

We then consider the case of 80% assist (3rd column, Fig. 3.2). If FA is set to 80% of R_{rs} and VA to 80% of E_{rs}, the ventilator contributes 80% of P_{res} and P_{el}, and hence P_{tot}, throughout inspiration (see shaded areas in the respective waveforms, Fig. 3.2). At any instant during inspiration, therefore, the proportionality of P_{aw} and P_{mus} is 4: 1. The P_{aw} waveform must therefore resemble the P_{mus} waveform. The latter has been amplified five times; for every 1 cmH$_2$O generated by the patient the ventilator generates 4 cmH$_2$O, resulting in a total pressure of 5.

Similar analysis can be carried out for other levels of assist. Thus, at 60% assist the proportionality is 1.5:1 and the amplification factor is 2.5. At 20% the proportionality and amplification factors are 0.25 and 1.25, respectively. In theory, therefore, the range of amplification can extend from zero (FA = 0, VA = 0) to infinity (FA = R_{rs}, VA = E_{rs}). This theoretical range is, however, limited in practice by ventilator response delays and by nonlinearities in resistive and elastic properties (see below).

3.2.1 Importance of Using Both FA and VA

FA and VA can obviously be applied separately. In fact, others have suggested the use of FA alone as a method of ventilatory support [5, 6]. The use of either FA or VA alone provides selective unloading of respiratory mechanics. However, P_{aw} will not be proportional to patient effort (P_{mus}). These methods of support, therefore, do not provide P_{aw} in proportion to instantaneous P_{mus} (i.e. PAV). The reason for this is shown in columns 4 and 5 of Fig. 3.2. With FA alone the P_{aw} waveform tracks flow. There is no support related to volume. The ventilator contribution is not a fixed fraction of P_{tot} (Fig. 3.2) and P_{aw} does not resemble P_{mus}. Since peak flow occurs well before the end of neural inspiration, maximum support is provided early on and is minimal towards end-inspiration where patient effort is maximal. With VA alone (last column, Fig. 3.2) the opposite occurs. The support lags behind patient effort, and there is little support at the beginning of inspiration. Furthermore, P_{aw} continues to increase for a while after P_{mus} has started to decrease at the end of neural inspiration (Fig. 3.2, last column).

Why is it useful to provide support in proportion to P_{mus} as opposed to selective unloading? Selective unloading might be useful in cases where ventilator dependence is related to pure selective mechanical abnormality (i.e. high resistance OR high elastance) with no muscle weakness. This situation is almost never encountered in ventilator-dependent patients. First, it is only the rare ventilator-dependent patient who can generate a maximum inspiratory pressure (MIP) that is >50 cmH_2O, and in many MIP is <40 cmH_2O. Given normal MIP values of 70–100 cmH_2O [7], inspiratory muscle weakness is an important contributor to ventilator dependence in virtually all patients, with the reasons being related to hyperinflation (in COPD and asthma [8]), sepsis [9], chronic heart disease [10], malnutrition [11], drugs [12] or simply disuse secondary to lengthy ventilator use. By amplifying muscle effort, PAV compensates for muscle weakness. Selective unloading reduces a specific load. However, the weak muscles may have difficulty coping with a normal load.

Second, pure resistive or elastic abnormalities are uncommon. Where the disease introduces primarily a pure elastic load (i.e. increased lung stiffness), the addition of an ET tube presents an added resistive load. Patients with obstructive diseases often face an additional elastic load related to dynamic hyperinflation [13].

The rationale behind PAV is that if the muscles are made (artificially) stronger they can cope with the increased load whether it is resistive or elastic. It is evident that through the application of PAV, where the disease is associated with predominantly high resistance the assist will necessarily include a relatively higher FA, and vice versa. Thus, preferential unloading of resistance or elastance continues to be included in PAV, but the presence of muscle weakness is also automatically dealt with.

3.2.2 Importance of FA and VA Being Less Than Patient's Resistance and Elastance

As long as FA<R_{rs} and VA<E_{rs} the patient must contribute a fraction of the total applied pressure (Fig. 3.2 and related text). Because with PAV P_{aw} is proportional to P_{mus}, any changes in P_{mus} result in qualitatively similar changes in P_{aw}. Thus when P_{mus} progressively decreases at the end of inspiration P_{aw} must also decrease. A point is reached where the sum of P_{mus} and P_{aw} becomes lower than P_{el}, which is highest near end-inspiration. At this point flow stops and the ventilator cycle is terminated.

When the gains of the FA and/or VA are greater than R_{rs} and/or E_{rs}, respectively, the ventilator-delivered pressure (P_{aw}) will exceed total pressure (P_{tot}) at some point in the inspiratory phase. With flow overassist, this point will occur early in inspiration whereas with volume overassist P_{aw} may not exceed P_{tot} until late in inspiration. Once P_{aw} exceeds P_{tot}, the requirement that the patient contribute to total pressure no longer exists and the ventilator acquires a life of its own. As the extent of overassist increases, the control of ventilator output (flow and volume) shifts progressively from patient to ventilator. With substantial overassist, the patient has little control over V_T and flow, and these become determined by the FA and VA settings and the volume and pressure limits on the ventilator.

The patterns observed during overassist vary considerably depending on which component (FA or VA) is excessive, the extent to which this component exceeds patient's resistance or elastance, and the extent of assist on the other component. At one extreme, there is the pattern associated with a large flow overassist (e.g. FA>3 R_{rs}). Here (Fig. 3.3), as soon as the ventilator is triggered flow increases in a rapidly accelerating manner. P_{aw} increases also rapidly as a result. Both increase until the cycle is terminated by a volume or P_{aw} limit.

Figure 3.4 shows the case at the other extreme, VA slightly above E_{rs} and FA = 0. Here, when the patient stops the inspiratory effort, flow fails to decrease to zero (since P_{aw} is >P_{el}), as would normally occur if VA is <E_{rs} (see above). Because inspiratory flow continues, volume continues to rise during neural expiration. Volume and, hence, P_{aw} continue to rise in an accelerating manner until: (a) the patient recruits expiratory muscles to force termination of inspiratory flow, (b)

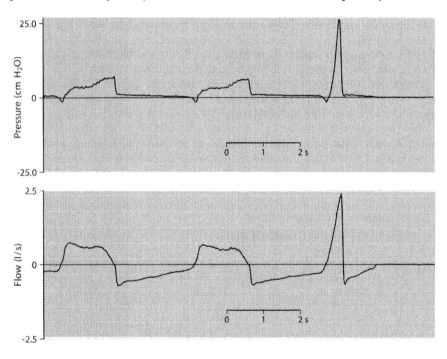

Fig. 3.3. Effect of increasing flow assist (FA) above patient's resistance. In the first two breaths FA and volume assist were at 50% of Rrs and Ers. FA was increased to 15 cm $H_2O/l/s$ (four times Rrs) between the second and third breaths. Note that flow and P_{aw} increase in a rapidly accelerating manner as soon as inspiratory flow begins. The cycle is terminated by a pressure limit on the ventilator (25 cmH$_2$O in this case). Note that flow pattern is entirely different from the normal pattern observed earlier and T_i is much shorter

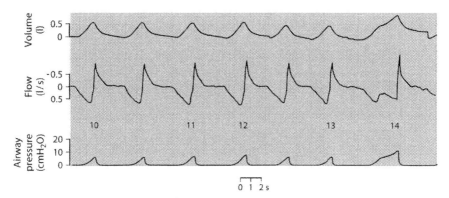

Fig. 3.4. Volume "runaway". In this sleeping patient volume assist (VA) was increased in small steps with flow assist being zero. The *numbers* above the airway pressure tracing are the values of VA. Note that at the transition between VA of 13 and 14 there is a pronounced change in pattern. Flow (inspiration down) fails to return to zero at the usual T_i (preceding breaths) and begins to increase again. This results in a characteristic saddle-shaped flow pattern, a long T_i and larger volume. From the response shown it can be surmised that the patient's Ers is between 13 and 14 cmH_2O/l

volume rises to a point where E_{rs} is no longer lower than VA on account of the nonlinear pressure-volume relation of the respiratory system [14], or (c) a volume or pressure limit is reached which aborts the cycle. The transition from a normal-looking breathing pattern to the characteristic pattern of saddle-shaped flow and a long T_i as a result of a minor increase in VA (i.e. as in Fig. 3.4) signifies that the VA setting is equal to the patient's E_{rs} This feature can be used to advantage to determine the patient's E_{rs}. With FA = 0, VA is increased in small steps until the characteristic transition is seen (i.e. Fig. 3.4). The VA setting at this point is E_{rs}. Furthermore, this characteristic pattern, representing minor volume overassist, may at times appear spontaneously and sporadically in occasional breaths during an otherwise normal-looking pattern. This again signifies that VA is very close to E_{rs}. The occasional "runaway" pattern occurs as a result of minor breath-by-breath changes in E_{rs} produced, for example, as a result of breath-by-breath changes in end-expiratory volume or in V_T in a patient where the P-V relation is nonlinear in the operating V_T range. When VA is very near average E_{rs}, some breaths with a below-average E_{rs} will be slightly overassisted.

As VA is further increased above E_{rs} and/or as FA is further added and increased, the pattern of overassist shifts progressively from that of Fig. 3.4 to that of Fig. 3.3. Examples are shown in Fig. 3.5. With all these patterns of overassist, the end of the ventilator cycle is no longer linked to the end of the patient's inspiratory effort and the cycle is terminated by machine-set limits or by the patient fighting the ventilator. These overassist patterns can be recognized by the fact that majority of the cycles are pressure or volume limited and, depending on which limiting mechanism is activated, peak pressure and/or V_T is monotonous as opposed to the variable P_{aw} or V_T observed when the patient controls ventilator output with properly adjusted PAV (i.e. $FA < R_{rs}$ and $VA < E_{rs}$).

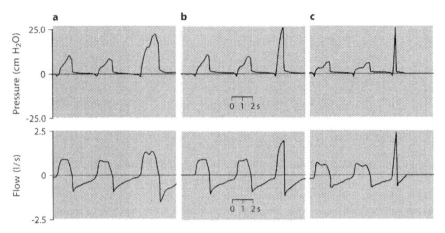

Fig. 3.5. Different patterns of "runaway". In all panels the first two breaths were supported at FA=50% Rrs and VA=50% Ers. A normal breathing pattern is seen. In the third breath FA and VA were altered. In the *left panel* (third breath) VA=Ers and FA=50% Rrs. Note that the pattern is similar to Fig. 3.4 but is somewhat more aggressive. In the *middle panel* VA remained at Ers and FA was 2 Rrs. In the *right panel* FA was increased further to 3 Rrs. In the last two examples the cycle was terminated by a pressure limit. Note that flow pattern is not similar to normal pattern in any of the panels. Flow and T_i can be adjusted at will by manipulating FA and VA in the range above the patient's Rrs and Ers

It should be pointed out that VA and/or FA have been proposed earlier as means to attain a target ventilator pressure [15], to attain a target V_T [16, 17], or to control $PaCO_2$ [18]. With all such applications the gains of FA and VA cannot be constrained to be below the patient's R_{rs} and E_{rs}, and the patient, as a result and by definition, has no control over ventilatory output. These other uses of FA and VA represent variants of pressure-cycled and volume-cycled ventilation and should not be confused with PAV [19], where no ventilatory or pressure targets are set.

3.3 Differences from Other Modes of Assisted Ventilation

A detailed discussion of the clinical and technical advantages and disadvantages of PAV relative to PSV and A/C ventilation is beyond the scope of this review. These will be mentioned only briefly. The interested reader is referred to several recent publications for further discussion [1, 4, 14, 20–22].

The main clinical/physiological advantages of PAV include: (a) assured synchrony between end of ventilator cycle and end of patient's inspiratory effort; (b) lesser likelihood of failed triggering efforts; (c) automatic adjustment of level of assist as ventilatory needs change as a result of changes in metabolic rate, temperature, acid-base status, sleep/wake cycle and behavioral factors; (d) a generally lower peak and mean airway pressure; (e) a generally lower V_T and hence the potential for less barotrauma; (f) lesser likelihood of hyperventilation; and (g) the ability to determine the patient's natural (desired) breathing pattern in the absence of distress, which may facilitate weaning (see below).

The main technical advantages of PAV include: (a) Ease of adjustment in the majority of patients, as there is only one variable (% assist) to be decided upon [14], and (b) greater tolerance of artifacts that may cause false triggering, thereby permitting the continued use of a sensitive triggering mechanism in the face of such noise (e.g. cardiac artifacts, hiccups).

The main clinical/physiological disadvantages include the fact that there is no guaranteed minimum ventilation (cf. A/C ventilation) or V_T (cf. A/C and PSV); $PaCO_2$ is likely to rise more in the presence of respiratory depression. Also, in some patients tidal volume can be quite small despite absence of distress (see below). Whether this may have adverse effects, in the long term, on gas exchange and respiratory mechanics is unknown.

The main technical disadvantages of PAV include: (a) sensitivity to leaks [14]; (b) need to know respiratory mechanics for proper adjustment; (c) difficulties in adjustment when pressure-volume and pressure-flow relations are grossly non-linear in the operating range (see below); (d) potential for overassist, which necessitates careful attention to pressure and volume limits [14]; (e) excessive sensitivity of degree of assist to uncompensated dynamic hyperinflation (see below).

PAV represents a major departure from conventional methods in the extent to which the caregiver can exercise control over ventilator output. The caregiver can determine only how hard or how little the patient is working. However, he/she cannot reliably influence the level of ventilation or breathing pattern. As with normal subjects [23] breathing pattern varies greatly among patients on PAV even with near-maximal assist ([24], see below). If the caregiver is unhappy with the tidal volume (too high or too low) or with $\dot{V}_E$ or frequency and attempts to increase or decrease the assist to bring these variables to what he/she is accustomed to, or feels appropriate, the patient will usually undertake an opposite action to maintain the same breathing pattern and $\dot{V}_E$ (see below). The adjustment to this "loss of control" is one of the major challenges facing caregivers when first using PAV.

3.4 Clinical Experience to Date

Several clinical studies have been completed. Some have been published, others are at different stages of the publication process and have been reported only in abstract form [4, 24–43]. The following is a summary of the findings most relevant to clinical application in the critical care setting.

3.4.1 Response to Different Levels of PAV

The response to different levels of PAV has been examined in a group of stable ventilator-dependent patients with assorted pathology [24], in patients with COPD where the response to different levels of PSV was also included [30], and in normal subjects while awake [36] and asleep [28]. In all cases PAV (% assist) was varied from the maximum (near 100% of E_{rs} and R_{rs}) to the minimum tolerable (i.e. with no clinical distress) level (0% in normals, 30%–60% assist in ventilator-dependent patients). The results in ventilator-dependent patients and in normals during sleep, were quite consistent. On average, tidal volume increased only marginally between minimum and maximum assist (Figs. 3.6 and 3.7). Respiratory rate changed little. Thus, under these conditions, increases in degree of assist result in down-regulation of P_{mus} so that V_T and $\dot{V}_E$ increase only marginally. This down-regulation of P_{mus} is almost certainly related to a small reduction in $PaCO_2$ between minimum and maximum assist.

The results were somewhat different in alert, awake subjects [36]. Although in the majority of subjects P_{di} and P_{mus} were down-regulated to a very low level as assist increased, resulting in only small increases in V_T and $\dot{V}_E$, in some subjects the pressure output of inspiratory muscles remained high at all levels of assist, despite marked hypocapnia. These subjects, then, had a substantial non-CO_2-dependent source of respiratory drive (likely the consciousness factor [44]). In these subjects the amplification produced by PAV in the face of persistently high P_{mus} resulted in marked increases in V_T and $\dot{V}_E$ with subsequent hypocapnia similar to PSV and A/C.

The conclusion that emerges from these studies is that when respiratory drive is dominated by CO_2 feedback (as during sleep, obtundation) V_T and $\dot{V}_E$ become fairly independent of level of assist, since $\dot{V}_E$ cannot increase by more that what is required to lower $PaCO_2$ by a few mmHg. In sleep [45] and under anesthesia [44] reductions in $PaCO_2$ by only a few mmHg cause down-regulation to zero (apnea). Where significant non-CO_2 sources to respiratory drive exist, down-regulation would be markedly attenuated, and V_T and $\dot{V}_E$ then become a function of level of

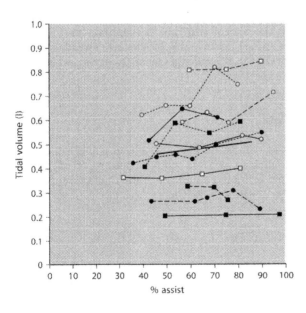

Fig. 3.6. Effect of progressively increasing level of PAV support on tidal volume. *x-axis*, Gain of volume assist as percentage of patient's elastance; *thin lines*, individual responses with lowest *x* value pertaining to lowest tolerable level of support; *thick line*, average response. From [24]

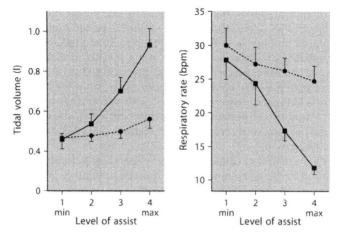

Fig. 3.7. Average response of tidal volume and ventilator rate with different levels of PAV and PSV in 11 ventilator-dependent patients with COPD. Minimum level of assist is that just above clinical distress in either mode. Maximum level was 90% assist in PAV and the level needed to achieve 10 ml/kg tidal volume in the case of PSV. Note that V_T increases progressively with PSV (thick line) but changes relatively much less with PAV (dotted line). The progressive decrease in rate with PSV was largely related to increasing number of efforts that failed to trigger the ventilator. From [30]

assist. Failure of V_T and $\dot{V}_E$ to increase substantially in the two patient groups studied [24, 30] therefore signifies that in these patients drive was predominantly CO_2 mediated. These patients were stable and, like most ICU patients, somewhat obtunded, albeit awake.

It may, accordingly, be expected that under other circumstances, where significant non-CO_2 sources of respiratory drive may exist, V_T and $\dot{V}_E$ may increase substantially with level of assist. Such situations may include patients with high metabolic rate, drive-promoting reflexes from the lung (? j receptors), severe metabolic acidosis, or patients who are very alert and/or agitated. In fact, the extent to which V_T and $\dot{V}_E$ increase with increasing assist may be a suitable test to determine the extent to which respiratory drive is related to non-CO_2 sources.

An important finding from the two ICU studies [24, 30] is that there was a very wide variability in desired V_T among patients (Fig. 3.6); V_T in the assist-insensitive range varied from 200 to 850 ml (3.4–14.1 ml/kg). All these patients were quite comfortable at their respective V_Ts and were able to increase their V_T to much higher levels on command. Thus, when V_T was small, this was not due to mechanical constraints; the V_T was that spontaneously selected by the patient's respiratory control.

A further relevant finding was that in some patients respiratory rate was quite high (up to 34 min^{-1}) despite high assist, comfort, and insensitivity to level of assist. This, again, indicates that high respiratory rates need not indicate distress. Since making this observation, we have successfully weaned several patients who were deemed weaning failures because every time they underwent a weaning trial from PSV or A/C their rate was found to be too high. When these patients were placed on high-level PAV their rate remained high, indicating that the high rate in these particular patients was not a marker of distress but represented the spontaneously selected pattern of breathing. Once this conclusion was reached, the patients were observed on zero assist for a few hours and, no change or distress being noted, were extubated. This successful outcome clearly applies to only a minority of patients with weaning difficulty, since in most cases a high rate during a weaning trial signifies distress [46]. PAV can be used to distinguish the two groups.

It must be pointed out that in the ventilator-dependent patients studied [24, 30] insensitivity of respiratory rate to level of assist applied only above a certain level of assist. In each patient, when assist was terminated or reduced below this point, rate increased along with appearance of clinical signs of distress. It follows that in every ventilator-dependent patient there is a range (range 1) over which rate decreases progressively with level of assist and a higher range (range 2) where it becomes fairly insensitive. We believe that respiratory rate in range 2 is the rate desired by the patient's control system, while range 1 signifies the patient's inability to attain the desired V_T, with the patient then compensating with rate. It is likely that range 1 is unsustainable. Until evidence to the contrary is produced, it is prudent to consider the patient as ventilator dependent until range 1 disappears (i.e. rate changes little as assist is gradually decreased to 0).

Finally, Fig. 3.7 shows the difference in response of COPD patients to varying levels of PAV and PSV [30]. Unlike the case with PAV, with PSV V_T increased, and respiratory rate decreased, progressively as a function of PSV level. The differences in respiratory rate response were largely artifactual and related to progressively more efforts failing to trigger the ventilator as PSV level increased; pressure continued well into neural expiration, thereby encroaching on time available for emptying before the next inspiratory effort. In fact, when patient's rate was counted considering the missed ventilator cycles (identified from transient dips in expiratory flow) there was no difference between PSV and PAV in response of respiratory rate to different levels of assist.

3.4.2 Peak Airway Pressure

One of the most consistent findings is that upon switching from a volume-cycled mode (SIMV, A/C) to PAV, peak P_{aw} decreases substantially even with very high levels of PAV assist [4, 31] (Fig. 3.8). Peak P_{aw} with high-level PAV assist (80%–90% of E_{rs} and R_{rs}) rarely exceeds 30 cmH$_2$O and is commonly less than 20 cmH$_2$O even with 5–10 cmH$_2$O of PEEP. This is true even in patients with moderately severe ARDS ($E_{rs} \approx 40$ cmH$_2$O). The reasons for the lower peak P_{aw} have been discussed in detail elsewhere [14] and include a usually smaller V_T, coincidence of end of machine cycle with maximum inspiratory pressure generated by the patient, lack of expiratory activity during the inflation phase, and occurrence of peak flow earlier in the inflation cycle.

Fig. 3.8. Response of peak airway pressure (*top*) and cardiac output (*bottom*) to alternation between volume-cycled assist/control (A/C) ventilation and proportional-assist ventilation (PAV). From [31]

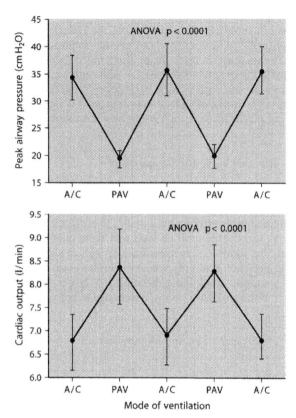

3.4.3 Noninvasive Use of PAV

The low peak P_{aw} requirement with PAV made it possible to attempt noninvasive support in patients with de novo acute respiratory failure (i.e. not acute or chronic) who were deemed to require urgent intubation and in whom the precipitating cause was felt to be correctable within 1–2 days (acute pulmonary edema, status asthmaticus, sepsis with ARDS, pneumonia). Eight of 11 patients were successfully supported and were spared intubation [25]. Noninvasive PAV is currently in routine use in our emergency room and medical ICU.

3.4.4 Hemodynamics in Septic Shock

Switching from A/C to PAV in eight patients with septic shock, on vasopressors, consistently resulted in an increase in cardiac output (Fig. 3.8). This was due to a greater stroke volume; heart rate did not change [31]. The increase in stroke volume is likely related to the slightly lower *mean* intrathoracic pressure (estimated to be only –1.7 cmH$_2$O despite the marked reduction in peak P_{aw}, Fig. 3.8), with a consequent increase in intrathoracic blood volume and, hence, ventricular preload. It should be pointed out that the reduction in mean intrathoracic pressure with PAV was due largely to greater inspiratory muscle pressure relative to A/C. The increase in mean inspiratory muscle pressure (P_I) was estimated to be 1.5 cmH$_2$O (range 0.7–5.0 cmH$_2$O). Although such an increase in P_I is insignificant in a person with normal respiratory muscles and represents an increase in tension time index of $\approx$2%, it may represent a significant stress, at least in some patients, given the abnormal respiratory muscle function in sepsis [9].

3.4.5 Effect on V_D/V_T and Oxygenation

Switching from A/C to PAV in a group of ventilator-dependent patients with assorted pathology had no effect, in the short term, on V_D/V_T or PaO$_2$/F$_I$O$_2$ ratio despite a significantly lower V_T [32]. The increase in V_D/V_T. expected from the lower V_T did not materialize. This was likely related to a reduction in zone 1 perfusion (due to lower transpulmonary pressure and greater pulmonary artery-to-pleural pressure gradient), which offset the expected increase related to a nearly fixed anatomic dead space becoming a larger fraction of V_T. The long-term impact of the smaller V_T on gas exchange is not yet known.

3.4.6 Importance of VA and FA Together

In a recent study, Navalesi et al. [26] confirmed several of the theoretical predictions and experimental findings described above in a group of ventilator-dependent patients with assorted pathology. They demonstrated that the use of VA alone (i.e. without FA), increases the resistive work of breathing, thereby confirming the importance of using both FA and VA (i.e. PAV), and that the patient's effort (P_{di}, P_{mus}) is down-regulated in a continuous fashion as the level of assist increases. In agreement with the study of Marantz et al. [24], V_T and V_E changed little as assist increased from 20% to 80% as a result of this down-regulation. Thus, V_T increased only by 15% at between 20% and 80% assist, whereas without down-regulation it would have more than doubled.

3.4.7 PAV Versus PSV

Ranieri et al. compared the response to an added dead space, which simulates an increase in ventilatory demand, when ventilator-dependent patients were on either PAV or PSV [27]. When on PAV, addition of dead space caused, as expected, an increase in assist, and the breathing pattern response consisted of an increase in V_T with little change in rate, a response that is similar to the response of normal subjects to increased CO$_2$ [47]. On PSV the response consisted of tachypnea with little change in V_T [27].

3.4.8 Long-term PAV Application In Ventilator-Dependent Patients

With the confidence gained in the locally constructed ventilators, several units were assigned to the intensive care areas and are currently operated by the regular respiratory therapists. For suitable patients (see below), and with the consent of the attending physician and patient, PAV is instituted and maintained throughout the duration of ventilatory support unless an exit criterion is met. Several dozen patients have been managed so far on PAV for extended periods (up to 10 days). The experience gained from these patients is incorporated into the practical approach outlined below.

3.5 Approach to the Clinical Use of PAV in Intubated, Critically III, Ventilator-Dependent Patients

3.5.1 Eligible Patients

Because spontaneous efforts are essential with PAV, central apnea and severe central depression are absolute contraindications. Severe central depression is recognized from lack of respiratory distress (e.g. accessory muscle use or tachypnea) in the face of respiratory or metabolic acidosis (e.g. pH<7.30).

Furthermore, until controlled studies are carried out to evaluate the safety of PAV (versus other modes) in cardiogenic shock and in the presence of serious arrhythmias, it is not advisable to use PAV when serious arrhythmias have occurred in the recent past or the patient has been in cardiogenic shock and is currently well controlled with conventional ventilation.

With the preceding exceptions, all patients can be placed on PAV, provided that the ventilator meets the requirements and personnel are readily available who are familiar with this mode and with the equipment.

3.5.2 The Ventilator

The ventilator should conform to certain minimum requirements with respect to mechanical performance, alarm and monitoring features and the presence of suitable back-up systems. These minimum requirements have been outlined elsewhere [14]. Using a ventilator with bare minimum requirements (The Winnipeg Ventilator) we have identified several technical problems that unnecessarily complicate the implementation of PAV. These will be discussed here. Hopefully, commercial PAV ventilators will incorporate features that obviate some or all of these difficulties, thereby greatly facilitating implementation.

Ventilator Response Characteristics

When the PAV assist is set at a given fraction of the patient's elastance and resistance the expectation is that the ventilator will assume this fraction of total pressure output, with the patient assuming the balance. This expectation can be met only if the ventilator faithfully follows the pressure waveform dictated by the settings. Thus, if 80% assist is dialed, P_{aw} should, ideally, track the following function at all times during inspiration:

$$P_{aw} = .8 \, \dot{V} \cdot R_{rs} + .8 \, V \cdot E_{rs}$$

These expectations are unrealistic, since all mechanical systems display response delays. These delays dictate that the assist received is less than the level intended. Clearly, the greater the response delay, the greater the discrepancy between actual and intended assist. Furthermore, for a given response delay, the shorter the inspiratory time the greater the discrepancy (Fig. 3.9). The degree of discrepancy between actual and intended assist is a function of the relative areas under the actual and intended pressure-time waveforms (Fig. 3.9). Thus, if the area under the actual waveform is 50% of the area under the intended waveform, the patient is receiving 50% of the intended assist (40% in the case of an intended 80%, etc.). Clearly, the better the response of the ventilator, the less the discrepancy. At times, respiratory distress or excessive patient work is present despite high levels of assist settings. Slow ventilator response can be one of the reasons. A procedure has been described earlier for measuring ventilator responsiveness [14]. This, however, requires removal of the ventilator from the patient for the sake of testing. Preferably, the ventilator itself should display the fraction of intended area that is actually being delivered. This would facilitate the identification of this problem, if present, as a cause of the patient's excessive work.

Poor Trigger Sensitivity

Delays in triggering cause the assist to begin after a finite fraction of the patient's inspiratory effort has elapsed. Triggering delays have an impact similar to that of poor ventilator response; the patient receives less assist than intended. Such delays may have three sources:

1. Maximum trigger sensitivity is still too insensitive: With PAV, the assist should, ideally, begin at the very onset of inspiratory effort. Because the assist will automatically terminate at the end of inspiratory effort, any delay in onset of assist reduces the fraction of neural T_i that is being assisted [14]. Apart from

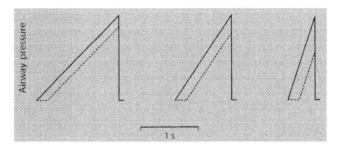

Fig. 3.9. Effect of delay in ventilator response on the degree of assist. *Solid lines* indicate desired pressure output, *dashed lines* indicate actual pressure output. A fixed delay of 200 ms was assumed. The patient receives less assist than intended, and the extent of the discrepancy increases as duration of inspiration decreases (note that the area between the solid and dashed lines becomes a bigger fraction of total area). From [14]

the impact of delays in onset of assist, the level of effort required to trigger the ventilator is not assisted throughout the breath. Thus, if the patient is required to generate 2 cmH$_2$O or to generate a flow of 15 l/min to trigger the assist, the assist will be applied to only a fraction of the patient's effort (i.e. actual effort minus trigger level) even after triggering starts [14]. Mitigating this vulnerability to poor trigger sensitivity is the fact that in the PAV mode trigger sensitivity can be increased substantially relative to other modes. This is because brief artifacts will not trigger a full breath [14]. For this reason, the range of trigger sensitivity on the ventilator should be wider to allow triggering to occur with minimal effort (e.g. 0.2 cmH$_2$O or flow of 2 l/min).

2. Leaks during expiration: In the presence of leaks during expiration, P$_{aw}$ may decrease below the PEEP level, causing false triggering. This is usually countered by decreasing trigger sensitivity to the point where false triggering does not occur. With PAV, expiratory time (T$_e$) can be quite variable. Accordingly, the extent to which P$_{aw}$ decreases below PEEP prior to onset of inspiratory effort, as a result of a leak, may vary depending on variability in T$_e$ and magnitude of leak. If trigger sensitivity is reduced to offset the leak with the longest T$_e$, trigger sensitivity will be good (i.e. high) in breaths following a long T$_e$ but may be poor in breaths following a short T$_e$. On average, therefore, trigger sensitivity may be suboptimal. This problem can be obviated by abandoning the use of fixed pressure or flow as the trigger level and moving to more intelligent methods which utilize the change in P$_{aw}$ or flow trajectory during expiration as the marker of inspiratory onset. Furthermore, modern ventilators are capable of measuring leaks. A display of the prevailing leak level can alert the user to this potential problem.

3. Dynamic hyperinflation (DH): The presence of DH can further delay triggering because the patient must first decrease expiratory flow to zero, using inspiratory muscles, before he/she can begin to lower pressure below PEEP, or generate inspiratory flow, to trigger the ventilator [48]. This problem can, again, be obviated by using intelligent algorithms for detection of onset of inspiratory effort.

Nonlinearity of the Pressure-Flow (P-V̇) Relation

When the P-V̇ relation is nonlinear in the operating range, resistance is not a constant but increases with flow rate. There is therefore no fixed R$_{rs}$ to rely on for the sake of adjusting the level of the flow-assist component of PAV. Because the patient's own resistance (R$_{pat}$) is quite independent of flow (i.e. R$_{pat}$ nearly constant), even with severe obstructive disease (e.g. Fig. 5 of ref. [49]), practically important nonlinearities are related to the ET tube and occur mostly when the ET tube is small (e.g. ≤7) and/or when flow rates are high [46, 50].

The practical difficulties imposed by a substantially nonlinear P-V̇ relation, in terms of setting the FA level, are as follows: Assume that total resistances at flow rates of 0.5, 1.0, and 1.5 l/s are 10, 17, and 24 cmH$_2$O/l/s, respectively. There is, in this case, no unique resistance value which can be used to set the flow-assist (FA) component of PAV. If one sets the FA gain based on the value at low flow, the assist may be too little if the patient wishes to generate a high flow (where actual resistance is much higher). On the other hand, if one chooses the resistance at a high flow as the guide to FA gain, flow overassist will result at low flow rates. Particularly when the volume assist is a large fraction of the patient's elastance, the flow overassist will promote flow "runaway" until a flow is reached where actual resistance equals the FA setting. Thus, if one sets the FA gain in the preceding example to 17 cmH$_2$O/l/s, a "runaway" situation will exist as long as flow is less than 1.0 l/s. Unless the patient actively opposes it, flow will increase until it reaches 1.0 l/s, even if the patient stops his or her own inspiratory effort. The ventilator then takes on a life of its own, helping to dictate flow rate, and this defeats the purpose of PAV.

The implementation difficulties related to nonlinear P-$\dot{V}$ relation can be obviated in one of three ways:

1. Using tracheal pressure, as opposed to external airway pressure, as the controlled pressure in the PAV algorithm. In this fashion ET tube resistance, the main source of nonlinearity, is automatically compensated for. The variable FA level of PAV can then be set taking only R$_{pat}$ into consideration.
2. The FA component of PAV may be made up of a tube-specific nonlinear component and a patient-related constant component. This solution does not take into account differences between in vitro and in vivo ET tube resistance [50].
3. Automatic determination, by the ventilator, of the pressure-flow relation in the operating flow range. The FA term in the PAV equation would then be a function of flow as determined by the established nonlinear P-$\dot{V}$ relation under operating conditions. This approach has the advantage of adjusting the assist level as resistive properties change (e.g. ET tube secretions, changes in bronchomotor tone, etc.).

Nonlinearity in the Elastic Pressure-VT Relation

The relation between respiratory system volume and elastic recoil is sigmoid, both in health and in disease [51]. In the mid 50%–60% of vital capacity the pressure-volume relation is linear (i.e. E$_{rs}$ nearly constant) and the elastance is least (compliance is highest). The system becomes stiffer at both ends. The majority of patients breathe in the linear midrange and E$_{rs}$ is nearly constant within the operating V$_T$ range. In others, the P-V relation is not linear within V$_T$. This creates some difficulties, since there is no fixed E$_{rs}$ value to use for setting the volume-assist component of PAV. The difficulties depend on whether the V$_T$ falls within the stiff upper range (high-end nonlinearity) or stiff lower range (low-end nonlinearity) of the sigmoid P-V relation.

High-end Nonlinearity. This occurs when end-inspiratory volume approaches the physiological ceiling of the respiratory system (total lung capacity, TLC). The clinical situations where this happens include: (a) severe dynamic hyperinflation, (b) excessive external PEEP, and (c) severe restrictive disease (e.g. severe ARDS), where the vital capacity is so reduced that the inspiratory capacity (difference between TLC and FRC), normally 2–3 l, is reduced to values within the usual V$_T$ range (0.4–0.8 l). Fig. 3.10, left, illustrates the case where the nonlinear upper range occurs within 0.6 l from FRC. As can be seen from the right panel, elastance (P$_{el}$/V$_T$) is constant only over the lower V$_T$ range and increases sharply in the higher range. The dashed line in the left panel represents volume assist (VA) of

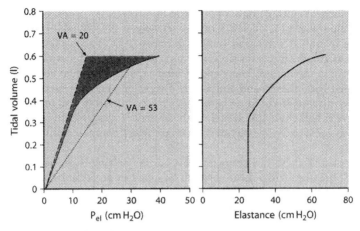

Fig. 3.10. Confounding effect of high-end nonlinearity in the pressure-volume relation on adjustment of volume assist (*VA*). The P-V curve (*left*) describes the case in a patient with severe restrictive disease. The P-V relation is linear over a small volume range (0.3 l); thereafter elastic recoil increases disproportionately. Calculated elastance (Pel/V_T) is constant at 25 cmH$_2$O/l up to a volume of 0.3 l. Thereafter it increases progressively as a function of volume. Setting VA as a percent of the elastance (e.g. 20 cmH$_2$O/l or 80% of the fixed E in the low volume range) results in underassist if the patient wishes higher volumes (note that width of the *shaded area*, representing patient's contribution, becomes a greater fraction of total elastic recoil pressure). To provide adequate assistance in a higher volume range by using a VA at 80% of elastance at V_T of 0.6 results in volume overassist at lower volumes (note assist line is to the right of the P-V relation). V_T will automatically runaway to the point of intersection of the VA and P-V lines unless the patient fights the ventilator. Under these conditions, V_T tends to become constant and not very responsive to changes in patient's efforts

80% of the patient's elastance in the low volume range. Because VA is constant while the P-V curve is not, the distance between the two lines (i.e. patient's contribution) increases disproportionally as a function of V_T. As long as V_T is less than 0.3 l, the patient is receiving, as intended, 80% assist. If the patient desires a larger V_T and makes more effort, the % assist decreases (width of shaded area/total recoil). The patient is thus less able to increase V_T beyond the range where E_{rs} is constant, and respiratory distress may result. If one responds by increasing VA, to take account of the higher elastance in the higher V_T range (dotted line), there will be volume overassist (ventilator providing more pressure than elastic recoil) through most of the V_T (note dotted line to the right of the P-V curve). Under these conditions VT is dictated to rise to the point of intersection of the dotted and solid lines, unless the patient fights the ventilator or a pressure limit is reached. The patient is no longer comfortably in control of V_T. In effect, in doing so, one has switched from patient-controlled V_T (i.e. PAV) to ventilator-controlled V_T.

Low-end Nonlinearity: Here the system is stiffest (least compliant) in the low range of V_T and becomes progressively less stiff as volume increases. This may occur under two broad circumstances: (a) Dynamic hyperinflation where elastic recoil pressure at end-expiration (i.e. onset of inspiration) is not zero but a finite positive value (Fig. 3.11, top, left, x intercept). Even if the P-V relation within V_T is linear the overall P-V relation (end-inspiratory P_{el}/V_T) is nonlinear; elastance decreases as volume increases (top right panel). (b) When end-expiratory volume occurs close to the natural lower end of vital capacity (residual volume). This is encountered with obesity and abdominal distension and in some cases of severe obstructive disease. In the latter case, the increase in elastance at low volume and its decrease at higher volume are related to reversible, progressive, volume-dependent airway closure: at low volumes there are fewer communicating alveoli, and vice versa.

The impact of these two abnormalities on PAV setting is the same. Clearly, if the patient breathes with a near constant V_T, one can determine elastance at this V_T (see below) and adjust VA to the desired % assist. With PAV, however, there is often substantial breath-by-breath variability, particularly in alert patients. This presents some problems in deciding on an appropriate VA. Assume that E_{rs} with the average V_T (0.4) was 28 cmH$_2$O (Fig. 3.11). VA is set at 90%, or 25 cmH$_2$O/l. At

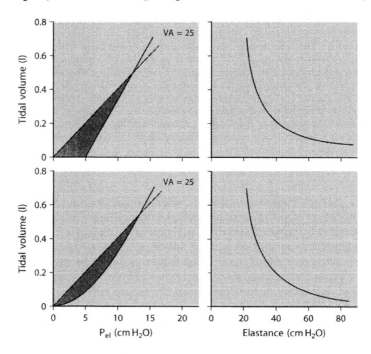

Fig. 3.11. Confounding effect of low-end nonlinearity in the P-V curve produced by dynamic hyperinflation (*top*, elastic recoil at end-expiration = 5 cmH$_2$O) or by breathing near the stiff lower range of vital capacity. Note that in either case elastance (Pel/V_T) decreases progressively as a function of V_T. Setting VA based on the high E at low volumes results in runaway (assist greater than elastic recoil) if patient takes a somewhat large breath. Setting VA based on the lower E at higher V_T avoids runaway but leaves smaller tidal volumes with little assist. *Shaded area* is patient contribution to elastic recoil. Note that patient receives considerably less assist early in the breath, when volume is low. See text for additional details

a V_T of 0.4, the patient is receiving 90% assist. However, the assist is less at volumes below 0.4 l. Furthermore, should the patient decide to take a deeper breath, the assist may exceed elastic recoil (dashed line crossing to the right of the solid line, Fig. 3.11, left) and a runaway develops which is terminated by the patient's active expiratory effort or by a machine pressure or volume limit. Reducing the assist to avert these occasional "runaway" breaths causes further underassist in the average and below-average V_T. A choice therefore has to be made between decreasing the level of assist or putting up with frequent beeping sounds as the ventilator limits the occasional "runaway" breath.

The technical implementation difficulties posed by nonlinear P-V relation can be obviated by suitable additions to ventilators. Ideally, the ventilator should be capable of determining the relation between V_T and elastic recoil over the operating volume range and providing VA as a % of this relation, including nonlinear relations.

3.5.3 Procedure

The procedure for placing a patient on PAV will clearly be affected by the features available on the ventilator. At the time of this writing it is not clear which of the facilitating features described in "The Ventilator" section (see before) will be available. Best- and worst-case scenarios will be described.

Best-Case Scenario

The best case is where the ventilator is equipped with automatic detection of onset of inspiration, automatic adjustment of trigger sensitivity, and automatic determination of the P-$\dot{V}$ and P-V relations in the operating range. In this case, one would simply set F_IO_2 and PEEP according to the usual criteria. Initially, pressure-limiting and volume-limiting levels are set at 40 cmH$_2$O and 15 ml/kg, respectively. All that remains is to set a % assist and default values for E and R to be used until the ventilator determines the P-$\dot{V}$ and P-V relations. A high assist value of 80% is recommended initially. This would be adjusted later (see Subsequent Management, below). The initial default values for E and R may be values determined earlier in the volume-cycled (see Worst-Case Scenario, below) mode, or empiric values. A suitable empiric value for E is 12 cmH$_2$O/l. At 80% assist the patient would receive a VA of 9.6 cmH$_2$O, which is about the average normal respiratory system elastance [51]. Alternatively, the default E value may be size dependent since compliance is size dependent (normal compliance = 0.02 predicted vital capacity/cmH$_2$O [51]). Thus, a reasonable default E value would be 1/predicted normal compliance. Since the patient's elastance will almost certainly be higher than normal, there is little likelihood of overassist, and this setting would provide a reasonable amount of support pending determination of the real P-V relations. Once the patient is switched to PAV a quick elastance can be determined using the end-expiratory occlusion (see below), and the default value is adjusted accordingly.

For the default R value, one can use the resistance of the ET tube at 0.5 l/s plus an assumed value of 3 cmH$_2$O/l/s for the patient's own resistance. Again, this would provide reasonable support with little likelihood of flow overassist (since 3.0 is the normal respiratory resistance [52]). If it is strongly suspected that the patient suffers from obstructive disease, a higher default value (e. g. ET tube + 8) may be used until the actual P-$\dot{V}$ relation is determined.

It should be emphasized that the choice of these default values is not terribly critical. A minor underestimation (e.g. 20%) of the patient's mechanics would have little consequence. A gross underestimation (e.g. 50%–70%) would result in underestimation of assist between onset of PAV and determination of actual P-$\dot{V}$ and P-V relations. Depending on how borderline the patient is, this may result in some clinical evidence of distress, at which point it would become obvious that the default values need to be increased. With the above-suggested default values the likelihood of substantial overassist is virtually nonexistent and, should it happen, the breath will be terminated by the relatively low pressure and/or volume limits.

Once the actual P-$\dot{V}$ and P-V relations are determined the desired % assist will be applied to these relations. The pressure and volume limits and the alarm settings are then readjusted according to prevailing peak P_{aw} and V_T, respectively (see steps 12 and 13, below).

Worst-Case Scenario

This procedure for the worst-case scenario is based on the one we used with the Winnipeg Ventilator and assumes that the ventilator has none of the automatic features described in "The Ventilator" section. Trigger sensitivity is adjusted manually, and VA and FA are dialed directly with no provision for nonlinear compensation. In this account it will be assumed that the patient was placed initially on a conventional mode and is being switched to PAV. Although institution of PAV immediately after intubation is not contraindicated, commonly the patient will not meet the eligibility criteria on account of excessive sedation or paralysis given prior to intubation or to control agitation following intubation (i.e. central depression).

3.6 What to Do

1. *Determine the patient's elastance and resistance.* This is done using conventional techniques. It is recommended, however, that measurements be carried out during a brief period of controlled mechanical ventilation (CMV). The patient is switched to assist-control ventilation, if not already on it, with a square flow pattern, and the backup rate is increased until no visible efforts are observed. This ensures relaxation and hence more reliable measurements. Calculate E_{rs} from ($P_{plateau}$ – PEEP)/V_T. $P_{plateau}$ should be measured early (e.g. 0.2 s) after the onset of the inspiratory hold since the relevant elastance for setting PAV is the dynamic elastance, determined as close as possible to the point of occurrence of zero flow. Calculate resistance (R_{rs}) from (P_{peak} – $P_{plateau}$)/$\dot{V}$. Again, $P_{plateau}$ should be measured early after the onset of inspiratory hold. It would be useful to determine R_{rs} at different flow rates (e.g. 0.5, 1.0, 1.5 l/s). This would facilitate setting the appropriate FA after the spontaneous

flow demand of the patient on PAV is known (see step 11 below). For this purpose, flow rate, in the CMV modes, is altered for 1–2 breaths and a 0.5-s inspiratory hold is obtained. R_{rs} is computed at the respective flow rates.

2. *Set the PAV controls.* Set the volume gain to approximately 80% of the patient's elastance [($P_{plateau}$ – PEEP)/V_T, in the CMV mode]. Set the flow assist to 80% of R_{rs} at 0.5 l/s. Use of a conservative flow of 0.5 l/s to initially estimate operating resistance avoids the development of flow "runaway", thereby making it possible to determine the flow desired by the patient (this would not be possible in the presence of flow "runaway". The estimated resistance can be adjusted subsequently once actual flow in PAV is estimated.*

3. *PEEP.* The use of PEEP with PAV is no different from its use with other modes and is guided by the need to maintain oxygenation and to counteract dynamic hyperinflation. The level selected prior to PAV, based on these indications, would then be retained. It should be remembered, however, that the use of external PEEP to counteract dynamic hyperinflation is effective only where dynamic hyperinflation is the result of flow limitation in the patient's airway and not due to high resistance in the ET tube or exhalation tubing (including the exhalation valve). Thus, in the presence of dynamic hyperinflation, every effort must be made to reduce the latter sources of resistance.

4. *Adjust the peak pressure limit* initially to 40 cmH$_2$O and the maximum tidal volume to 1.2 l. These can be readjusted later as needed (see below). A T_I limit of 3.0 s should be selected if an external control is available.

5. *Switch to PAV.*

6. *Adjust trigger sensitivity to the level just necessary to eliminate repetitive triggering during expiration* (automatic cycling).

7. *Look for evidence of volume overassist.* There should be no "runaway" if the patient's elastance on PAV is similar to that measured earlier on CMV. At times, however, elastance is lower on PAV, so 80% of the elastance determined under CMV may be higher than actual elastance on PAV. The reasons for these differences vary but may be related to a smaller V_T on PAV in the face of the nonlinear pressure-volume relation near FRC, to less auto-PEEP on PAV, or to the presence of expiratory activity during the inspiratory hold in the pre-PAV measurements (thereby causing overestimation of elastance values).

In the alert patient, volume overassist is identified from the visible activation of the expiratory muscles prior to cycling off. The patient also may, upon questioning, indicate that the pressure delivered is too much for his or her liking (even though actual pressure may be low by usual criteria). In this case, the gain of the volume assist is reduced to a level deemed comfortable by the patient.

In the obtunded patient, volume overassist should be suspected when the inspiratory phase is terminated by one of the limiting variables (peak pressure, V_T, T_I; see step 4 above). Here the problem may be either volume overassist or high ventilatory demand by the patient. The volume-assist level should be decreased

---

* Actual flow rate on PAV can be determined from the direct flow display, when available, or from the displayed values of $\dot{V}_E$ and T_I/T_{TOT}. Thus average inspiratory flow ($\dot{V}_I$) is given by $\dot{V}_E$ (T_I/T_{TOT}). For example, if $\dot{V}_E$ is 12 l/min and T_I/T_{TOT} is 0.4, $\dot{V}_I$ is 30 l/min or 0.5 l/s.

gradually (i.e., over 1–2 min). In the former case (overassist), there will be a step change in breathing pattern (large reduction in V_T and/or T_I) as volume assist is reduced below a certain level, with the new levels remaining fairly stable as the assist is reduced further. This is the reverse of the "runaway" procedure illustrated in Fig. 3.4. In the case of high ventilatory demand, this will not occur.

8. *Measure elastance on PAV.* The reason for repeating this measurement has been outlined above. Two methods can be used.

In the *inspiratory hold method* (Fig. 3.12) the expiratory line is occluded during an inspiration, and the occlusion is maintained through part of the ensuing expiration. A well-defined pressure plateau is seen, particularly in obtunded patients. Elastance is determined from ($P_{plateau}$ – PEEP)/V_T, where V_T is the specific tidal volume whose expiration was occluded (note that with PAV, tidal volume is quite variable). Where there is appreciable breath-by-breath variability in V_T, one should attempt to obtain data from small and large breaths. This could identify nonlinearities in the P-V relation which would help to explain situations in which excessive patient effort or respiratory distress is present despite a seemingly high level of support (see below).

As shown in Fig. 3.12 (the fourth inspiration), and unlike the case with CMV or A/C, plateau pressure is higher than peak pressure. This occurs because plateau pressure reflects total elastic recoil, whereas the ventilator provides only a fraction of elastic recoil during the inspiratory phase. The higher the level of volume assist, the closer peak and plateau pressures are to each other.

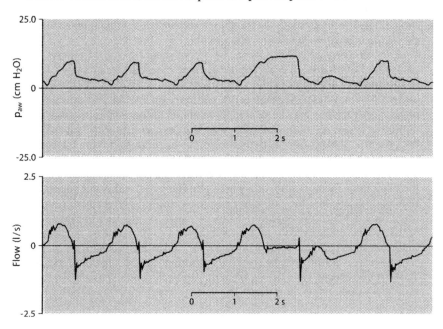

Fig. 3.12. Tracings showing inspiratory-hold method of determining elastance on PAV. The expiratory line was occluded during the fourth inspiration, and occlusion was maintained for approximately 1 s into expiration. Note that the plateau pressure is greater than the peak pressure

The only circumstance where peak pressure may exceed plateau pressure is where the flow-assist level is high relative to the elastic assist (e.g. in a patient with very high resistance and low elastance). In this case, peak pressure is dominated by the flow assist.

In the "*runaway*" method, with FA at zero, the level of volume assist is slowly increased until a level is reached where the ventilator fails to reset at the usual inspiratory time (i.e. that observed at lower levels of support) (Fig. 3.4). The rationale for this approach has been explained earlier (see Fig. 3.4 and related text). The advantage of this approach over the inspiratory-hold technique is that no computation is required. The volume-assist level at the point of the "runaway" is essentially the patient's elastance. The results of the two methods are very similar; however, this method is suitable only for obtunded patients; alert patients tend to activate expiratory muscles and terminate the cycle soon after the onset of the hold, making it difficult to recognize the characteristic pattern of minimum overassist (e.g. Fig. 3.4).

9. *Adjust volume assist to 80% of the elastance measured on PAV.*
10. *Observe the patient's ventilation, breathing pattern, peak flow and airway pressure.*
11. *Adjust flow assist to 80% of R_{rs} at the prevailing average flow rate* (see footnote 2).
12. *Reset the pressure and volume limits to be somewhat above the prevailing peak pressure and V_T.* Note that with PAV there can be substantial breath-by-breath differences in these variables. Set the limits to permit the patient the full range of his or her desired V_T, as indicated by the spontaneous variability.
13. *Set the alarms based on the prevailing breathing pattern.* For example, the low-pressure and low-V_T alarms can be set at 50% of average peak pressure and average V_T.

3.7 What to Expect

3.7.1 Usual Response

When eligibility criteria are adhered to, the ventilator is technically satisfactory, and the preceding procedure for initiating PAV is followed, the majority of patients experience no difficulty following the transition. Some inspiratory effort is evident, but there is no distress. Breathing pattern varies considerably among patients, with some electing slow, deep breathing and others breathing in a rapid, shallow pattern (see above). In the absence of respiratory distress, shallow breathing represents the preferred pattern by the patient's own control system. The treating physician may decide, however, that this pattern is not in the best interest of the patient. Until studies have been done to assess this issue, switching back to conventional ventilation or continued observation under PAV, with monitoring of hemodynamics and oxygenation, and return to conventional ventilation in the event of deterioration are both reasonable approaches.

Except in obtunded patients, there is usually substantial breath-by-breath variability in V_T, respiratory rate, and flow rate, and spontaneous sighing is common

(Fig. 3.13). Airway pressure reflects these changes (Fig. 3.13). This variability is normal [53, 54]. Prevailing peak airway pressure will almost invariably be lower, and usually much lower, than with AMV if a standard V_T (8–12 ml/kg) was used previously. Whether or not it will be lower than PSV depends on what PSV level was used previously.

When F_IO_2 is matched, PaO_2 will usually be within a few mmHg (in either direction) relative to the pre-PAV level. $PaCO_2$ usually will increase immediately upon switching to PAV, but pH remains normal (>7.35). The extent of increase in $PaCO_2$ depends on how much the patient was overventilated relative to his or her target $PaCO_2$ prior to PAV. With PAV, the patient selects his or her $PaCO_2$, whereas with other methods, $PaCO_2$ is determined largely by ventilator settings. Provided that pH is normal, the patient is comfortable, and the increase in $PaCO_2$ is not progressive, some increase in $PaCO_2$ is acceptable and indicates that the patient was overventilated previously. In the usual case, blood pressure and heart rate change little upon switching to PAV.

3.7.2 Respiratory Distress

In a minority of patients evidence of excessive inspiratory effort (accessory muscle use, intercostal indrawing) with or without clinical distress continues or appears (if patient is switching from another mode) despite seemingly adequate PAV support (e.g. >80% of E and R). There are several possible reasons for this:
1. Poor mechanical response of the ventilator
2. Poor trigger sensitivity related to inappropriate setting of this function, to leaks, or to dynamic hyperinflation
3. Nonlinearities in the P-$\dot{V}$ and/or P-V relation
4. The presence of a high, non-CO_2-related source of respiratory drive: From a large number of observations made during studies with normals and patients under a variety of circumstances, we are convinced that down-regulation of respiratory muscle output, and hence relief of distress by mechanical ventilation, is mediated largely via reduction in $PaCO_2$. Unloading per se, without concomitant reduction in $PaCO_2$, does not materially reduce respiratory effort. It follows that when the source of excessive respiratory drive is not CO_2 relat-

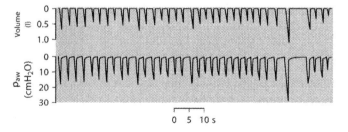

Fig. 3.13. Example of volume and airway pressure tracings during PAV (constant gain throughout). Note the considerable breath-by-breath variability, including a "sigh" with a brief post-sigh apnea. From [14]

ed, reducing $PaCO_2$ by increasing ventilator support will not be very effective in relieving the distress. Patients who display high non-CO_2-related respiratory drive include agitated patients and patients with systemic sepsis, severe metabolic acidosis, high metabolic rate, and shock of any cause.

Approach to Respiratory Distress on PAV

1. The presence of high, non-CO_2-related respiratory drive is easily recognized when $\dot{V}_E$ is high (e.g. >15 l/min) despite normal or low $PaCO_2$. Often the mechanics are not very abnormal. These patients will continue to work hard no matter which mode they are ventilated with. Until the primary abnormality responsible for the increased drive is corrected, sedation with or without paralysis is the most effective way to reduce ventilatory demand. Although judicious administration of sedatives with continued use of PAV, along with careful monitoring of pH and hemodynamics, is a feasible option, it would be prudent under these conditions to switch the patient to another mode with which the physician is more familiar. Because of the exquisite sensitivity of pH to $PaCO_2$ in the presence of severe metabolic acidosis, if the use of sedative plus PAV is elected in the presence of severe metabolic acidosis a low ventilation alarm should be set at the ventilation level consistent with a tolerable pH. Should ventilation decrease below this level due to excessive sedation, the patient is switched to another mode in which $\dot{V}_E$ is not so vulnerable to patient effort (e.g. A/C).
2. Look for evidence of delayed triggering. Note the extent of delay between the first visible inspiratory effort on the patient's thorax and the sound signifying onset of inspiratory flow from the ventilator. When triggering is excellent, the delay between the two signals is so small as to be imperceptible. A trained observer can identify undesirable delays using this simple technique. Alternatively, the airway pressure signal or expiratory flow signal (if available) should be inspected to see the time lag between the point at which there is a clear inflection in the tracing in an inspiratory direction (regardless of whether pressure is still above PEEP or flow is still expiratory) and the point of triggering (Fig. 3.14). Should delays exist, recheck to make sure that trigger sensitivity is just below the level that results in autocycling. If delays still exist, increase external PEEP in small steps. Should this reduce the delay, increase PEEP further. Should increasing PEEP result in no further reduction in delay and the delay is still excessive (e.g. >0.3 s), it will be concluded the dynamic hyperinflation cannot be offset by external PEEP (i.e. main resistance is in tubing). If patient's effort continues to be high, consider switching to a mode that is not so vulnerable to uncompensated dynamic hyperinflation. It should be pointed out that this difficulty can be obviated by suitable additional features on the ventilator.
3. In the absence of significant triggering delay or excessive drive, the problem is either a poor ventilator response or nonlinearities in the P-$\dot{V}$ and P-V relation. An indication of nonlinearities in the P-V relation may already exist from inspiratory hold manoeuvres at different V_T (see step 8 above). Suction ET tube to make sure that secretions are not increasing its resistance. Increase FA level gradually until evidence of flow runaway appears (high flow acceleration at the

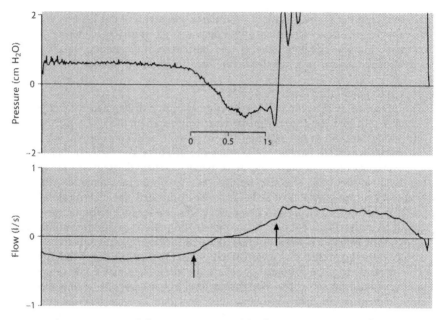

Fig. 3.14. Airway pressure and flow tracings at transition between expiration and inspiration. Pressure scale greatly amplified (±2 cmH₂O). Onset of inspiratory effort is identified from sharp change in trajectory of P_{aw} or flow with the change being in an inspiratory direction (*first arrowhead*). Note the substantial delay between onset of inspiratory effort and triggering (*second arrowhead*). The delay between first arrowhead and zero flow crossing is related to intrinsic PEEP. The delay between zero flow crossing and triggering is related to poor ventilator trigger sensitivity

beginning of inspiration with a very early peak, Figs. 3.3, 3.5). Decrease FA to just below this level. At this point flow should not rise precipitously to an early peak. If excessive respiratory effort continues, increase VA gradually until volume runaway occurs. This will first appear in the occasional breath (breath terminated by pressure or volume limit along with a beeping sound). Further increases cause runaway more frequently. VA should be set to the level just below the runaway point. If effort continues to be high, it must be concluded that the extent of nonlinearities is such that high level unloading cannot be offset by linear FA and VA algorithms or that there is a ventilator malfunction in the PAV mode. Switch to another mode.

3.7.3 Progressive Respiratory Acidosis

The development of progressive hypercapnia and acidosis despite seemingly adequate PAV support and in the absence of respiratory distress is unequivocal evidence of central depression. Although such patients are usually identifiable prior to the institution of PAV and do not meet eligibility criteria, in some cases one cannot be sure about the adequacy of the patient's ventilatory control system in advance. PAV can be instituted, with close monitoring of ventilation and blood gas tensions, as a test to assess the patient's respiratory control. If there is no obvious reason for central depression (e.g. sedatives, CNS pathology), consider the possibility that the patient was previously (i.e. prior to the current episode which led to intubation) in chronic respiratory failure and that the $PaCO_2$ was artificially driven down earlier during the use of another mode (CMV, A/C, PSV). Such patients tend to retain their high CO_2 set point for a long time, even after artificially normalizing $PaCO_2$. When weaning is attempted, or upon switching to PAV, respiratory output is very low until $PaCO_2$ approximates their high CO_2 set point. If this scenario is suspected, and particularly if it becomes known for sure that the patient was in chronic respiratory failure earlier, it would be reasonable to let $PaCO_2$ rise, accepting a low pH (within limits), as long as the patient shows no complications related to acute respiratory acidosis (drowsiness, arrhythmias) and there is no respiratory distress. Often $PaCO_2$ and pH will stabilize at a new level (e.g. $PaCO_2$ 70–80, pH 7.25–7.30), the pH corrects later, and the patient is found to be weanable soon after.

3.7.4 Hemodynamic Deterioration

In my experience with over 200 patients, I encountered only one patient who developed angina upon switching from AMV to PAV. This resolved promptly upon reinstitution of AMV. We have not observed clinically significant hypotension to develop after switching to PAV in any patient. In fact, in septic shock we have observed that BP improves (see earlier). The lack of significant hemodynamic deterioration in our experience may be related to our practice, so far, of not instituting PAV in any patient with recent myocardial infarction or who is in cardiogenic shock, or in patients with recent significant arrhythmias. In these patients it is theoretically possible that the higher distending pressures associated with conventional ventilation may facilitate left ventricular function and that a switch to PAV may result in decreased cardiac output with attendant hypotension, arrhythmias, or angina. The development of any of these complications upon a switch from conventional ventilation to PAV should contraindicate the use of PAV and cause one to consider the presence of very marginal left ventricular function, if that has not already been established.

3.8 Subsequent Management

One of the major advantages of PAV is that ventilator output faithfully reflects many important patient variables. The ventilator thus serves as an accurate monitor of the patient's ventilation and tidal volume demands, and its rate is an accurate reflection of the patient's own respiratory rate. This feature should be used to advantage in the clinical management of the patient. Thus a high level of ventilation reflects a high ventilatory demand and is not due to too much tidal volume setting (as in AMV) or pressure setting (as in PSV). Such an occurrence should prompt an investigation into the causes of a high respiratory drive, without the need to first experiment with reducing the level of assist, as is the case with other modes. A change in machine rate signifies a corresponding change in the patient's rate. This cannot be taken for granted with other modes, where synchrony between the end of the machine cycle and the end of a patient's inspiration is less assured. Thus an increase in machine rate from an average of 20–30/min with PAV reflects a substantial change in respiratory drive and possibly imminent, if not existent, distress. The same change with PSV (or AMV) may simply reflect improved synchrony between the patient and the ventilator due, for example, to a somewhat larger effort per breath [21]. With properly adjusted PAV, changes in ventilatory demand are both obvious (from monitored $\dot{V}_E$) and largely compensated for (since machine assist increases with increasing effort). The development of respiratory distress on previously satisfactory PAV settings indicates with greater certainty that something significant has occurred to respiratory mechanics (including tubing) or ventilator performance. Distress developing with other modes may simply be due to an increase in demand which rendered a previously satisfactory setting unsatisfactory.

In the usual case, ventilation, V_T, and P_{aw} are expected to vary from time to time with demand. This complicates the process of setting up the alarms. Some experience with PAV and with the specific patient is required to set the alarms such that safety is ensured while the alarms are not frequently and unnecessarily beeping.

By their very nature, patients in intensive care units on mechanical ventilation are susceptible to many respiratory, cardiovascular, metabolic, and psychiatric complications in the course of their stay. These complications may occur with any mode of ventilation, and the patient on PAV is clearly not immune to them. The purpose of the next section is to alert the reader to developments that are unique to the mode (e.g. no. 1 below) and to provide a guide, based on limited information available so far, or advice about when to abandon PAV in favour of a more conventional mode. Unless so stated, recommendation to switch to another mode need not signify that PAV is deleterious under the circumstance. Rather, it simply means that we do not know whether it is beneficial, harmful, or indifferent relative to other modes, and prudence dictates that under these conditions the patient should be switched. These recommendations may thus change as clinical experience expands. Decision-making with respect to some of the following occurrences is expected also to be facilitated in the future with availability of ventilators that automatically monitor leaks, ventilator performance, and changes in respiratory mechanics.

1. The alarms reflecting breath termination by one of the machine's set limits (P_{aw}, V_T, T_I) may sound very frequently or with every breath. This indicates either a substantial increase in ventilatory demand or a "runaway" situation. The latter may be due to a new leak or to the assist becoming greater than the patient's elastance or resistance. Should this occur, end-inspiratory occlusion is performed. Leaks are identified from difficulty in maintaining pressure during the occlusion. If a satisfactory plateau can be obtained, elastance is recomputed. If E is lower than the gain of volume assist, then a "runaway" exists (volume-assist gain was increased or patient's elastance decreased rel-

ative to previous levels). If measured E is higher than the volume-assist gain, then the increase in peak pressure and V_T (and hence the activation of machine limits) is due to increased ventilatory demand. Readjust the machine limits and alarms.

2. Respiratory distress develops. This should indicate a machine malfunction, a change in respiratory mechanics due to medical (e.g., pneumothorax, pulmonary edema, etc.) or technical causes (including partial blockage of tubing, ET tube sliding into a main-stem bronchus, etc.), a change in level of auto-PEEP, anxiety, or other medical problems frequently associated with distress (shock, embolus, etc.). Although such complications are not related to PAV, it would be prudent, for the time being, to switch the patient to a conventional mode while the cause is investigated. It is also advisable to monitor respiratory mechanics at intervals in order to detect changes in mechanics before they have progressed to the point of causing distress. The frequency of such measurements should depend on the likelihood of such changes taking place.

3. Deterioration occurs in gas exchange (i.e. PaO_2 at a given F_IO_2). In the patient whose spontaneously selected V_T on PAV is within the currently accepted range (e.g. >8 ml/kg), the deterioration is clearly not related to PAV per se, and management should be along the usual lines. In patients who insist on breathing with a small V_T on PAV the situation is somewhat different. Although the deterioration may be unrelated to PAV, a contribution of the small V_T cannot be excluded. Until the results of more definitive studies to assess the net impact of the small V_T on morbidity become available, it is prudent to switch such patients to a conventional mode.

4. Hypoventilation and respiratory acidosis occur. The de novo appearance of respiratory acidosis without distress indicates the development of central depression. The most likely cause is excessive sedation. If hypoventilation is significant (e.g. pH <7.30), the patient may be placed temporarily on a conventional mode until the effect of the sedative abates. The previously given dose should be noted and avoided in the future. Should undistressed respiratory acidosis develop in the absence of sedative intake, a medical reason for central depression should be sought, and PAV is discontinued until this is corrected.

5. Hemodynamic instability may occur. The de novo appearance of shock, arrhythmias, or angina in a patient already on PAV for hours or days cannot be attributed to PAV. Nonetheless, the use of PAV beyond this point should be reconsidered. Where the problem is likely to be cardiac in origin, PAV may not be an appropriate mode, although direct information in this regard is lacking. PAV has been shown to be superior, from the hemodynamic standpoint, in septic shock. The occurrence of this complication while the patient is on PAV should not call for a switch to conventional ventilation unless, of course, heavy sedation and/or paralysis is indicated to combat agitation or to reduce ventilatory demand, in which case PAV would have to be discontinued. The situation in hypovolemic shock is likely similar to that in septic shock, although this needs to be confirmed experimentally.

6. Agitation: Sedatives are not contraindicated when PAV is used. However, particularly when the response of a given patient to sedatives is not known, the

dose should be titrated initially until the amount required to attain the desired effect without severe depression is learned. Since backup systems must always be available on PAV delivery systems, the inadvertent use of an excessive amount should not be hazardous.

The frequency with which the preceding complications are encountered clearly depends on the type of patient managed with PAV. Patients with naturally unstable medical conditions are more likely to sustain one or more of these complications. It is prudent for medical personnel who contemplate using PAV to begin with fairly stable patients until they have acquired sufficient understanding of, and experience with, this unconventional mode, where the patient, and not the care giver, determines ventilation and pattern. Only then should they proceed to use it on unstable patients.

3.9 Weaning

A high level of support (e.g. 70%–90% of E and R) is recommended throughout the acute phase of the illness unless the patient indicates that he or she is receiving too much pressure. Although the amount of patient work at this level of support is small, it is almost certainly above the level required to prevent disuse. Once the underlying medical condition is brought under control, the level of support is decreased gradually. Some reserve should be allowed, however, to meet changing metabolic needs and moderate changes in mechanics. Thus it would be appropriate to maintain volume and flow assist somewhat higher (e.g. 20% of E and R) than the minimum level tolerated by the patient. This minimum level can be tested at intervals, as the patient recovers, by gradually reducing the level of assist in steps, each lasting 10–20 min.

3.10 References

1. Younes M (1992) Proportional assist ventilation, a new approach to ventilatory support: theory. Am Rev Respir Dis 145:114–120
2. Remmers JE, Gautier H (1976) Servorespirator constructed from a positive pressure ventilator. J Appl Physiol 41:252–256
3. Daubenspeck JA, Pichon D, Knuth KV, Bartlett D jr, St John WM (1988) An inexpensive servorespirator based upon regulation of a shunt resistance. Respir Physiol 73:87–96
4. Younes M, Puddy A, Roberts D, Light RB, Quesada A, Taylor K, Oppenheimer L, Cramp H (1992) Proportional assist ventilation: results of an initial clinical trial. Am Rev Respir Dis 145:121–129
5. Poon CS, Ward SA (1986) A device to provide respiratory mechanical unloading. IEEE Trans Biomed Eng 33:361–365
6. Schulze A, Schaller P, Gehrhardt B, Madler H-J, Gmyrek D (1990) An infant ventilator technique for resistive unloading during spontaneous breathing. Results in a rabbit model of airway obstruction. Pediatr Res 28:79–82
7. Black LF, Hyatt RE (1969) Maximal respiratory pressures: normal values and relationship to age and sex. Am Rev Respir Dis 99:696–702
8. Rochester DF, Braun NMT (1985) Determinants of maximal inspiratory pressure in chronic obstructive pulmonary disease. Am Rev Respir Dis 132:42–47

9. Boczkowski J, Aubier M (1995) The respiratory muscles in sepsis. In: Roussos C (ed) The thorax. Lung biology in health and disease, vol 85, chap 51. Dekker, New York, pp 1483–1513

10. McParland C, Krishnan B, Wang Y, Gallagher CG (1992) Inspiratory muscle weakness and dyspnea in chronic heart failure. Am Rev Respir Dis 146:467–472

11. Lewis MT, Belman MJ (1988) Nutrition and the respiratory muscles. Clin Chest Med 9:337–348

12. Aldrich TK, Prezant DJ (1990) Adverse effect of drugs on the respiratory muscles. Clin Chest Med 11: 177–189

13. Younes M (1990) Load responses, dyspnea and respiratory failure. "State of the art." Chest 97:595–685

14. Younes M (1994) Proportional assist ventilation. In: Tobin M (ed) Principles and practice of mechanical ventilation. McGraw-Hill, New York, pp 349–370

15. Harries JR, Tyler JM (1964) Mechanical assistance to respiration in emphysema. Am J Med 36:68–78

16. Stawitcke FA, Mordan WJ, Jimison HB, Piziali R, Ream AK (May 15, 1984) Medical ventilator device parametrically controlled for patient ventilation. U.S. Patent 4,448,192

17. Etherington TJ, Greene JG, Poon CS, Storsved M (1988) A new means of ventilation. The Negative Impedance Respirator. Biomed Sci Instrum 24:209–215

18. Huang KA(1985) A microprocessor-based servo-respirator with synchronized airflow pattern. MSc Thesis, North Dakota State University of Agriculture and Applied Science, Fargo, ND

19. Younes M (1992) Proportional assist and negative impedance ventilation (letter to the editor). Am Rev Respir Dis 146:1642–1643

20. Younes M (1991) Proportional assist ventilation and pressure support ventilation: similarities and differences. In: Update in Intensive Care and Emergency Medicine, vol 15. Springer, Berlin Heidelberg New York, pp 361–380

21. Younes M (1993) Patient–ventilator interaction with pressure–assisted modalities of ventilatory support. Semin Respir Med 14:299–322

22. Younes M (1995) Interactions between patients and ventilators. In: Roussos C (ed) The thorax. Lung biology in health and disease, vol 85, chap 81. Dekker, New York, pp 2367–2420

23. Jammes Y, Auran Y, Gouvermet J, Delpierre S, Grimaud C (1979) The ventilatory pattern of conscious man according to age and morphology. Bull Eur Physiopathol Respir 15:527–540

24. Marantz S, Patrick W, Webster K, Roberts D, Oppenheimer L, Younes M (1996) Response of ventilator-dependent patients to different levels of proportional assist (PAV). J Appl Physiol 80:397–403

25. Patrick W, Webster K, Ludwig L, Roberts D, Wiebe P, Younes M (1996) Noninvasive positive-pressure ventilation in acute respiratory distress without prior chronic respiratory failure. Am J Respir Crit Care Med 153:1005–1011

26. Navalesi P, Hernandez P, Wongsa A, Laporta D, Goldberg P, Gottfried SB (1996) Proportional assist ventilation in acute respiratory failure: effects on breathing pattern and inspiratory effort. Am J Respir Crit Care Med 154:1330–1338

27. Ranieri VM, Giuliani R, Mascia L, Grasso S, Petruzzelli V, Puntillo N, Perchiazzi G, Fiore T, Brienza A (1996) Patient ventilator interaction during acute hypercapnia: pressure support vs proportional assist ventilation. J Appl Physiol 81:426–436

28. Meza S, Giannouli E, Younes M (1995) Ventilatory response to inspiratory muscle unloading with PAV (proportional assist) during sleep. Am J Respir Crit Care Med 151:A639

29. Giannouli E, Webster K, Patrick W, Roberts D, Younes M (1994) Determination of dynamic hyperinflation in patients on synchronized (assist) methods of ventilatory support. Am J Respir Crit Care Med 149:A72

30. Giannouli E, Webster K, Roberts D, Younes M (1999) Response of ventilator-dependent patients to different levels of pressure support and proportional assist. Am J Respir Crit Care Med 159:1716–1725

31. Patrick W, Webster K, Wiebe P, Roberts D, Light B, Oppenheimer L, Kassum D, Younes M (1993) Effect of proportional assist ventilation on the hemodynamics of patients in septic shock. Am J Respir Crit Care Med 147:A611
32. Mettias M, Mendoza M, Wiebe P, Younes M, Light B (1993) Effect of proportional assist ventilation (PAV) vs controlled mandatory and pressure support ventilation (CMV, PSV) on gas exchange in patients with hypoxemic respiratory failure. Clin Invest Med 16:B23
33. Georgopoulos D, Webster K. Mitrouska I, Bshouty Z, Younes M (1995) Effect of inspiratory muscle unloading on the ventilatory response to CO_2 Am J Respir Crit Care Med 151:A639
34. Rimmer KP, Rose MS, Hecker Js, Whitelaw WA (1995) Effect of proportional assist ventilation on ventilatory response to CO_2 Am J Respir Crit Care Med 151:A639
35. Chrusch C, Bauerle O, Younes M (1996) The effect of proportional assist ventilation (PAV) on exercise endurance time in COPD. Am J Respir Crit Care Med 153:A171
36. Hernandez P, Maltais F, Gursahaney A, LeBlanc P, Navalesi P, Gottfried SB (1996) Proportional assist ventilation (PAV) improves exercise performance in severe COPD. Am J Respir Crit Care Med 153: A172
37. Appendini L, Purro A, Patessio A, Zanaboni S, Polese G, Donner CF, Rossi A (1996) CPAP improves ventilatory assistance with proportional assist ventilation (PAV) in COPD patients. Am J Respir Crit Care Med 153:A380
38. Mendez M, Fernandez R, Younes M (1996) Changes in respiratory motor output with different levels of volume-cycled, pressure support and proportional assist ventilation in normal subjects. Am J Respir Crit Care Med 153:A375
39. Puntillo F, Vitale N, Grasso S, Mascia L, Giuliani R, Tunzi P, Cicale P, DeLuca Tupputi L, Fiore T, Ranieri M (1996) Compensation for increase in elastic load during pressure assisted modes (part 1). Am J Respir Crit Care Med 153:A373
40. Grasso S, Puntillo F, Mascia L, Ancona G, Fiore T, Bruno F, Slutsky AS, Ranieri M (2000) Compensation for increase in respiratory workload during mechanical ventilation. Pressure support versus proportional-assist ventilation. Am J Respir Crit Care Med 161:819–826
41. Gursahaney A, Mirkovic T, Hernandez P, Navalesi P, Laporta D, Goldberg, P, Gottfried SB (1996) Comparison of airway opening and tracheal pressure regulated forms of proportional assist ventilation (PAV). Am J Respir Crit Care Med 153:A372
42. Gursahaney A, Mirkovic T, Hernandez P, Laporta D, Goldberg P, Gottfried SB (1996) Proportional assist ventilation (PAV) improves breathing pattern and inspiratory effort in acute respiratory failure (ARF). Am J Respir Crit Care Med 153:A372
43. Appendini L, Purro A, Zanaboni S, Patessio A, Spada E, Carone M, Polese G, Ganassini A, Donner CF, Rossi A (1996) Effects of endotracheal tube (ET) on patient-ventilator interactions during proportional assist ventilation (PAV) in COPD patients. Am J Respir Crit Care Med 153:A373
44. Fink BR, Hanks EC, Ngal EH, Papper EM (1963) Central regulation of respiration during anesthesia and wakefulness. Ann NY Acad Sci 190:892–899
45. Skatrud SJ, Dempsey JA (1983) Interaction of sleep state and chemical stimuli in sustaining rhythmic ventilation. J Appl Physiol 55:813–22
46. Tobin M (1990) Weaning from mechanical ventilation. Curr Pulmonology 11:47–105
47. Hey EN, Lloyd BB, Cunningham DJC, Jukes MGM, Bolton DPG (1966) Effects of various respiratory stimuli on the depth and frequency of breathing in man. Respir Physiol 1:193–205
48. Marini JJ (1990) Lung mechanics determination at the bedside: instrumentation and clinical application. Respir Care 35:669–696
49. Guerin C Coussa ML, Eissa NT, Corbeil C, Chasse M, Braidy J, Matar N, Milic-Emili J (1993) Lung and chest wall mechanics in mechanically ventilated COPD patients. J Appl Physiol 74:1570–1580
50. Wright PE, Marini JJ, Bernard GR (1989) In vitro versus in vivo comparison of endotracheal tube airflow resistance. Am Rev Respir Dis 140:10–16
51. Agostoni E, Mead J (1964) Statics of the respiratory system. In: Handbook of physiology. Respiration, sect 3, vol 1, chap 13. Am Physiol Soc., Washington DC, pp 387–409

52. Mead J, Agostoni E (1964) Dynamics of breathing. In: Handbook of physiology. Respiration, sect 3, vol 1, chap 14. Am Physiol Soc., Washington DC, pp 411–427
53. Newsom-Davis J, Stag. D (1975) Interrelationships of the volume and time components of individual breaths in resting man. J Physiol (Lond) 245:481–498
54. Tobin MJ, Mador MJ, Guenther SM, et al (1988) Variability of resting respiratory drive and timing in healthy subjects. J Appl Physiol 65:309–317

4 Influence of Ventilator Performance on Assisted Modes of Ventilation

J.-C. Richard and L. Breton

4.1 Introduction

More recent generations of ventilators that are based on state-of-the-art technology tend to be better adapted to the wide range of ventilatory situations usually observed in critically ill patients. They differ from previous generations in many technical aspects, particularly pressurization working principles: e.g., pressurized gas source, piston, turbine, compressor bellows, Venturi system, flow-regulation systems based on microprocessors. These features associated with new software now permit manufacturers to provide attractive modes of ventilation. The rationale claimed for the development of these sophisticated ventilators is to allow a better adaptation of machines to patients' needs. Nevertheless, studies aiming at comparing currently available ventilator performance in vitro as well as in vivo are relatively scarce. In routine practice, respiratory failure under mechanical ventilation is more often attributed to a patient's worsening or to inadequate ventilatory settings, whereas poor technical performance related to the ventilator itself is rarely cited. Recently, several studies have stressed the clinical impact of technical differences regarding either the trigger or the delivered flow.

In this chapter we emphasize the importance of ventilator performance in clinical situations where assisted modes are used, such as in the weaning process. We will also review the ways in which ventilators can be compared.

4.2 Physiological Aspects of Patient-Ventilator Interactions

Respiratory volume displacement needed for gas exchange, and related to either negative pressure (P_{mus}) generated by the patient during spontaneous breathing or positive pressure (P_{appl}) provided by the ventilator during MV, can be described at each instant by the equation of motion:

$$P_{mus} + P_{appl} = (Flow \times R_{tot}) + (Volume \times E_{st}) + PEEPi$$

where R_{tot} represents the resistance and E_{st} the elastance of the respiratory system. In other words, the pressure needed to generate a given flow, and then a volume, has to overcome resistive pressure (Flow $\times$ R_{tot}) and elastic recoil pressure (Volume $\times$ E_{st}), added to the inspiratory threshold load related to intrinsic PEEP (PEEPi).

From a clinical point of view, the situation in which the breathing pattern is completely controlled by the ventilator because of sedation and muscle paralysis (i.e., P_{mus} is abolished) is opposite to the situation where the patient is breathing spontaneously without any ventilatory support ($P_{appl} = 0$). Most of the time, the patient is not able to sustain the breathing effort alone, and the total pressure applied to the respiratory system (P_{tot}) depends on both the negative pressure generated by the patient and the positive pressure provided by the ventilator. Both systems, the ventilator and the patient, should be synchronized as closely as possible in order to improve ventilatory assist and minimize patient-ventilator asynchrony. These particular characteristics emphasize the importance of patient-ventilator interactions. The breathing pattern is determined by the patient's ventilatory drive, inspiratory flow demand, and inspiratory time, which characterize the patient, whereas the trigger system, the delivered flow (that may be pressure or flow limited) and the cycle variable that terminates the breath will characterize the response of the ventilator. Ventilator performance may often interfere with the patient's breathing pattern.

4.3 Clinical Aspects of Ventilator Performance

4.3.1 Inspiratory Triggering Function

The triggering systems refer to the technical function which has been incorporated into the ventilator to detect patient inspiratory effort. Regardless of the type of breath, whether flow or pressure targeted, triggering the ventilator is a key feature of any assisted mode of ventilation.

Technical Aspects of Triggering Function

During controlled ventilation mode, ventilatory breaths are time triggered, which means that the mandatory breath is delivered after a fixed time, depending on respiratory rate setting. In contrast, during assisted ventilation, the breath may be flow or pressure triggered, which means that the signal detected by the ventilator to initiate the breath is either inspiratory flow or a negative pressure generated by the patient. Several systems combining flow and pressure thresholds have also been developed to improve sensitivity without compromising reliability and to minimize the risk of self-triggering. Volume triggering can also be accomplished but is not widely used at present. Among the factors shown to influence inspiratory effort during the assisted mode of ventilation is the effort required to trigger the ventilator. In this area, significant advances have been made in producing more responsive ventilators, which are better adapted to the patient's individual needs. With flow-triggering systems the patient breathes throughout an open circuit leading to less inspiratory effort than with pressure-triggering systems in which the circuit is closed. Almost all the available triggering systems have been investigated either under laboratory test conditions or in physiological studies. Also, a better understanding of patient ventilator asynchrony or interactions has recently emphasized the clinical importance of the triggering systems.

Influence on Inspiratory Effort

Numerous studies have demonstrated that flow triggering is associated with a reduction in breathing effort as compared with pressure triggering. In a lung model study, Sassoon et al. demonstrated that the response time with the Puritan Bennett 7200ae (PB7200ae) was significantly shorter during flow-trigger (FT) than during pressure-trigger (PT) (Sassoon and Gruer 1995). The same group also demonstrated a reduction in respiratory effort associated with FT in the same ventilator (Sassoon et al. 1992). However, the operation system of this ventilator associated with FT or PT differs in several points which concern not only the trigger but also inspiratory flow delivery. Therefore, the influence of the triggering system on physiological indexes is difficult to interpret. A similar issue has been reported to explain discrepancies regarding the physiological evaluation of CPAP in three recent ICU ventilators where, in one system, an additional pressure support was automatically applied (Calzia et al. 1998).

The trigger working principle of several ventilators has been previously described in detail (Branson and Campbell 1998; Sassoon and Gruer 1995). Although a significant benefit related to FT was not consistently found in all studies, sufficient evidence exists to support the favorable effects of such systems. Recently, Aslanian et al. tested the hypothesis that the clinical impact of both FT and PT could be influenced by the mode of ventilation (Aslanian et al. 1998). The experimental part of this study revealed significant differences in airway pressure-time product among the nine ventilators tested. Current ventilators have exhibited significantly better performance (i.e., lesser airway pressure fall and shorter time delay related to the triggering phase) as compared with the older systems. In the clinical part of this study, FT was compared with PT during assist-control ventilation (ACV) and pressure-support ventilation (PSV) delivered by a PB7200ae. During ACV, inspiratory flow was set at 50 l/min and the tidal volume (Vt) was set as measured during PSV. Interestingly, FT was associated with a significant reduction of all breathing effort indexes during PSV, whereas no difference was found between the two triggering systems during ACV (Fig. 4.1). These results suggest that the small beneficial effects of FT on breathing effort may depend on factors as diverse as patient inspiratory demand, ventilatory mode, or settings, as well as on underlying disease.

Bench-Test Evaluation

Bench-test evaluation permits the comparison of numerous ventilators in standardized conditions regardless of confounding physiological factors. Although the clinical relevance of lung model findings has been demonstrated, studies evaluating the performance of currently available ventilators are relatively scarce. Using a spontaneously breathing lung model, Bunburaphong et al. tested the performance of nine bi-level pressure ventilators compared with the Puritan Bennett 7200ae (Bunburaphong et al. 1997). In six of the nine bi-level pressure ventilators tested, the time delay required to trigger the breath was significantly shorter than that measured in the Puritan Bennett 7200ae with the FT. Interestingly, this latter ventilator was outperformed by all of the bi-level ventilators as regards the trigger pressure fall. This feature could be explained, at least in part, by the substantial flow-by provided by turbine-based systems.

In an active lung model, we recently compared 22 ventilators including seven new-generation ventilators, six of the previous generation, and nine piston or turbine based (Table 4.1) (Richard et al. 2000). Triggering sensitivity was assessed by measuring time delay and pressure fall during two levels of simulat-

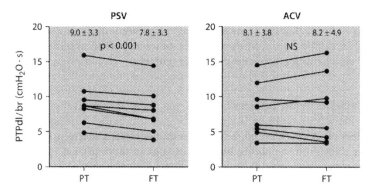

Fig. 4.1. Comparison of the effects of pressure triggering (*PT*) and flow triggering (*FT*) on inspiratory effort during pressure-support ventilation (*PSV*) and assist-control ventilation (*ACV*). Individual values for transdiaphragmatic pressure-time product per breath (PTPdi/br). FT was associated with a consistent reduction in inspiratory effort in PSV, while no significant difference was found during ACV. (From Aslanian et al. 1998, with permission)

Table 4.1. Tested ventilators according to generation and working principles

New-generation ventilators
  Horus (Taema; Antony Cedex, France)
  Evita II (Drägerwerk AG, Lübeck, Germany)
  Evita II Dura (Drägerwerk AG, Lübeck, Germany)
  Evita IV (Drägerwerk AG, Lübeck, Germany)
  NPB 840 (Nellcor Puritan-Bennett Corp; Carlsbad, Calif.)
  Gallileo (Hamilton Medical, Rhäzüns, Switzerland)
  Siemens Servo 300 (SV 300; Siemens-Elema, Solna, Sweden)

Previous-generation ventilators
  Siemens Servo 900C (SV 900 C; Siemens-Elema, Solna, Sweden)
  Adult Star (Infrasonics, San Diego, Calif.)
  Nellcor Puritan-Bennett 7200ae (Nellcor Puritan-Bennett Corp; Carlsbad, Calif.)
  Bird 8400ST (Bird Products Corp., Palm Springs, Calif.)
  Bear 1000 (Bear Medical Systems, Riverside, Calif.)
  Hamilton Veolar (Hamilton Medical, Rhäzüns, Switzerland)

Piston- or turbine-based ventilators
  BiPAP S/T-D30 (Respironics Inc; Murrysville, Pa.)
  BiPAP Vision (Respironics Inc; Murrysville, Pa.)
  T Bird (Bird Products Corp., Palm Springs, Calif.)
  O'NYX (Pierre Medical; Verrieres le Buisson, France)
  Quantum PSV pressure-support ventilator (Healthdyne; Marietta, Ga.)
  NPB 740 (Nellcor Puritan-Bennett Corp; Carlsbad, Calif.)
  Respicare (Drägerwerk AG, Lübeck, Germany)
  Hellia (Saime, Savigny Le Temple, France)

ed inspiratory drive. As regards time delay, all new-generation ventilators out-performed the previous-generation group and six of the nine piston- or turbine-based systems, whereas no difference was found regarding pressure fall except in two previous-generation and one turbine ventilators. Whatever the condition tested (PEEP=5 cmH$_2$O or ZEEP), no difference was found within the new-generation ventilator group regarding time delay or pressure fall. These results suggest that newer technologies implemented on recent commercialized ventilators have substantially improved their performance regarding trigger sensitivity, in spite of very heterogeneous operation algorithms.

4.3.2 Inspiratory Flow Delivery

Regardless of the mode used, it has been demonstrated that ventilatory support depends mainly on the ability of the ventilator to meet patient inspiratory flow demand, especially when the patient exhibits high inspiratory drive. In contrast to ACV, during which inspiratory flow is preset, PSV theoretically allows the flow to increase according to the demand. PSV is a widely used mode of partial ventilatory support that has been proposed for acute respiratory failure and the weaning process (Brochard 1994; Brochard et al. 1994). From a physiological point of view, PSV reduces not only the respiratory muscle load but also the oxygen cost of breathing (Brochard et al. 1989).

Clinical Impact
The importance of inspiratory flow in reducing inspiratory workload regardless of the ventilatory mode has been emphasized in a study comparing assisted volume (ACV) with assist pressure-controlled ventilation (PCV) (Cinnella et al. 1996). Vt was kept constant while the effects on work of breathing (WOB) of PCV and ACV (at high and low inspiratory flow, respectively) were tested. The results suggest that a pressure-targeted mode more effectively reduced respiratory effort as compared with ACV in low mean inspiratory flow condition, suggesting that the theoretical ability of PCV to deliver flow whatever the inspiratory demand could be of major importance. In a group of COPD patients, Bonmarchand et al. demonstrated that modifying inspiratory flow rate by adjusting the pressure ramp, despite a similar pressure-support level set on the ventilator, significantly affected WOB (Bonmarchand et al. 1996). In these series PSV was delivered by an ICU ventilator on which the time required to reach the pressure level target could be adjusted (0.1–1.5 s). In these 11 selected COPD patients it was found that the higher the flow rate, the lower the respiratory effort (Fig. 4.2a). However, it has been also demonstrated in ventilator-dependent patients that increasing inspiratory flow rate above an "optimal level" led to higher respiratory rate, shorter inspiratory time, and smaller Vt and may also increase dyspnea (Corne et al. 1997; Laghi et al. 1999; MacIntyre and Ho 1991; Manning et al. 1995). Under these circumstances, optimization of patient-ventilator interaction may be carried out not simply by increasing inspiratory flow "as much as possible", but by setting the ventilator to obtain inspiratory flow "as close as possible" to real patient flow requirements.

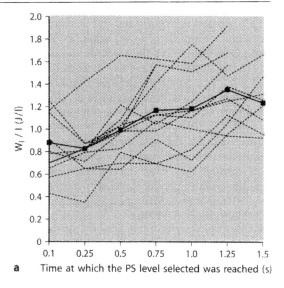

a   Time at which the PS level selected was reached (s)

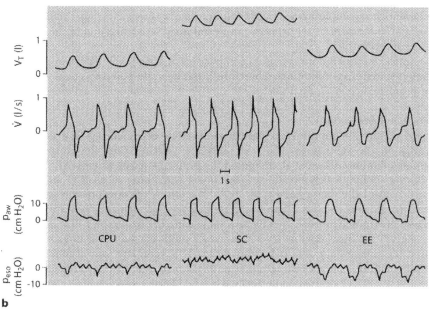

Fig. 4.2. a Effects of pressure ramp settings on inspiratory work of breathing performed per liter of ventilation (W_I/l). The lower the pressure ramp, the higher the work of breathing. Individual data are shown and the *boldface lines* and *squares* represent the variation of the mean values. (From Bonmarchand et al. 1996, with permission). **b** Tracings of tidal volume (V_T), flow, airway pressure (P_{aw}) and esophageal pressure (P_{eso}) in a representative patient ventilated during 15 cmH_2O of pressure-support ventilation with three different ventilators: CPU-1 (*CPU*), Servo 900 C (*SC*) and Engström Erica (*EE*). Esophageal pressure swings which represent the inspiratory effort significantly differ among the ventilators. (From Mancebo J, et al. 1995a, with permission)

PSV is based on algorithms and working principles that may differ considerably from one ventilator to the other, leading to potentially heterogeneous technical performance. For these reasons, several authors have attempted to assess the clinical impact of these technical differences. Mancebo et al. compared the effects of PSV (15 cmH$_2$O) delivered by three different ICU ventilators on breathing pattern and WOB (Mancebo et al. 1995a). The significant differences they found were related mainly to various pressure ramps associated with the different working principles (Fig. 4.2b). In another study, these authors demonstrated that at a similar maximal pressure level during assisted breathing through a mouthpiece, conventional PSV (pressure-limited and flow-cycled) ventilators outperformed the older intermittent positive-pressure breathing ventilators (flow-limited and pressure-cycled) where maximal inspiratory flow was limited (i.e., CPU1, Ohmeda, Maurepas, France; Monaghan 505, Monaghan, Plattsburgh, NY) (Mancebo et al. 1995b).

Home bi-level pressure-support ventilators (BIPAP) were compared with a single ICU ventilator specifically designed for PSV with regard to their ability to relieve respiratory workload in a group of seven difficult-to-wean patients (Lofaso et al. 1996). The esophageal pressure-time product (PTP) was found to be 30% higher in the home devices. In the same study, a bench evaluation showed that the ICU ventilators outperformed the BIPAP ventilators as regards trigger sensitivity, speed of attainment of set pressure, and expiratory resistance, and in the occurrence of rebreathing.

Clinical studies did not permit a comparison of several ventilators under different standardized conditions. Therefore, it has been proposed to assess ventilator performance in a lung model.

Bench-Test Evaluation

Based on the assumption that patient respiratory effort during PSV depends greatly on the ventilator's ability to meet the patient's peak flow inspiratory demand, Bunburaphong et al. compared the performance of nine BIPAP ventilators in a spontaneously breathing lung model with those of an ICU ventilator (NPB 7200ae) (Bunburaphong et al. 1997). The effects of three pressure-support levels (5, 10, and 15 cmH$_2$O) and four inspiratory flow demands on inspiratory airway pressure area were investigated. Increasing the inspiratory flow demand for a given pressure-support level induced a significant reduction in ventilatory assist (i.e., inspiratory area reduction) in the ICU ventilator and in four BIPAP ventilators (Fig. 4.3). Interestingly, as regards the inspiratory airway pressure area, most of the BIPAP devices outperformed the PB7200ae and were able to meet the simulated inspiratory flow demand increase.

Using a similar approach, we compared 22 ventilators in their ability to reach and maintain the set pressure-support level (5, 10, and 15 cmH$_2$O) at, respectively, low, moderate, and high simulated inspiratory drive (corresponding to 0.1, 0.6, and 1.2 l/s). To evaluate ventilatory assist, we measured the net inspiratory area based on the airway pressure (P$_{aw}$) trace at 0.3 and 0.5 s. These criteria were chosen because it had been shown that the essential part of the inspiratory effort is often performed at the onset and in the early phase of inspiration. Thus, we assumed that the initial efficacy of pressurization was a crucial feature to be

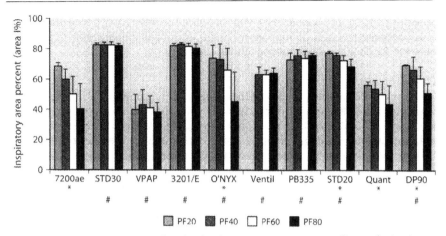

Fig. 4.3. Inspiratory area computed under the airway pressure trace according to the inspiratory flow demand for the different tested ventilators. Most of the bi-level pressure ventilators outperformed the PB7200ae, especially in cases of high inspiratory flow demand. *PF*, inspiratory flow demand; *asterisks*, $p<0.05$ among different PF; #, $p<0.05$ ventilators vs 7200ae. (From Bunburaphong et al. 1997, with permission)

assessed (Cinnella et al. 1996). As regards area 0.3, which was the most sensitive index to differentiate ventilators, all "new-generation" and the majority of the turbine-based machines outperformed the "previous-generation" systems. Since the clinical impact of initial flow rate related to pressure slope has been demonstrated for pressure-limited modes, these results obtained in vitro suggest that recent ICU and also piston- and turbine-based ventilators could be more adapted to the patient's needs than the older ones. These results may be particularly relevant to clinical situations associating high inspiratory demand, respiratory mechanical impairment, and moderate levels of pressure support (i.e., weaning or noninvasive ventilation).

4.3.3 Expiratory Triggering Function (Switch-off) and Expiratory Flow

PSV is a form of assisted ventilation during which neither the respiratory rate nor the inspiratory time is set by the physician. As previously discussed, the patient determines his own breathing frequency by the triggering function, while inspiratory time determination is more complex and depends on several factors (MacIntyre and Ho 1991).

Technical Aspects
From a technical point of view, breath termination during PSV occurs when the cycle variable is reached. In most ventilators, this variable is either a percentage of peak flow or a set cycling flow. Under these circumstances, the inspiratory time (Ti) is determined exclusively by the time required for the exponential declining flow to reach the flow threshold value, thus determining the mechanical Ti. Since

patient-ventilator asynchrony has been shown to be often associated with inadequacy between mechanical and neural Ti, the advantage of being able to individually set the flow threshold value could be useful.

Clinical Impact

This hypothesis was tested by MacIntyre et al. in a group of 33 mechanically ventilated patients allocated to receive PSV with different combinations of initial flow rate and breath termination criteria (MacIntyre and Ho 1991). The authors demonstrated that changes in PSV termination criteria from 50% to 25% of peak flow had minimal effects on synchrony, while changes in inspiratory flow rate profoundly affected the ventilatory pattern. Interestingly, Santos and Mancebo showed that changes in cycling-off criteria modified the breathing pattern with no impact in inspiratory muscle effort (Santos and Mancebo 2000). In contrast to invasive ventilation, the leaks that occur at the end of inspiration during noninvasive ventilation (NIV) could interfere with flow cycle criteria, leading to potentially prolonged mechanical Ti and asynchrony. Calderini et al. demonstrated that in the presence of air leaks, a time-cycled expiratory trigger improved patient-ventilator synchrony compared with flow cycling (Calderini et al. 1999).

In PSV, patient-ventilator asynchrony may also be associated with ineffective inspiratory efforts (Fabry et al. 1995; Nava et al. 1995). It has been demonstrated that "missed breaths" are associated with dynamic hyperinflation related to high pressure-support levels which could be reduced by lowering pressure-support level. A similar phenomenon has been described in patients with prolonged time constant due to COPD (Jubran et al. 1995). Although this issue has never been specifically addressed, differences in expiratory circuits and valve resistance reported in vitro as well as in vivo could also be responsible for potential excessive expiratory work load and asynchrony (Lofaso et al. 1998).

4.4 Clinical Application During the Weaning Process

4.4.1 Influence of the Ventilator

It has recently been shown that, more than 40% of the time under mechanical ventilation (MV) is spent trying to wean the patient from the ventilator. Assist-control modes of ventilation have been claimed to facilitate the weaning process in patients with difficulties in tolerating MV discontinuation. Because PSV is widely used either during the period devoted to the weaning process or to test the patient's ability to breath spontaneously, the previously mentioned discrepancies related to the heterogeneous technical performance of ventilators may affect the weaning course. In fact, during the weaning period, the association of high respiratory demand, mechanical impairment, and moderate pressure-support levels may have deleterious clinical consequences due to the differences in ventilator performance. Although this issue has never been specifically addressed, in the light of the comparative bench-test results, we can not rule out that the ventilator design may affect the clinical response to a pressure support of 7 cmH$_2$O trial.

Thus, ventilator design may influence the decision-making process concerning extubation. Considering the types of ventilators currently available, the use of newer-generation machines for difficult-to-wean patients makes sense not only because of their monitoring capabilities but also because of their better technical performance.

4.4.2 Further Prospects

The incorporation of microprocessors into ventilator technology, associated with more efficient demand valves, now makes it possible to program machines to deliver gas with virtually any flow or pressure profile. These significant technical advancements have enabled manufacturers to develop new modes of ventilation which permit better synchrony between the ventilator and the patient's breathing pattern. In this situation, the ventilator should be able to recognize any instantaneous change in ventilatory requirements and in respiratory mechanics (input). Also, the mode of ventilation depends on the specific algorithm that will adapt the delivered flow pattern (output) to the patient input. An additional factor is the ability of the system to be automatically regulated, which means that the ventilator output continuously attempts to adjust the input signal according to a controlled algorithm. This approach recently implemented with ventilators has been termed "closed-loop technology". To date, numerous closed-loop systems have been developed to better synchronize the ventilatory support with the patient's own respiratory control.

4.5 Conclusion

Assisted modes of ventilation are currently widely used, not only at the onset and during respiratory failure, but also at any stage of the weaning process (Esteban et al. 1994). Major technical improvements have been made by manufacturers in producing ventilators that are better adapted to patients' needs. In the new generation of ventilators, recent advancements that concern all three phases of breath delivery – triggering, flow delivery, and cycling functions – allow a more effective assist and better patient-ventilator synchrony.

Acknowledgements. The authors wish to thank Laurent Brochard for reviewing the manuscript and for his helpful advice. Richard Medeiros also provided valuable editorial assistance.

4.6 References

Aslanian P, El Atrous S, Isabey D, Valente E, Corsi D, Harf A, Lemaire F, Brochard L (1998) Effects of flow triggering on breathing effort during partial ventilatory support. Am J Respir Crit Care Med 157:135–143

Bonmarchand G, Chevron V, Chopin C, Jusserand D, Girault C, Moritz F, Leroy J, Pasquis P (1996) Increased initial flow rate reduces inspiratory work of breathing during pressure support ventilation in patients with exacerbation of chronic obstructive pulmonary disease. Intensive Care Med 22:1147-1154

Branson RD, Campbell RS (1998) Triggering the ventilator. Curr Opin Crit Care 4:48-58

Brochard L (1994) Pressure support ventilation. In: Tobin MJ (ed) Principles and practice of mechanical ventilation. McGraw-Hill, New York, pp 239-257

Brochard L, Harf A, Lorino H, Lemaire F (1989) Inspiratory pressure support prevents diaphragmatic fatigue during weaning from mechanical ventilation. Am Rev Respir Dis 139:513-521

Brochard L, Rauss A, Benito S, Conti G, Mancebo J, Rekik N, Gasparetto A, Lemaire F (1994) Comparison of three methods of gradual withdrawal from ventilatory support during weaning from mechanical ventilation. Am J Respir Crit Care Med 150:896-903

Bunburaphong T, Imanaka H, Nishimura M, Hess D, Kacmarek RM (1997) Performance characteristics of bi-level pressure ventilators: a lung model study. Chest 111:1050-1060

Calderini E, Confalonieri M, Puccio PG, Francavilla N, Stella L, Gregoretti C (1999) Patient-ventilator asynchrony during noninvasive ventilation: the role of expiratory. Intensive Care Med 25:662-667

Calzia E, Lindner KH, Stahl W, Martin A, Radermacher P, Georgieff M (1998) Work of breathing, inspiratory flow response, and expiratory resistance during continuous positive airway pressure with the ventilators EVITA-2, EVITA-4 and SV 300. Intensive Care Med 24:931-938

Cinnella G, Conti G, Lofaso F, Lorino H, Harf A, Lemaire F, Brochard L (1996) Effects of assisted ventilation on the work of breathing: volume-controlled versus pressure-controlled ventilation. Am J Respir Crit Care Med 153:1025-1033

Corne S, Gillespie D, Roberts D, Younes M (1997) Effect of inspiratory flow rate on respiratory rate in intubated ventilated patients. Am J Respir Crit Care Med 156:304-308

Esteban A, Alía I, Ibañez J, Benito S, Tobin MJ (1994) Modes of mechanical ventilation and weaning. A national survey of Spanish hospitals. The Spanish Lung Failure Collaborative Group. Chest 106:1188-1193

Fabry B, Guttmann J, Eberhard L, Bauer T, Haberthür C, Wolff G (1995) An analysis of desynchronization between the spontaneously breathing patient and ventilator during inspiratory pressure support. Chest 107:1387-1394

Jubran A, Van de Graaff WB, Tobin MJ (1995) Variability of patient-ventilator interaction with pressure support ventilation in patients with chronic obstructive pulmonary disease. Am J Respir Crit Care Med 152:129-136

Laghi F, Karamchandani K, Tobin M (1999) Influence of ventilator settings in determining respiratory frequency during mechanical ventilation. Am J Respir Crit Care Med 160:1766-1770

Lofaso F, Brochard L, Hang T, Lorino H, Harf A, Isabey D (1996) Home versus intensive care pressure support devices. Experimental and clinical comparison. Am J Respir Crit Care Med 153:1591-1599

Lofaso F, Aslanian P, Richard JC, Isabey D, Hang T, Corriger E, Harf A, Brochard L (1998) Expiratory valves used for home devices: experimental and clinical comparison. Eur Respir J 11:1382-1388

MacIntyre NR, Ho LI (1991) Effects of initial flow rate and breath termination criteria on pressure support ventilation. Chest 99:134-138

Mancebo J, Amaro P, Mollo JL, Lorino H, Lemaire F, Brochard L (1995a) Comparison of the effects of pressure support ventilation delivered by three different ventilators during weaning from mechanical ventilation. Intensive Care Med 21:913-919

Mancebo J, Isabey D, Lorino H, Lofaso F, Lemaire F, Brochard L (1995b) Comparative effects of pressure support ventilation and intermittent positive pressure breathing (IPPB) in non-intubated healthy subjects. Eur Respir J 8:1901-1909

Manning HL, Molinary EJ, Leiter JC (1995) Effect of inspiratory flow rate on respiratory sensation and pattern of breathing. Am J Respir Crit Care Med 151:751-757

Nava S, Bruschi C, Rubini F, Palo A, Iotti G, Braschi A (1995) Respiratory response and inspiratory effort during pressure support ventilation in COPD patients. Intensive Care Med 21:871-879

Richard JC, Carlucci A, Langlais N, Jaber S, Fougère S, Harf A, Brochard L (2001) Evaluation of assisted ventilation among three different generations of ventilators. (submitted)

Santos JA, Mancebo J (2000) Effects of different cycling-off criteria (COC) during pressure support ventilation (PSV) (abstract). Am J Respir Crit Care Med 161:A462

Sassoon CS, Gruer SE (1995) Characteristics of the ventilator pressure- and flow-trigger variables. Intensive Care Med 21:159–168

Sassoon CS, Lodia R, Rheeman CH, Kuei JH, Light RW, Mahutte CK (1992) Inspiratory muscle work of breathing during flow-by, demand-flow, and continuous-flow systems in patients with chronic obstructive pulmonary disease. Am Rev Respir Dis 145:1219–1222

5 Application of Tracheal Gas Insufflation for Critical Care Patients

L. Blanch, G. Murias, P.V. Romero, R. Fernandez, and A. Nahum

5.1 Introduction

Lung-protective mechanical ventilatory strategies have been proposed for acute respiratory distress syndrome (ARDS) [1,2]. These strategies typically involve the use of small tidal volume to avoid high alveolar pressures at end-inspiration and alveolar overdistension, and the use of high positive end-expiratory pressure (PEEP) levels to keep alveoli open at end-expiration, thus maintaining alveolar recruitment. Such ventilatory strategies may involve a decrease in alveolar ventilation and a significant rise in $PaCO_2$. This strategy has been called permissive hypercapnia. Mechanical ventilation strategies designed to protect the lungs from excessive stretch resulted in improvements in several important clinical outcomes in patients with acute lung injury and in patients with ARDS [3–5]. Unfortunately, CO_2 retention must sometimes occur over brief intervals, which leads to unacceptably severe respiratory acidosis.

Although permissive hypercapnia is generally well tolerated, it may not be acceptable in some patients in whom lung and brain injury coexist. On the basis of recent data [4], it would be advantageous to use a lung-protective strategy without respiratory acidosis. Tracheal gas insufflation (TGI) is an adjunct to mechanical ventilation that allows ventilation with small tidal volumes while CO_2 is satisfactorily cleared [6]. Pioneering studies in healthy experimental animals [7] and in human beings with respiratory failure [8] demonstrated that the expiratory flushing of proximal dead space decreased minute ventilation with no change in $PaCO_2$. Recent work has shown that conventional mechanical ventilation aided by TGI may represent a novel ventilatory strategy that succeeds in limiting both the distending forces acting on the lung and the level of $PaCO_2$ elevation that invariably occurs during permissive hypercapnia [9–12].

5.2 Physiologic Effects of TGI

The lung has several compartments with different implications on gas exchange. The physiologic dead space is comprised of conducting airways (instrumental and anatomic dead space) and alveoli that are well ventilated but receive minimal blood flow. In the second, or intrapulmonary shunt compartment, little or no gas exchange takes place because alveoli are perfused but not ventilated. Gas exchange takes place in the third compartment, which contains alveoli that are both ventilated and perfused. Because the anatomic dead space remains relatively constant as tidal volume is reduced, low tidal volumes are associated with a high ratio of dead space to tidal volume [13]. Tracheal gas insufflation, applied together with conventional mechanical ventilation, effectively reduces the size of the dead space compartment and improves overall CO_2 elimination by replacing the anatomic dead space, normally laden with CO_2 during expiration, with fresh gas. As a consequence, less CO_2 is recycled to the alveoli during the next inspiration and the ventilatory efficiency of each tidal respiration is improved. Therefore, TGI reduces anatomic dead space and increases alveolar ventilation for a given frequency and tidal volume combination [6, 13–17].

The main effect of TGI is to flush the dead space from the carina to the Y of the ventilator circuit. However, TGI also has a distal effect that contributes to removing CO_2. The distal effect region consists of a jet area extending from the catheter tip and a turbulent region extending beyond the jet towards the alveoli. The extent of the jet and turbulence regions is related to flow velocity at the catheter tip, and velocity is directly related to flow rate and inversely related to the internal diameter of the TGI catheter [14]. Although the distal effect enhances CO_2 removal, the presence of the catheter and the jet effect oppose expiratory flow, favoring autoPEEP [5, 14, 18].

5.3 Working and Technical Aspects

5.3.1 Flow Delivery

Tracheal gas can be delivered throughout the respiratory cycle, during the expiration or only during a specific portion of the expiratory period. Continuous-flow TGI is the easiest method to implement but has the potential to cause complications. Continuous-flow TGI could increase delivered tidal volume, airway and alveolar pressure and total PEEP with both pressure-control (PCV) and volume-control ventilation (VCV). Moreover, in PCV when the ventilator flow reaches zero, the continuous flow from the continuous TGI increases VT and airway pressures. A similar phenomenon occurs during end-inspiratory pauses in VCV. These increases happen because the exhalation valve of the ventilator is not active during the inspiratory phase [19]. Overpressurization can be identified by examining the airway pressure tracing [13] and can be remedied by placing a pressure relief valve in the ventilator circuit to dissipate insufflated flow that produces excess pressure [20]. Phasic expiratory TGI has also been extensively studied [21]. Expiratory TGI appears to be as effective as continuous TGI and avoids some of the potential problems that continuous TGI can cause. Imanaka et al. [19] have shown in a lung model that the marked increases in system pressures and volumes caused by continuous TGI could be avoided with expiratory-phase TGI and volume-adjusted TGI.

5.3.2 Catheter Design and Placement

Currently, there is no standard method of introducing an insufflation catheter into the trachea. In most human studies, a small-caliber catheter has been introduced through an angled side-arm adapter attached to the endotracheal tube and positioned above the carina [6, 13, 14, 22] or incorporated into the wall of the endotracheal tube [12, 23–25]. The presence of a catheter inside the endotracheal tube may increase both inspiratory and expiratory resistance, particularly when small endotracheal or tracheostomy tubes are used.

Boussignac et al. [26] designed a TGI endotracheal tube that allows gas to be injected through capillaries imbedded in the tube thus eliminating the inside catheter. The Boussignac tube allowed successful bypass and washout of the endotracheal dead space and ensured adequate gas exchange with lower insufflation pressures [27]. The fact that clinicians do not know what patients would be suitable for TGI application, and the potential risks associated with endotracheal tube replacement [28] constitute limitations against the routine use of the Boussignac tube. Kolobow et al. [29] have developed a reverse-thrust catheter that directs gas flow from the distal to the proximal part of the endotracheal tube, creating a Venturi effect. The inverted flow is less effective in accomplishing expiratory flushing compared with straight flow but it has the advantage of avoiding hyperinflation. Finally, endotracheal tubes used for one-lung anesthesia have been used successfully to provide selective TGI in experimental models of acute lung injury [30].

Recommended catheter position appears to be at 1–3 cm from the carina [9]. Placement can be done blindly and by estimating the position from a chest X-ray or under bronchoscopic guidance. Moving the catheter further down enhances gas mixing but can cause hyperinflation or damage to the mucosa of the tracheobronchial tree. Finally, heating and humidification of the insufflated gas is advisable.

5.4 Efficiency of CO_2 Removal

Experimental studies in healthy animals have shown that TGI allowed reduction of $PaCO_2$ during hypoventilation [7, 22, 31, 32]. This effect occurred similarly when the origin of hypoventilation was caused either by a decrease in minute ventilation or by an increase in respiratory rate at constant minute ventilation. Application of TGI allowed a decrease in tidal volume and a 25% reduction in airway pressures. In an experimental model of ARDS, Nahum et al. [33] found that increasing CO_2 elimination with 10 l/min of TGI allowed reduction of $PaCO_2$ from 55 mmHg to 45 mmHg whereas tidal volume was kept constant. However, the efficacy of TGI on $PaCO_2$ diminishes when an increased alveolar component dominates the total physiologic dead space. Nahum et al. [34] demonstrated that allowing $PaCO_2$ to rise to supranormal levels (a permissive hypercapnia strategy) counteracted the detrimental effect of increased alveolar dead space on the CO_2 removal efficacy of TGI.

Carbon dioxide elimination efficiency is also determined by the position of the tracheal catheter, flush volume and timing of the tracheal gas flow (continuous or expiratory). Nahum et al. [31] found that CO_2 elimination efficiency was greater when the distal tip of the TGI catheter was positioned 1 cm above the carina than when the catheter was placed more proximally.

The volume of gas injected per breath during expiration is the determinant of TGI efficiency. In a series of experiments, Ravenscraft et al. [9] found that, with or without lung deflation, the volume of gas flushed during the expiratory period determines the effectiveness of TGI, provided that inspired minute ventilation remains unchanged and end-expiration is included in the catheter flush period. Increasing catheter flow in clinical situations where only a brief expiratory time is available may maintain TGI efficiency. In fact, Nakos et al. [35] observed an inverse correlation between respiratory rate and $PaCO_2$, which indicates that longer expiratory times (or lower breathing frequencies) favor TGI efficiency (defined as reductions in $PaCO_2$ and VD/VT). Moreover, for the same catheter injection flow rate and duration, the efficiency of TGI is much higher when catheter flushing is performed late in expiration [13]. This investigation demonstrated that TGI efficiency is improved by including the end-expiratory segment of the cycle. If TGI is applied only early during expiration, the injected fresh gas is swept out with the discharging alveolar gas. TGI during late expiration flushes CO_2 from the anatomic dead space that would normally remain to be rebreathed on the next inspiration.

5.5 TGI in Patients with End-Stage Pulmonary Disease

Continuous insufflation of fresh gas (oxygen/air) through an intratracheal catheter has been used in patients with end-stage pulmonary disease to provide continuous oxygen therapy and to decrease oxygen flow requirements [36–39]. In patients with end-stage lung disease, TGI provides a method for oxygen delivery and confers the additional benefits of decreasing dyspnea and increasing exercise tolerance [40]. The physiologic basis for these changes appears to relate to alterations in breathing pattern and gas exchange efficiency.

Bergofsky and Hurewitz [36] studied the physiologic effects of airway insufflation in tracheostomized spontaneously breathing patients with chronic CO_2 retention. A continuous flow of 4–5 l/min delivered to the tracheostomy tube produced a reduction in dead space, tidal volume, and minute ventilation without affecting $PaCO_2$ in the acute state, and maintained or reduced $PaCO_2$, presumably due to reductions in dead space, in the chronic state. These authors also found a reduction in the oxygen consumption and CO_2 production associated with airway insufflation in patients with the most severe form of chronic obstructive pulmonary disease (Fig. 5.1). The decrease in metabolic rate without a change in $PaCO_2$ suggested a reduction in the work of breathing during TGI in spontaneously breathing patients. Interestingly, Hurewitz et al. [37] found that the application of airway insufflation for patients with advanced obstructive and restrictive lung disease produced either a reduction in minute ventilation with minimal changes of alveolar ventilation, or no variations in minute ventilation associated with an increase in alveolar ventilation. These different responses to dead space reduction suggest that the breathing pattern is CO_2-driven in a subgroup of chronic patients, while other patients exhibit a breathing pattern modulated by factors such as lung parenchymal receptors, diaphragmatic tension, and/or hyperinflation [40–42].

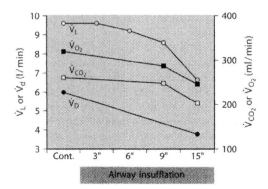

Fig. 5.1. Effect of airway insufflation in a patient with severe chronic obstructive lung disease. The decrease in minute ventilation (V_L) induced by airway insufflation was accompanied by a parallel decrease in oxygen consumption (VO_2) and carbon dioxide production (VCO_2). (From [36] with permission)

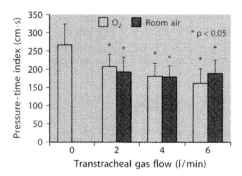

Fig. 5.2. Transtracheal delivery of oxygen or air reduced the pressure-time index of the diaphragm in five patients with end-stage pulmonary disease. (From [38] with permission)

In addition to the effects on gas exchange, minute ventilation, and dead space, TGI resulted in a decrease in the oxygen cost of breathing in spontaneously breathing patients. Benditt et al. [38] found that transtracheally administered gas reduced the oxygen cost of breathing, estimated by the pleural pressure time index, and changed the respiratory pattern of the diaphragm (diaphragm tension time index) to a less demanding pattern (Fig. 5.2). These findings helped to explain the improvements in exercise tolerance and decreased dyspnea and supported the use of transtracheal gas therapy for indications other than oxygenation.

5.6 TGI in Patients with ARDS

A number of studies have been published on the effect of TGI in patients receiving mechanical ventilation. The majority of the studies have been performed in patients with ARDS and focused on demonstrating a reduction in tidal volume and subsequently on airway pressure while $PaCO_2$ was maintained constant, or a reduction in the $PaCO_2$ during permissive hypercapnia [9–12, 43]. Despite the fact that TGI in human beings receiving mechanical ventilation was first tested in 1969 [8], level I studies are still lacking.

In patients with ARDS, part of the dead space resides in the alveoli as alveolar dead space. The alveolar gas originating from those ventilated but hypoperfused lung regions is CO_2-poor, diminishing the impact of washing proximal dead space free of CO_2 on alveolar ventilation. A permissive hypercapnia strategy increases the amount of CO_2 that can be removed from the proximal anatomic dead space and counterbalances the decreased CO_2 removal efficacy of TGI caused by increased alveolar dead space [6]. Several studies [10, 12, 44] have shown that one of the most important features of TGI is to maintain normocapnia or a given level of $PaCO_2$ while tidal volume is decreased, allowing a reduction in minute ventilation. TGI can thereby be used to decrease the forces acting on the lung, thus minimizing ventilator-induced lung injury in ARDS patients.

During permissive hypercapnia in ARDS patients, Kalfon et al. [43] found that expiratory washout of 15 l/min was extremely useful to reduce $PaCO_2$ by 30% and to increase PaO_2 significantly from 205 mmHg to 296 mmHg. The reduction of $PaCO_2$ was accompanied by an increase in plateau pressure from 26 cmH_2O to 32 cmH_2O. A significant increase in airway pressure and in lung volumes is a well-known side effect of TGI and correlates with the flow used [31, 45]. When insufflation of gas is limited to the expiratory phase, tidal volume remains virtually unchanged during volume control ventilation, but airway pressures can still increase through expiratory flow limitation and autoPEEP. Increase in lung volume caused by TGI application is a serious limitation of the technique and should be avoided. Solutions to minimize expiratory TGI-induced autoPEEP include using lower TGI flows, delivering TGI during PCV, and optimizing mechanical ventilation during TGI application. During PCV, a TGI-induced increase in airway pressure automatically results in a decrease in the tidal volume, and the lack of expiratory TGI-induced autoPEEP is associated with a reduction in the efficiency of CO_2 elimination [46]. Likewise, if TGI flow is reduced, the ability to clear CO_2 will also be diminished.

Optimization of mechanical ventilation appears to be a suitable method of delivering a pressure-limited ventilatory strategy combined with TGI while avoiding autoPEEP and the deleterious effects of hypercapnia in patients with severe ARDS. Richecoeur et al. [12] demonstrated that the combination of increasing respiratory rate to the limit of autoPEEP, removing the tubing connecting the Y-piece to the endotracheal tube, and an expiratory washout of 15 l/min produced a significant reduction in $PaCO_2$ from 84 mmHg during conventional ventilation to 45 mmHg. The combination of expiratory washout and optimization of mechanical ventilation invariably originated autoPEEP but the concomitant decrease in external PEEP allowed a constant total PEEP and plateau pressures during the different treatments (Fig. 5.3). In the study of Richecoeur et al. [12] oxygenation did not improve, suggesting that expiratory TGI per se has no direct effect on alveolar recruitment when autoPEEP does not induce an increase in mean airway pressure.

The effect of different gas mixtures (helium and oxygen) during TGI application has been studied in patients with respiratory failure [47]. Helium is an inert gas that has a much lower density than oxygen or air. When given at the same flow rate as a nitrogen/oxygen mixture, a helium/oxygen mixture produces a much lower Reynolds number and laminar flow [48]. In the study by Pizov et al. [47], TGI with helium was more effective than TGI with oxygen in treating hypercar-

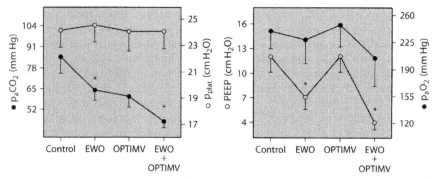

Fig. 5.3. Changes in PaCO$_2$, inspiratory plateau airway pressure (P_{plat}), PEEP, and PaO$_2$ induced by optimized mechanical ventilation (*OPTIMV*), expiratory washout (*EWO*), and the combination of OPTIMV and EWO in six patients with severe ARDS. Extrinsic PEEP had to be reduced by 5.3±2.1 cmH$_2$O during EWO and by 7.3±1.3 cmH$_2$O during the combination of OPTIMV and EWO, whereas it remained unchanged during OPTIMV alone. Plateau pressure did not significantly change, suggesting that lung hyperinflation was not produced. In patients with severe ARDS, the combination of OPTIMV and EWO had additive effects and resulted in PaCO$_2$ levels close to normal values. (From [12] with permission)

bia, since the use of helium leads to a lesser increase in airway pressure accompanying the decrease in PaCO$_2$. Since the combination helium/oxygen for TGI application has the potential to decrease PaO$_2$, precautions should be taken with the use of helium, particularly in patients who require high FiO$_2$ values to provide adequate oxygenation.

5.7 Weaning

Liberation from mechanical ventilation is an easy process for most patients. In recent clinical trials, between 60% and 80% of patients were extubated directly from full ventilatory support [49–51]. However, in patients with prolonged ventilatory support, weaning can be difficult. Failure of the respiratory muscle pump is probably the most common cause of failure to wean from mechanical ventilation. Indeed, COPD patients who subsequently fail a trial of weaning exhibit not only an almost immediate rapid and shallow breathing when ventilatory support is discontinued but also a progressive worsening of pulmonary mechanics with inefficient CO$_2$ clearance, in comparison to those COPD patients who are successfully extubated after the spontaneous breathing trial. Deterioration in respiratory system mechanics in patients who fail the weaning trial is characterized by an increase in intrinsic PEEP, and by inspiratory resistance and a decrease in dynamic lung compliance [52]. Thus, inefficient CO$_2$ clearance in the failing group appeared to be a consequence of worsening pulmonary mechanics with increased energy expenditure and rapid shallow breathing, since the decrease in tidal volume inevitably caused an increase in dead space ventilation. In this context, TGI could have a role as an adjunct to wean patients from the ventilator.

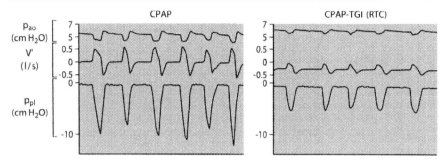

Fig. 5.4. Representative recordings of airway opening pressure (P_{ao}), flow (V'), and pleural pressure (P_{pl}) during CPAP alone and during CPAP with tracheal gas insufflation (*TGI*) at 10 l/min of insufflation flow through a reverse-thrust catheter. CPAP plus TGI reduced respiratory rate, minute ventilation, and the effort of breathing. (From [53] with permission)

Cereda et al. [53] studied the effect of TGI combined with continuous-flow positive airway pressure (CPAP) on the effort of breathing in spontaneously breathing sheep with acute lung injury. They found that the beneficial physiologic effects of TGI on minute ventilation and gas exchange were followed by a decrease in the inspiratory work of breathing (Fig. 5.4). Remarkably, no additional benefit was observed from raising insufflation flow from 10 l/min to 15 l/min. These authors attributed the beneficial effect of TGI with CPAP on effort of breathing to a favorable balance between decreased ventilatory requirement and low work load superimposed by the apparatus and TGI. In fact, when CPAP is delivered with a mechanical ventilator combined with TGI, additional inspiratory effort is required to overcome the insufflation flow and trigger the ventilator valves. In a bench study, Hoyt et al. [54] nicely showed that TGI might interfere with ventilator triggering at low peak inspiratory flow rates. These findings suggested that weak patients may fail to open the demand valve of the CPAP system during TGI at high catheter flow rates (Fig. 5.5).

Based on the hypothesis that TGI has the potential for decreasing anatomic dead space, enhancing gas mixing, and possibly reducing the work of breathing, several authors have tested the effects of TGI on lung function in patients undergoing weaning from mechanical ventilation. A study by Nakos et al. [35] showed that tidal volume, minute ventilation, $PaCO_2$, and physiologic dead space were reduced in a flow-dependent manner when gas was delivered through an oral-tracheal tube. Moreover, they found that a distal position of the TGI catheter was more effective than the proximal one and the results were less effective in patients with tracheostomy. Interestingly, the improvement in ventilatory efficiency resulting from the functional reduction of dead space allowed for a decrease in $PaCO_2$ at the same respiratory rate and at lower tidal volume. These data suggest that the inspiratory work of breathing was also reduced, since tidal volume was significantly reduced. In preliminary work [55], we studied the effects of expiratory TGI during CPAP on six ready-to-wean patients. Expiratory TGI of 8 l/min produced a decrease in the pressure time product of the diaphragm in five of six patients, a reduction in tidal volume, and no changes in respiratory rate and $PaCO_2$. Data from these studies [24, 47] suggest that expiratory TGI might help patients with difficulties during weaning.

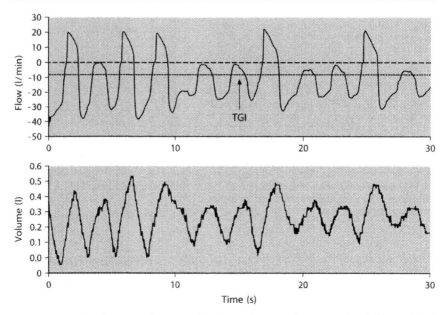

Fig. 5.5. Flow and inductive plethysmographic lung volume tracing in a mechanically ventilated patient (PSV of 4 cmH$_2$O) during pan-expiratory TGI of 8 l/min. In six of 11 breaths, TGI flow meets the patient's inspiratory flow demand and provides the total inspiratory volume for the breath, and the ventilator is not triggered. (From [54] with permission)

5.8 Monitoring During TGI

TGI is a simple and apparently safe method of reducing both minute ventilation and PaCO$_2$. Regardless of the approach used, TGI has the potential to alter volumes and airway and alveolar pressure and requires careful monitoring of delivered volumes and pressures to ensure safe clinical application and to evaluate the effect on lung function. Moreover, the position of the TGI catheter inside the endotracheal tube should be carefully controlled. The presence of a catheter inside the endotracheal tube may increase both inspiratory and expiratory resistances, particularly when small endotracheal or tracheostomy tubes are used [6, 13, 14, 22]. Lucangelo et al. [56] studied the airflow resistance of a 2.7-mm external diameter catheter placed inside endotracheal tubes of various sizes, and found resistance markedly increased at the different tube sizes and flows tested.

During continuous TGI, total tidal volume is the sum of ventilator-derived volume plus the additional volume delivered by TGI. The difference between the preprogrammed ventilator tidal volume and the ventilator-delivered volume plus the contribution of volume from the TGI catheter can adversely affect the ability of the ventilator to monitor pressures and volumes, calibrations, and leak detections and may cause the ventilator to sound the alarm continuously. The measurement of autoPEEP by the end-expiratory occlusion technique may bring about a dramatic elevation of lung volume if TGI flow is not simultane-

Fig. 5.6. Representative exhalation capnograms in two patients without TGI and with TGI at 6 l/min insufflation flow. A greater reduction in end-tidal CO_2 ($P_{ET}CO_2$) from the $P_{ET}CO_2$ base value corresponded with a larger reduction in $PaCO_2$. At a given insufflation flow, efficiency to clear CO_2 is a function of the time available to flush proximal dead space. (From [9] with permission)

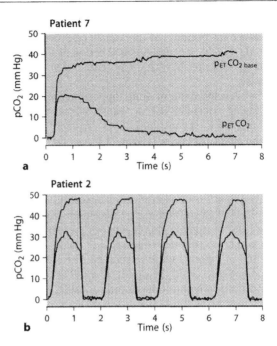

ously interrupted. The same effect will be seen with continuous TGI during end-inspiratory occlusions [6, 22].

The efficacy of TGI may be monitored by capnography. The observation of exhalation capnograms provides an indicator of the effect of TGI on the CO_2 concentration of the gas remaining in the proximal anatomic dead space compartment at the onset of inspiration (Fig. 5.6) [9, 11]. Although in patients with respiratory failure end-tidal ($P_{et}CO_2$) is a poor estimate of $PaCO_2$ [57, 58], changes in $P_{et}CO_2$ induced by TGI correlated significantly with changes in $PaCO_2$, justifying routine measurement of $P_{et}CO_2$ during TGI application as a marker of its effectiveness [9, 11, 34].

5.9 Potential Complications

Delivering catheter gas at higher flows must be examined with regard to the need for humidification and the potential for tracheal damage with long-term use. The presence of a catheter inside the endotracheal tube may complicate suction of respiratory secretions and sputum removal.

TGI has the potential to increase end-expiratory lung volume in a flow-dependent fashion or depending on catheter design [15, 31, 32, 43]. Catheter flow can increase alveolar pressure in three ways [6]. First, part of the momentum of the discharging jet stream is transferred to the alveoli. Second, placement of the catheter decreases the cross-sectional area of the trachea available for expiratory flow, effectively increasing expiratory resistance. Third, catheter flow through the endotracheal tube, expiratory circuit, and expiratory valve during expiration builds a back pressure at the airway opening that impedes expiratory flow from the lung. Finally, a complete obstruction of the outflow can cause overinflation of the lungs in seconds, with the potential of pneumothorax or hemodynamic compromise.

The development of lung hyperinflation can be effectively controlled by decreasing external PEEP to counterbalance the increase in autoPEEP, so that the total PEEP is kept constant [12]. Overpressurization can be identified by examining the airway pressure tracing [13] and can be remedied by placing a pressure-relief valve in the ventilator circuit to dissipate insufflated flow that produces excess pressure [20]. Other authors have designed systems that allow increase of CO_2 clearance without the risks of hyperinflation. De Robertis et al. [23] studied the combination of aspiration of anatomic and instrumental dead space in the late phase of expiration and replacement with fresh gas through the inspiratory line of the ventilator. This aspiration system allowed reductions in airway pressure and tidal volume while keeping $PaCO_2$ constant in healthy human beings [24] and in patients with ARDS [25]. The aforementioned aspiration system has the potential to avoid the problems associated with jet streams of gas or with gas humidification without developing autoPEEP.

5.10 Conclusion

Tracheal gas insufflation is a promising technique to complement mechanical ventilation. TGI is very effective during permissive hypercapnia in patients with ARDS, diminishing the complications associated with both mechanical ventilation and respiratory acidosis. Furthermore, some studies suggest that weaning aided by TGI may allow a reduction in a patient's respiratory demands. However, routine use of TGI in intensive care still warrants further investigation to improve technical problems and to demonstrate clinical benefit with randomized trials in patients receiving mechanical ventilation or those with weaning difficulties.

5.11 References

1. Dreyfuss D, Saumon G 1998) Ventilator induced lung injury. Lessons from experimental studies. Am J Respir Crit Care Med 157:294–323
2. International Consensus Conferences in Intensive Care Medicine (1999) Ventilator-associated lung injury in ARDS. Am J Respir Crit Care Med 160:2118–2124
3. Amato MBP, Barbas CS, Medeiros DM, Magaldi RB, Schettino GP, Lorenzi-Filho G, Kairalla RA, Deheinzelin D, Muñoz C, Oliveira R, Takagaki TY, Carvalho CR (1998) Effect of a protective-ventilation strategy on mortality in the acute respiratory distress syndrome. N Engl J Med 338:347–354
4. Acute Respiratory Distress Syndrome Network (2000) Ventilation with lower tidal volume as compared with traditional tidal volumes for acute lung injury and the acute respiratory distress syndrome. N Engl J Med 342:1301–1308
5. Ranieri VM, Suter P, Tortorella C, De Tulio R, Dayer JM, Brienza A, Bruno F, Slutsky AS (1999) Effect of mechanical ventilation on inflammatory mediators in patients with acute respiratory distress syndrome: a randomized controlled trial. JAMA 282:54–61

6. Nahum A, Marini JJ, Slutsky AS (1998) Tracheal gas insufflation. In: Marini JJ, Slutsky AS (eds) Physiological basis of ventilatory support. Dekker, New York, pp 1021–1045

7. Stresemann E, Sattler FP (1969) Effect of washout of anatomic dead space on ventilation, pH and blood gas composition in anesthetized dogs. Respiration 26:116–121

8. Stresemann E, Votteri BA, Sattler FP (1969) Washout of anatomical dead space for alveolar hypoventilation. Respiration 26:425–434

9. Ravenscraft SA, Burke WC, Nahum A, Adams AB, Nakos G, Marcy TW, Marini JJ (1993) Tracheal gas insufflation augments CO_2 clearance during mechanical ventilation. Am Rev Respir Dis 148:345–351

10. Nakos G, Zakinthinos S, Kotanidou A, Tsagaris H, Roussos C (1994) Tracheal gas insufflation reduces the tidal volume while $PaCO_2$ is maintained constant. Intensive Care Med 20:407–413

11. Saura P, Lucangelo, Blanch L, Artigas A, Mas A, Fernandez R (1996) Factores determinantes de la reducción de la $PaCO_2$ con la insuflación de gas traqueal en pacientes con lesión pulmonar aguda. Med Intensiva 20:246–251

12. Richecoeur J, Lu Q, Vieira SRR, Puybasset L, Kalfon P, Coriat P, Rouby JJ (1999) Expiratory washout versus optimization of mechanical ventilation during permissive hypercapnia in patients with severe acute respiratory distress syndrome. Am J Respir Crit Care Med 160:77–85

13. Ravenscraft SA (1996) Tracheal gas insufflation: adjunct to conventional mechanical ventilation. Respir Care 41:105–111

14. Adams AB (1996) Tracheal gas insufflation. Respir Care 41:285–292

15. Kirmse M, Fujino Y, Hromi J, Mang H, Hess D, Kacmarek RM (1999) Pressure-release tracheal gas insufflation reduces airway pressures in lung injured sheep maintaining eucapnia. Am J Respir Crit Care Med 160:1462–1467

16. Nahum A, Ravenscraft SA, Adams AB, Marini JJ (1995) Inspiratory tidal volume sparing effects of tracheal gas insufflation in dogs with oleic acid-induced lung injury. J Crit Care 10:115–121

17. Imanaka HM, Kirmse M, Mang D, Hess D, Kacmarek RM (1999) Expiratory phase tracheal gas insufflation and pressure control ventilation in lung lavage sheep with permissive hypercapnia: effects of TGI flow direction and inspiratory time. Am J Respir Crit Care Med 159:49–54

18. Slutsky A, Menon A (1987) Catheter position and blood gases during constant-flow ventilation. J Appl Physiol 62:513–519

19. Imanaka H, Kacmarek RM, Riggi V, Ritz R, Hess D (1998) Expiratory phase and volume adjusted tracheal gas insufflation: a lung model study. Crit Care Med 26:939–946

20. Gowski DT, Delgado E, Miro AM, Tasota FJ, Hoffman LA, Pinsky MR (1997) Tracheal gas insufflation during pressure control ventilation: effect of using a pressure relief valve. Crit Care Med 25:145–152

21. Blanch L (2001) Clinical studies of tracheal gas insufflation. Respir Care 46:158–166

22. Dorne R, Liron L, Pommier C (2000) Insufflation tracheale de gaz associee a la ventilation mecanique pour l'epuration du CO_2. Ann Fr Anesth Reanim 19:115–127

23. De Robertis E, Sigurdur E, Sigurdsson E, Drefeldt B, Jonson B (1999) Aspiration of airway dead space. A new method to enhance CO_2 elimination. Am J Respir Crit Care Med 159:728–732

24. De Robertis E, Servillo G, Jonson B, Tufano R (1999) Aspiration of dead space allows normocapnic ventilation at low tidal volumes in man. Intensive Care Med 25:674–679

25. De Robertis E, Servillo G, Tufano R, Jonson B (2000) Aspiration of dead space allows normocapnia at small tidal volumes and adequate PEEP in ARDS. Am J Respir Crit Care Med 161:A387

26. Boussignac G, Bertrand C, Huguenard P (1988) Etude preliminaire d'une nouvelle sonde d'intubation endotracheale. Conv Med 7:111–113

27. Pinquier D, Pavlovic Boussignac G, Aubier M, Beaufils F (1996) Benefits of the low pressure multichannel endotracheal ventilation. Am J Respir Crit Care Med 154:82–90

28. Valles J (1999) Prevention of nosocomial pneumonia in patients with acute respiratory distress syndrome. In: Mancebo J, Blanch L (eds) Syndrome de detresse respiratoire aigue en reanimation. Elsevier, Amsterdam, pp 252–264

29. Kolobov T, Powers T, Mandava S, Aprigliano M, Kawaguchi A, Tsuno K, Mueller E (1994) Intratracheal pulmonary ventilation (ITPV): control of positive end-expiratory pressure at the level of the carina through the use of a novel ITPV catheter design. Anesth Analg 78:455–461

30. Blanch L, Van der Kloot TE, Youngblood M, Murias G, Naveira A, Adams A, Shapiro R, Nahum A (1999) Selective tracheal gas insufflation (TGI) improves lung function in unilateral lung injury. Am J Respir Crit Care Med 159:A366

31. Nahum A, Ravenscraft SA, Nakos G, Burke WC, Adams AB, Marcy TW, Marini JJ (1992) Tracheal gas insufflation during pressure-control ventilation. Effect of catheter position, diameter, and flow rate. Am Rev Respir Dis 146:1411–1418

32. Burke WC, Nahum A, Ravenscraft SA, Nakos G, Adams AB, Marcy TW, Marini JJ (1993) Modes of tracheal gas insufflation. Comparison of continuous and phase-specific gas injection in normals dogs. Am Rev Respir Dis 148:562–568

33. Nahum A, Chandra A, Niknam J, Ravenscraft SA, Adams AB, Marini JJ (1995) Effect of tracheal gas insufflation on gas exchange in canine oleic acid-induced lung injury. Crit Care Med 23:348–356

34. Nahum A, Shapiro RS, Ravenscraft, SA, Adams AB, Marini JJ (1995) Efficacy of expiratory tracheal gas insufflation in a canine model of lung injury. Am J Respir Crit Care Med 152:489–495

35. Nakos G, Lachana A, Prekates A, Pneumatikos J, Guillaume M, Pappas K, Tsagiris H (1995) Respiratory effects of tracheal gas insufflation in spontaneously breathing COPD patients. Intensive Care Med 21:904–912

36. Bergofsky EH, Hurewitz AN (1989) Airway insufflation: physiologic effects on acute and chronic gas exchange in humans. Am Rev Respir Dis 140:885–890

37. Hurewitz AN, Bergofsky EH, Vomero E (1991) Airway insufflation. Increasing flow rates progressively reduce dead space in respiratory failure. Am Rev Respir Dis 144:1229–1232

38. Benditt J, Pollock M, Roa J, Celli B (1993) Transtracheal delivery of gas decreases the oxygen cost of breathing. Am Rev Respir Dis 147:1207–1210

39. Hoffman LA, Johnson JT, Wesmiller SW, et al (1991) Transtracheal delivery of oxygen: efficacy and safety for long-term continuous theraphy. Ann Otol Rhinol Laryngol 100:108–115

40. Wesmiller SW, Hoffman LA, Sciurba FC, et al (1990) Exercise tolerance during nasal cannula and transtracheal oxygen delivery. Am Rev Respir Dis 141:789–791

41. Tobert DG, Simon PM, Stroetz RW, Hubmayr R (1997) The determinants of respiratory rate during mechanical ventilation. Am J Respir Crit Care Med 155:485–492

42. Georgopoulos D, Mitrouska I, Webster K, Bshouty Z, Younes M (1997) Effects of inspiratory muscle unloading on the response of respiratory motor output to CO_2. Am J Respir Crit Care Med 155:2000–2009

43. Kalfon P, Umamaheswara GS, Gallart L, Puybasset L, Coriat P, Rouby JJ (1997) Permissive hypercapnia with and without expiratory washout in patients with severe acute respiratory distress syndrome. Anesthesiology 87:6–17

44. Kuo PH, Wu HD, Yu CJ, Yang SC, Lai YL, Yang PC (1996) Efficacy of tracheal gas insufflation in acute respiratory distress syndrome with permissive hypercapnia. Am J Respir Crit Care Med 154:612–616

45. Nahum A, Ravenscraft SA, Nakos G, Adams AB, Burke WC, Marini JJ (1993) Effect of catheter flow direction on CO_2 removal during tracheal gas insufflation in dogs. J Appl Physiol 75:1238–1246

46. Findlay GP, Dingley J, Smithies MN, Kalfon P, Rouby JJ (1998) Expiratory washout in patients with severe acute respiratory distress syndrome. Anesthesiology 88:835–836

47. Pizov R, Oppenheim A, Eidelman LA, Weiss YG, Sprung CL, Cotev S (1998) Helium versus oxygen for tracheal gas insufflation during mechanical ventilation. Crit Care Med 26:290–295

48. Jaber S, Fodil R, Carlucci A, Boussarsar M, Pigeot J, Lemaire F, Harf A, Lofaso F, Isabey D, Brochard L (2000) Noninvasive ventilation with helium-oxygen in acute exacerbations of chronic obstructive pulmonary disease. Am J Respir Crit Care Med 161:1191–1200

49. Brochard L, Rauss A, Benito S, Conti G, Mancebo J, Rekik N, et al (1994) Comparison of three methods of gradual withdrawal from ventilatory support during weaning from mechanical ventilation. Am J Respir Crit Care Med 150:896–903
50. Esteban A, Frutos F, Tobin MJ, Alia I, Solsona JF, Vallverdu I, Fernandez R, et al (1995) A comparison of four methods of weaning patients from mechanical ventilation. N Engl J Med 332: 345–350
51. Ely EW, Baker AM, Dunagan DP, Burke HL, Smith AC, Kelly PT, Johnson MM, Browder RW, Bowton DL, Haponik EF (1996) Effect on the duration of mechanical ventilation of identifying patients capable of breathing spontaneously. N Engl J Med 335: 1864–1869
52. Jubran A, Tobin MJ (1998) Discontinuation of ventilatory support. In: Marini JJ, Slutsky AS (eds) Physiological basis of ventilatory support. Dekker, New York, pp 1283–1313
53. Cereda MF, Sparacino M, Frank A, Trawoger R, Kolobov T (1999) Efficacy of tracheal gas insufflation in spontaneously breathing sheep with lung injury. Am J Respir Crit Care Med 159:845–850
54. Hoyt JD, Marini JJ, Nahum A (1996) Effect of tracheal gas insufflation on demand valve triggering and total work during continuous positive airway pressure ventilation. Chest 110:775–783
55. Murias G, Fernandez R, Romero PV, Nahum A, Blanch L (2000) Expiratory tracheal gas insufflation reduces minute ventilation during continuous positive airway pressure. Am J Respir Crit Care Med 161:A387
56. Lucangelo U, Blanch L, Artigas A, Fernandez R (1995) Resistencia al flujo aereo sobreañadida por los diferentes materiales del circuito ventilatorio de pacientes en ventilacion mecanica. Med Intensiva 19:125–129
57. Blanch L, Fernandez R, Saura P, Baigorri F, Artigas A (1994) Relationship between expired capnogram and respiratory system resistance in critically ill patients during total ventilatory support. Chest 105:219–223
58. Hess D (1990) Capnometry and capnography: technical aspects, physiologic aspects, and clinical applications. Respir Care 35: 557–576

6 What a Clinician Should Do When a Patient "Fights the Ventilator"

C.G. Alex, P.J. Fahey, and M.J. Tobin

6.1 Introduction

"Fighting the ventilator" is a phrase used to describe a ventilator-supported patient who displays agitation and/or respiratory distress. Such "fighting" is common at the time of intubation and initiation of mechanical ventilation, and is due largely to the anxiety that is to be expected under these circumstances. However, the development of "fighting" in a previously calm patient suggests the likelihood of a new, and potentially serious complication (Table 6.1). Excessive agitation needs to be approached in a systematic manner since it can threaten the life of a ventilator-supported patient [1].

6.2 Recognition of the Problem

Since ventilator-supported patients are often cognitively impaired or semiconscious and their speech is usually prohibited by the presence of a tracheal tube [2], communicating the development of new symptoms is very difficult. Sudden respiratory embarrassment usually results in the development of dyspnea, which in turn may be manifested as anxiety or agitation in the ventilator-supported patient [3]. By asking directed questions or requesting a patient to provide a written description of his or her complaint, an attendant can derive a considerable amount of information. The major physical signs of respiratory distress include tachypnea, diaphoresis, nasal flaring, recruitment of the accessory muscles (scalenes and sternomastoids), recession of the suprasternal/supraclavicular/intercostal spaces, rib cage abdominal asynchrony and paradox, tracheal tug, abnormal auscultatory findings, tachycardia, arrhythmias, and hypotension [4]. In some patients, a generalized increase in muscle tone may be the only evidence of discomfort [1]. If mechanical ventilation is being delivered in an assisted mode, it is important to check for synchronization between movement of the patient's chest wall and delivery of gas from the ventilator.

In addition to symptoms and signs of respiratory distress, the physician may utilize several cardiorespiratory variables that are usually monitored [4]. Alterations in the pattern of breathing can be very helpful. A sudden increase in respiratory rate is an extremely sensitive sign of respiratory embarrassment [5], but further assessment is necessary to determine the precise cause of the dis-

Table 6.1. Causes of sudden respiratory distress in a patient receiving mechanical ventilation

Patient-related causes	Ventilator-related causes
Artificial airway problems	System leak or circuit malfunction
Secretions	Inadequate F_iO_2
Pneumothorax	Inadequate ventilator support
Bronchospasm	
Pulmonary edema	
Pulmonary embolism	
Dynamic hyperinflation	
Abnormal respiratory drive	
Alteration in body posture	
Drug-induced problems	
Abdominal distension	
Agitation	
Patient-ventilator asynchrony	

turbance. Although a comment is often made about shallow respirations, it is important to note that clinical estimation of tidal volume is notoriously unreliable [6]. It is important to check for asynchronous or paradoxical motion of the rib cage and abdomen, since this indicates an increase in respiratory load [7, 8]. An arterial blood gas (ABG) sample should be obtained, but there can be a considerable time lag between drawing the sample and obtaining the result, and deterioration in ABGs may occur late in the evolution of acute respiratory failure. As a result, continuous monitoring of oxygenation with a pulse oximeter is desirable in a ventilator-supported patient. However, patients with a high baseline arterial oxygen tension (PaO_2) may develop considerable deterioration in gas exchange without much change in oxygen saturation because their levels are located on the flat portion of the O_2 dissociation curve [4]. Capnography or end-tidal carbon dioxide (CO_2) monitoring is helpful in detecting esophageal intubation (absent end-tidal CO_2 tracing) or sudden pulmonary embolism or air embolism (sudden decrease in end-tidal CO_2 level), but it does not reliably reflect arterial CO_2 tension ($PaCO_2$) in patients with underlying lung disease [9]. Monitoring changes in respiratory compliance can be very helpful in diagnosing the cause of sudden distress in a ventilator-supported patient. The contour of the airway pressure tracing (Fig. 6.1) provides important information regarding the appropriateness of the ventilator settings and patient comfort [10], and a check should be made to see if the patient has developed intrinsic positive end-expiratory pressure or auto-PEEP [11]. Electrocardiography, arterial pressure, and pulmonary artery pressure monitoring provide useful information regarding cardiovascular performance.

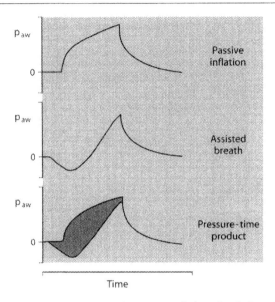

Fig. 6.1. Airway pressure (P_{aw}) tracings during controlled mechanical ventilation in a completely relaxed patient (*top*) and during an assisted breath (*middle*). The shaded area in the *bottom* tracing is the pressure-time product of the inspiratory muscles calculated as the difference in area subtended by the P_{aw}-time curve in the presence (*middle*) and absence (*top*) of inspiratory muscle activity. (From [74])

6.3 General Principles of Management

The cardinal principle of management is to ensure oxygenation and the delivery of adequate ventilation to the patient [3]. This takes precedence over everything else, although at the same time one should begin to try to determine the underlying cause. The general principles of management are listed in Table 6.2.

Once the patient has been disconnected from the ventilator, manual ventilation should be initiated with a self-inflating bag containing 100% oxygen. If the distress resolves, the problem is due to the ventilator. If the distress continues, the problem is patient based. A rapid physical examination should be performed and the physiologic indices being monitored should be assessed in an attempt to determine the cause of the respiratory distress. The patency of the patient's airway should be assessed, and passage of a suction catheter will help in determining the presence of a blocked airway or large quantities of secretions. If death appears imminent, one needs to consider and treat the most likely causes, such as airway obstruction or tension pneumothorax, before undertaking further diagnostic studies. Once the patient has been stabilized, a more detailed assessment can be undertaken and a more comprehensive management plan initiated.

Table 6.2. General principles of management of sudden respiratory distress in a ventilator-supported patient

1. Disconnect the patient from the ventilator.
2. Initiate manual ventilation using a self-inflating bag containing 100% oxygen.
3. Perform a rapid physical examination and assess monitored indices.
4. Check patency of the airway (pass a suction catheter).
5. If death is imminent, consider and treat the most likely causes, such as pneumothorax and airway obstruction.
6. Once the patient is stabilized, undertake a more detailed assessment and management plan.

6.4 Specific Causes of Sudden Respiratory Distress

Conditions that can cause sudden respiratory distress in a ventilator-supported patient are listed in Table 6.1. As mentioned above, the persistence or resolution of distress upon disconnecting the patient from the ventilator and the institution of manual ventilation with a self-inflating bag containing 100% O_2 is helpful in determining whether the underlying problem is patient or ventilator based.

6.4.1 Artificial Airway Problems

Problems with artificial airways are a particularly important source of trouble, and several factors may be responsible.

Migration of the Endotracheal Tube
Endobronchial intubation may occur in up to 20% of ventilated patients [12, 13]. A recent prospective study assessing the incidence and risk factors of endotracheal tube misplacement demonstrated that misplacement was best predicted by a longer duration of endotracheal intubation and the occurrence of cardiac arrest requiring cardiopulmonary resuscitation [13]. Endobronchial intubation is usually due to excessive neck movement and/or inadequate external fixation of the endotracheal tube [3, 14]. Neck flexion causes an endotracheal tube to move an average of 1.9 cm (range 0–3.1 cm) towards the carina [14]. Main-stem intubation occurs more often on the right side, probably because the right main-stem bronchus forms a less acute angle with the trachea than does the left main-stem bronchus. While breath sounds are typically reduced over the atelectatic lung, this is a very unreliable sign [12]. If endobronchial intubation is suspected, the endotracheal tube should be pulled back a few centimeters, the chest should be re-auscultated, and the position of the tube confirmed by X-ray.

Migration of an endotracheal tube above the vocal cords can result in sudden distress accompanied by a decrease in tidal volume, the ability to phonate, and the escape of air through the nose and mouth. This is usually due to excessive neck movement and/or inadequate tube fixation. Neck extension causes an endotracheal tube to move an average of 1.9 cm away from the carina [14].

6.4.2 Cuff Herniation

Occlusion of a tracheal tube may result from herniation of the cuff over the end of the tube. This most commonly occurs following changes in the posture of the head and neck or changes in position of the tube. It may result in an increase in airway pressure, an increased resistance during manual ventilation, a decrease in tidal volume, difficulty in passing a suction catheter, and the presence of an abnormal musical sound during inspiration [3]. Deflation of the cuff produces immediate relief.

6.4.3 Cuff Rupture

Manifestations of cuff rupture include abnormal upper airway sounds suggestive of leakage around the cuff, failure to withdraw the same volume of air that was used to inflate the cuff, a decrease in delivered tidal volume, an inability to maintain the set level of PEEP, and aspiration of saliva, vomitus or food. Management consists of replacing the defective tube.

6.4.4 Endotracheal Tube Obstruction

Kinking of an endotracheal tube is a relatively uncommon complication and is associated with the use of soft-rubber nasotracheal tubes and with changes in the position of the head and neck. The problem is prevented by avoiding tube traction and excess tube length and is usually corrected by slight manipulation of the head, neck, or tube. Biting of the endotracheal tube occasionally occurs and is managed by placing a bite block and, if necessary, by increasing sedation. Occlusion of an endotracheal tube may result from a variety of foreign bodies ranging from dried lubricant [15] to avulsion of the nasal turbinates during nasotracheal intubation [16].

6.4.5 Tracheomalacia

Dilatation of the tracheal lumen from softening of the tracheal cartilage may occur with prolonged intubation and regional ischemia from cuff pressures which exceed tracheal perfusion pressure. Signs are similar to those associated with cuff rupture. Dilatation of the tracheal air column on chest X-ray also may indicate tracheomalacia. Prevention is the best management, where proper monitoring of cuff pressure is important.

6.4.6 Innominate Artery Rupture

Erosion of the innominate artery has been reported to occur in 0.4%–4.5% of tracheostomies performed [17] and has an extremely high mortality [18]. The clinical presentation may be quite dramatic, with blood gushing from the tracheal tube, or it may be heralded by a "sentinel bleed." If this sign is recognized, the cuff should be overinflated in an attempt to achieve tamponade. An index finger should be inserted into the stoma in an attempt to compress the artery against the sternum [3, 17, 18]. If this is successful, a blood transfusion should be administered while the patient is being transported to the operating room for ligation of the vessel [18].

6.4.7 Tracheoesophageal Fistula

Tracheoesophageal fistula is a rare complication due primarily to ischemia of the tracheal wall secondary to pressure by a tube or an overinflated cuff [19]. Patients with this complication typically have had both a tracheal tube and a nasogastric tube in place for a prolonged time [20]. The inability to deliver a preset tidal volume despite a functional cuff is a characteristic finding in this setting.

6.5 Secretions

Airway secretions can cause problems by being too dry or too copious in amount. Since a tracheal tube bypasses the upper airway, which normally heats and humidifies inspired gas, secretions may become excessively dry and encrusted and result in significant blockage of the tracheal tube over a relatively short period of time [21]. Obstruction of a tracheal tube should be suspected if difficulty is experienced during passage of a suction catheter. Excessive secretions can lead to mucus plugging and atelectasis. To avoid this problem, careful bronchial toilet and frequent suctioning are necessary in patients with copious secretions. If atelectasis occurs and fails to resolve with conservative measures, bronchoscopy should be undertaken.

6.6 Pneumothorax

Sudden respiratory distress in a ventilator-supported patient should always arouse suspicion of a pneumothorax [22]. Although peak airway pressure is probably not a direct determinant of alveolar rupture, it is easy to measure and appears to be a useful indicator of the risk of a pneumothorax. In one study, no patient whose peak inspiratory pressure was less than 60 cmH$_2$O developed barotrauma, whereas it occurred in 43% of those with pressures greater than 70 cmH$_2$O [23]. In a recent study using multivariate analysis [24], pneumothorax was found to correlate with acute respiratory distress syndrome (ARDS) and not with elevated peak or plateau pressures. The authors concluded that previous reports of the association of barotrauma and airway pressures were most likely related to the occurrence of elevated pressures in ARDS. Clinical manifestations of pneumothorax include respiratory distress, hyperresonance, tracheal deviation to the contralateral side, decreased breath sounds, a decrease in thoracic compliance (both static and "dynamic") (Table 6.3), and cardiovascular collapse.

Table 6.3. Patterns of alteration in thoracic pressure-volume relationships

Parameter	Case 1		Case 2	
	1 h ago	Now	1 h ago	Now
Tidal volume (ml)	600	600	600	600
Plateau pressure (cmH^{2}O)	10	10	10	30
Peak pressure (cmH$_2$O)	20	40	20	40
Static compliance (ml/cmH$_2$O)	60	60	60	20
"Dynamic compliance" (ml/cmH$_2$O)	30	15	30	15

Interpretation: In case 1, because plateau pressure is unchanged, suspect an airway problem. In case 2, because plateau pressure is increased and there is no increase in the gradient between peak and plateau pressures, suspect a pneumothorax, main-stem intubation, or atelectasis.

If a pneumothorax is suspected and death is imminent, a 14-gauge needle attached to a liquid-filled syringe should be inserted into the second intercostal space. If the patient is stable, however, a chest X-ray should be performed first to verify the diagnosis before inserting a chest tube.

6.7 Bronchospasm

Bronchospasm is a common cause of sudden respiratory distress. It results in dyspnea, wheezes, and clinical evidence of increased work of breathing. Peak airway pressure will be increased, resulting in a decrease in the "dynamic characteristic", while static compliance shows little or no change (Table 6.3) [4]. Management consists of the administration of inhaled bronchodilator agents.

6.8 Pulmonary Edema

Pulmonary edema is an important cause of sudden distress, and the reader is referred elsewhere for reviews of this common condition [25, 26]. Cardiac and noncardiac causes need to be considered, and if the distinction is difficult to make, passage of a pulmonary artery catheter may be necessary.

6.9 Pulmonary Embolism

Typical manifestations of acute pulmonary embolism include dyspnea, tachypnea, chest pain, fever, hemoptysis, pleural rub, and features of deep-vein thrombosis [27]. The presence of normal thoracic compliance in a hypoxemic patient with sudden respiratory distress is an important diagnostic clue. However, clinical manifestations are neither sensitive nor specific, and pulmonary angiography is negative in more than 50% of suspected cases. Diagnostic tests include ventilation-perfusion scan, pulmonary angiography, and impedance plethysmography (to detect venous thrombosis). Therapy usually consists of heparin followed by warfarin.

6.10 Dynamic Hyperinflation

Ventilator-supported patients commonly display tachypnea and have increased respiratory resistance and/or abnormal pulmonary compliance, all of which predispose to the development of dynamic hyperinflation [28, 29]. This hyperinflation is associated with the presence of positive recoil pressure at the end of expiration (i.e., auto-PEEP) [30, 31].

Hyperinflation may cause significant patient discomfort, because it decreases the efficiency of force generated by the respiratory muscles and increases the work of breathing by forcing the patient to breathe at the upper and less compliant portion of the pressure-volume curve of the lung. Also, inwardly directed elastic recoil of the chest wall with hyperinflation poses an additional elastic load [32, 33]. To initiate inspiratory air flow, a patient must generate a negative pressure equal in magnitude to the opposing elastic recoil pressure (i.e., level of auto-PEEP). Likewise, a patient with substantial auto-PEEP attempting to trigger a mechanical ventilator will need to generate a negative pressure equal in magnitude to the level of auto-PEEP in addition to the set minimum circuit pressure drop before a ventilator-assisted breath is initiated [34]. This is one of the factors that may account for the not infrequent observation of a patient who is unable to trigger a ventilator despite obvious respiratory effort (Fig. 6.2) [35].

Measures to decrease the amount of auto-PEEP include bronchodilator therapy, decreasing the minute ventilation by controlling fever or pain, using a large-bore endotracheal tube, and minimizing the ratio of inspiratory time to expiratory time by increasing inspiratory flow rate or using nondistensible tubing in the ventilator circuit [36]. In the patient with auto-PEEP who has difficulty in triggering a ventilator, the addition of external PEEP can be helpful. This allows triggering of the ventilator when alveolar pressure falls below the level of external PEEP, rather than below zero [30, 31, 33, 37–39]. This may seem paradoxical since external PEEP, which is commonly used to induce hyperinflation in patients with microatelectasis, is being used to decrease the work of breathing induced by hyperinflation consequent to auto-PEEP. This paradox can be explained by employing the analogy of a waterfall [33]. The height of the waterfall represents the critical closing pressure of airways in patients with auto-PEEP and COPD (Fig. 6.3). Thus, elevating downstream pressure, such as with external PEEP, has no influence on either expiratory airflow or the pressure upstream (auto-PEEP) from the site of critical closure (upper panel, Fig. 6.3). This situation exists until downstream pressure is elevated to a value equal to the critical closing pressure (middle panel, Fig. 6.3). However, once downstream pressure is elevated above the critical closing pressure (height of the waterfall), the pressure upstream increases immediately and hyperinflation is worsened (lower panel, Fig. 6.3). Although external PEEP can help in decreasing respiratory work, it is important to keep in mind that it does not decrease the accompanying hyperinflation and its detrimental effect [32].

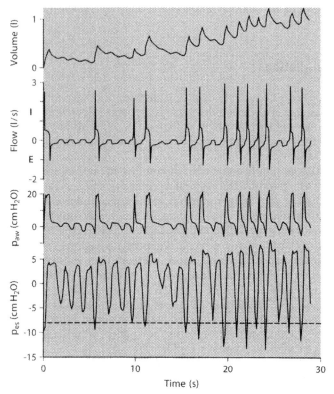

Fig. 6.2. Recordings of tidal volume, flow airway pressure (P_{aw}), and esophageal pressure (P_{es}) in a patient with chronic obstructive pulmonary disease receiving pressure-support ventilation. Note that nearly half of the patient's inspiratory efforts did not trigger the ventilator. When the patient generated a P_{es} more negative than –8 cmH$_2$O (indicated by the *dashed horizontal line*), triggering occurred. (Reproduced with permission from [75])

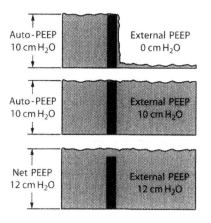

Fig. 6.3. The analogy of a waterfall over a dam (indicated by the *solid block*) is used to explain the effect of external PEEP ("upstream pressure") during expiration. See text for discussion. (Reproduced with permission from [33])

6.11 Abnormalities of Respiratory Drive

An increase or decrease in respiratory center output may lead to sudden deterioration in respiratory status.

6.11.1 Inadequate Respiratory Output

Respiratory drive may be decreased as a result of acute neurological disorders, heavy sedation, or metabolic alkalosis. Although drive per se may not be decreased, it may be inadequate to maintain a satisfactory level of alveolar ventilation if there is a sudden increase in ventilatory demands or in mechanical load.

6.11.2 Elevated Respiratory Output

Respiratory drive may be elevated as a result of pain, anxiety, hypoxic and/or hypercapnic stimulation, peripheral sensory receptor stimulation, increased ventilatory demands, medications, early sepsis, or improper ventilatory settings. In addition, excessive respiratory drive may result in severe respiratory alkalosis, which, in turn, may cause arrhythmias, hypotension, cerebral vasoconstriction, and seizures [40–43].

6.12 Alteration of Body Posture

An alteration in body posture can cause as much as a 30% fall in PaO_2 [44, 45], especially in patients with unilateral lung disease. This fall may be due to changes in the distribution of ventilation and perfusion in the healthy and damaged zones of the lung.

6.13 Drug-Induced Distress

Hypoxemia may result from worsening of ventilation-perfusion relationships secondary to bronchodilators or vasodilators (e.g., nitroglycerin, nitroprusside). Aminoglycoside antibiotics have the potential to aggravate neuromuscular blockade and may produce respiratory embarrassment [46]. High levels of theophylline may produce agitation and/or seizures [47].

6.14 Abdominal Distension

Abdominal distension may produce elevation of the diaphragm, basilar atelectasis, and deterioration in ventilation-perfusion relationships. Massive gastric distension, or "meteorism", can produce gastric rupture [48]. This condition also may occur as the result of a tracheoesophageal fistula. Insertion of a small-bore nasogastric tube helps to prevent or alleviate this complication. Massive colonic distension without small intestinal dilatation or distal obstruction (Ogilvie's syndrome) has been described in patients receiving mechanical ventilation [49]. Perforation of an overdistended cecum is often the first evidence of this complication. Accordingly, abdominal X-rays should be obtained in patients with abdominal distension, and colonoscopy should be considered when the cecal diameter exceeds 9 cm.

6.15 Agitation

Ventilator-supported patients develop agitation as a result of four major conditions: pain, anxiety, delirium, and dyspnea [1]. Untreated pain and anxiety can lead to insomnia and delirium. These problems are aggravated by the discomfort of dyspnea, which may result from injudicious ventilator settings such as improper trigger sensitivity and/or inspiratory flow settings (see below). It is important to follow a systematic approach when evaluating a patient for the source of pain or anxiety, as simple problems may be overlooked while a search is conducted for a more esoteric source of distress.

6.16 Ventilator-Related Problems

If manual ventilation with an anesthesia bag containing 100% O_2 relieves the respiratory distress, this suggests that the ventilator is the source of the problem (Table 6.1).

6.16.1 Leak in the System

Malfunction of the ventilator may result from the tubing being connected to the wrong outlet, a poor fit or uncoupling of connections, or obstruction of the circuit due to kinks, intraluminal fluid, or a malfunctioning valve. If this is suspected, the ventilator should be replaced, while each component of the defective ventilator is checked against the schematic circuit diagram.

6.16.2 Inadequate Inspired Fraction of Oxygen (F_IO_2)

If delivered tidal volume is adequate, and distress is relieved by manual ventilation, then a fault in the F_IO_2 setting should be suspected. This can be verified by obtaining an independent direct measurement of F_IO_2.

6.16.3 Inadequate Ventilator Support

The appropriateness of ventilator modes and settings is commonly evaluated in terms of improvements in PaO_2 and $PaCO_2$. However, monitoring of gas exchange does not provide information as to whether the respiratory muscles are being adequately rested. If ventilator support is provided at an insufficient level, it may contribute to the development of respiratory muscle fatigue or delay its reversal. Unfortunately, simple monitoring techniques that can quantitate a patient's active respiratory muscle contractions during mechanical ventilation do not exist. In addition, investigations have not been conducted to determine the optimal level of respiratory muscle rest. Intuitively, total rest might appear appropriate in a patient who is likely to have respiratory muscle fatigue. However, too much rest may produce disuse atrophy and weakness of the respiratory muscles [50]. In addition, the use of neuromuscular blocking agents may damage the respiratory neuromuscular apparatus (see below).

6.17 Patient-Ventilator Asynchrony

Many of the problems previously discussed interfere with synchronization of a patient's respiratory rhythm with that of the ventilator. An inappropriate ventilator mode or improper selection of ventilator settings also can contribute to the development of such asynchrony.

6.17.1 Ventilator Mode Considerations

A major goal of mechanical ventilation is to reduce the work of breathing. This is accomplished by a smooth synchronization between the inspiratory and expiratory phases of a patient's effort and the respective cycling of the ventilator. The characteristics of patient-ventilator interaction with common modes of mechanical ventilation are incompletely defined, although certain aspects have been reported.

Despite appropriately selected settings during assist-control ventilation, patients still perform about one third of the work of the ventilator during passive conditions [51, 52]. With intermittent mandatory ventilation (IMV), it was believed that the degree of respiratory muscle rest was proportional to the number of mandatory breaths delivered by the ventilator. However, recent studies [53, 54] have demonstrated that the respiratory center is unable to adapt to this type of intermittent unloading. At IMV rates of 14 breaths/min or less, the inspiratory effort is increased to a level likely to induce respiratory muscle fatigue. This occurs not only with the intervening spontaneous breaths but also with the ventilator-assisted breaths. During pressure support, the algorithm used to cycle between inspiration and expiration may cause patients to activate their expiratory muscles while the ventilator is inflating the chest. Cycling from inspiration to expiration during pressure support is based on a decrease in inspiratory flow, usually to a level of 25% of peak inspiratory flow. Patients with airway obstruction have a long time constant, and therefore require more time for the inspiratory flow to fall to this threshold. Consequently, mechanical inflation may persist into neural expiration [55]. To counteract such neural-mechanical asynchrony, patients may activate their expiratory muscles at a time when the ventilator is inflating the chest. This expiratory muscle activity during ventilator inflation thus may cause patients to fight the ventilator.

6.17.2 Improper Trigger Sensitivity Setting

Most mechanical ventilators employ pressure triggering, whereby a decrease in circuit pressure is achieved by a patient's inspiratory effort. This is required to initiate either a ventilator-assisted breath in assist-control, IMV, or pressure-support ventilation modes or to permit spontaneous breathing between IMV breaths or during continuous positive airway pressure. From a practical standpoint, it is difficult to employ a trigger setting more sensitive than −1 to −2 cmH₂O without causing the ventilator to autocycle. As the trigger mechanism is made less sensitive, a patient's work of breathing increases significantly (Fig. 6.4) [52].

Recently, flow triggering has been introduced as an alternative to pressure triggering. On the Puritan-Bennett 7200ae ventilator (PS 7200ae; Puritan-Bennett, Carlsbad, Calif.) this is termed "flow-by", because a continuous base flow is used [56, 57]. The Siemens Servo 300 (SV300; Siemens-Elema, Solna, Sweden), another microprocessor-based ventilator, also employs flow triggering. The flow sensitivity (usually set at 2 l/min) is computed as the difference between the base flow within the circuit (usually set at 5–20 l/min) and the patient's exhaled flow. In other words, sensitivity is equivalent to the magnitude of flow diverted from the exhalation circuit into the patient's lungs. The trigger phase refers to the time from the onset of inspiratory effort to the onset of inspiratory flow and is considerably less with flow triggering than with pressure triggering. In addition, work of inspiration is less with flow triggering than with pressure triggering [58, 59].

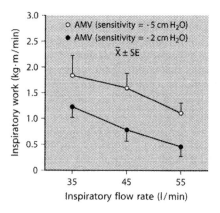

Fig. 6.4. The effect of changing trigger sensitivity from −2 cmH₂O (*closed circles*) to −5 cmH₂O (*open circles*) on rate of inspiratory work of breathing in ten critically ill patients receiving assist-control ventilation. At all inspiratory flow settings, work was significantly greater at the higher sensitivity setting. Values represent mean ±SE. (Adapted with permission from [52])

6.17.3 Improper Inspiratory Flow Setting

In addition to a proper trigger sensitivity, optimal synchronization of a patient's inspiratory efforts with the ventilator depends on the proper selection of the flow, volume, and timing settings on the ventilator. Employment of a flow setting that does not meet the ventilatory demands will cause patients being ventilated in the assist-control mode to pull against their own pulmonary impedance and that of the ventilator, resulting in a marked increase in active inspiratory work (Fig. 6.5) [52, 53]. This is likely to be a greater problem in patients with a heightened respiratory drive or high minute ventilation [53].

Deliberate prolongation of inspiratory time, as in the case of inverse-ratio ventilation, can be very uncomfortable. Heavy sedation and, frequently, neuromuscular blockade are necessary to combat the resulting patient-ventilator asynchrony.

6.18 Pharmacotherapy

Pharmacological agents are commonly employed when a specific cause of acute distress cannot be detected and corrected (Table 6.1) and reassurance provides no relief. The primary classes of agents that are used to allay distress include opiate analgesics, benzodiazepines, and neuromuscular blocking agents.

When approaching a patient in distress, it is important first to consider the need for pain relief, since sedative agents do not provide analgesia. Morphine sulfate remains the most popular analgesic for ventilator-supported patients. Although diazepam (Valium) is still widely employed, it should probably be avoided, because the slow elimination of its active metabolites may hinder the weaning process [60, 61]. More appropriate benzodiazepines include lorazepam (Ativan) and midazolam hydrochloride (Versed).

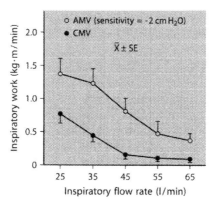

Fig. 6.5. The effect of changing inspiratory flow rate on rate of inspiratory work of breathing during controlled mechanical ventilation (*closed circles*) and assist-control ventilation (*open circles*). At all flow rates, the work of breathing was significantly greater during assist-control ventilation than during controlled ventilation. During both modes of mechanical ventilation, work increased as flow rate was decreased. Values are mean ±SE. (Adapted with permission from [52])

When a patient's severe agitation does not respond to other measures, neuromuscular blockade can be helpful. The respiratory muscles normally consume only 1%–2% of total body O_2 consumption [62, 63], but this can increase to as much as 55% in some patients who require ventilator support [64]. An O_2 cost of breathing of this magnitude markedly diminishes the availability of O_2 for delivery to other body systems. In this situation, vulnerable tissue beds may become ischemic, especially if O_2 delivery is compromised. In such instances, neuromuscular blockade and controlled mechanical ventilation can lead to a decrease in O_2 consumption and improvement in arterial oxygenation [65, 66].

On the other hand, neuromuscular blocking agents have several disadvantages. Their use masks a patient's complaints and physical findings. Unrecognized disconnection of the ventilator circuit may occur and produce apnea with catastrophic hypoxemia. Elimination of cough predisposes to the development of atelectasis. Finally, prolonged paralysis after discontinuation of a neuromuscular blocking agent is a worrisome adverse effect, since it leads to longer periods of ventilator dependency, increased morbidity, and greater hospital costs [67, 68].

This latter effect has been reported in up to 70% of certain patients who received prolonged administration of pancuronium or vecuronium [69–71]. Recent reports have linked prolonged paralysis with the concomitant use of corticosteroids and aminosteroidal neuromuscular blocking agents for patients with acute severe asthma [72]. Once thought to be without adverse effects, atracurium, a nonsteroidal neuromuscular blocking agent has now been reported to be associated with prolonged weakness in patients who received corticosteroids [73].

Efforts to minimize prolonged weakness after the use of neuromuscular blocking agents should include close monitoring of the level of neuromuscular blockade with peripheral nerve stimulation. Dissipation of neuromuscular blockade on a daily basis to assess a patient's clinical status is also important.

As a result of the various toxicities, neuromuscular blocking agents should be employed only as a last resort in a patient who demonstrates severe patient-ventilator asynchrony or uncontrollable high peak airway pressures.

6.19 Conclusion

Sudden distress in a ventilator-supported patient is a true medical emergency. The first rule is to ensure adequate ventilation and oxygenation. The patient should be disconnected from the ventilator and manually ventilated with 100% oxygen. While this is being performed, a systematic effort should be made to determine the cause of the distress and correct it.

6.20 References

1. Hansen-Flaschen JH (1992) The agitated patient in respiratory failure. In: Fishman AP (ed) Update: pulmonary diseases and disorders. McGraw Hill, New York, pp 383
2. Manzano JL, Lubillo S, Henriquez D, Martin JC, Perez MA, Wilson DJ (1993) Verbal communication of ventilator-dependent patients. Crit Care Med 21:512–517

3. Hudson LD (1982) Diagnosis and management of acute respiratory distress in patients on mechanical ventilators. In: Moser KM, Spragg RG (eds) Respiratory emergencies. Mosby, St. Louis, pp 201–213
4. Tobin MJ (1988) State of the art: respiratory monitoring in the intensive care unit. Am Rev Respir Dis 138:1625–1642
5. Browning IB, D'Alonzo GE, Tobin MJ (1990) Importance of respiratory rate as an indicator of respiratory dysfunction in patients with cystic fibrosis. Chest 97:1317–1321
6. Semmes BJ, Tobin MJ, Snyder JV, Grenvik A (1985) Subjective and objective measurement of tidal volume in critically ill patients. Chest 87:577–579
7. Tobin MJ, Guenther SM, Perez W, Lodato RF Mador MJ, Allen SJ, Dantzker DR (1987) Konno-Mead analysis of ribcage-abdominal motion during successful and unsuccessful trials of weaning from mechanical ventilation. Am Rev Respir Dis 135:1320–1328
8. Tobin MJ, Perez W, Guenther SM, Lodato RF, Dantzker DR (1987) Does ribcage abdominal paradox signify respiratory muscle fatigue? J Appl Physiol 63:851–860
9. Hoffman RA, Krieger BP, Kramer MR, Segel S, Bizousky F, Gazeroglu H, Sackner MA (1989) End-tidal carbon dioxide in critically ill patients during changes in mechanical ventilation. Am Rev Respir Dis 140:1265–1268
10. Marini JJ (1990) Strategies to minimize breathing effort during mechanical ventilation. Crit Care Clin 6:635–661
11. Pepe PE, Marini JJ (1982) Occult positive end-expiratory pressure in mechanically ventilated patients with airflow obstruction. Am Rev Respir Dis 126:155–170
12. Brunel W, Coleman DL, Schwartz DE, Peper E, Cohen NH (1989) Assessment of routine chest roentgenograms and the physical examination to confirm endotracheal tube position. Chest 96:1043–1045
13. Kollef MH, Legare EJ, Damiano M (1994) Endotracheal tube misplacement: incidence, risk factors, and impact of a quality improvement program. South Med J 87:248–254
14. Conrardy PA, Goodman LR, Lainge F, Singer MM (1976) Alteration of endotracheal tube position: flexion and extension of the neck. Crit Care Med 4:8–12
15. Hosking MR, Lennon RL, Warner MA, Gray JR, Masley R, De Luca LA, et al (1989) Endotracheal tube obstruction: recognition and management. Milit Med 154:489–491
16. Ripley JF, McAnear JT, Tilson HE (1984) Endotracheal tube obstruction due to impaction of the inferior turbinate. J Oral Maxillofac Surg 42:687–688
17. Myers EN, Carrau RL (1991) Early complications of tracheostomy: incidence and management. Clin Chest Med 12:589–595
18. Gelman JJ, Aro M, Weiss SM (1994) Tracheo-innominate artery fistula. J Am Coll Surg 179:626–634
19. Harley HRS (1972) Ulcerative tracheoesophageal fistula during treatment by tracheostomy and intermittent positive pressure ventilation. Thorax 27:338
20. Wood DE, Mathisen DJ (1991) Late complications of tracheostomy. Clin Chest Med 12:597–609
21. Shelly MS (1992) Inspired gas conditioning. Respir Care 37:1070–1080
22. Albeda SM, Gefter WR, Kelley MA, Epstein DM, Miller WT (1983) Ventilator-induced subpleural air cysts: clinical, radiographic, and pathologic significance. Am Rev Respir Dis 127:360–365
23. Peterson GW, Baier H (1983) Incidence of pulmonary barotrauma in a medical ICU. Crit Care Med 11:67–68
24. Gammon RS, Shin MS, Groves RH, Hardin JM, Hsu C, Buchalter SE (1995) Clinical risk factors for pulmonary barotrauma: a multivariate analysis. Am J Respir Crit Care Med 152:1235–1240
25. Matthay MA (1985) Pathophysiology of pulmonary edema. Clin Chest Med 6:521–545
26. Albert RK (1987) Pulmonary edema. Curr Pulmonol 8:1–16
27. Hirsh J, Hull RD, Raskob GE (1986) Clinical features and diagnosis of venous thrombosis. J Am Cardiol 8:114B–127B
28. Kimbal WR, Leith DE, Robins AG (1982) Dynamic hyperinflation and ventilator dependence in chronic obstructive pulmonary disease. Am Rev Respir Dis 126:991–995

29. Vinegar A, Sinnett EE, Leith DE (1979) Dynamics mechanisms determine functional residual capacity in mice, *Mus musculus*. J Appl Physiol 46:867–871
30. Rossi A, Gottfried SS, Zocchi L, Higgs BD, Lennox S, Calverly PMA, Begin P, Grassino A, Milic-Emili J (1985) Measurement of static compliance of the total respiratory system in patients with acute respiratory failure during mechanical ventilation: the effect of intrinsic positive end-expiratory pressure. Am Rev Respir Dis 131:672–677
31. Smith TC, Marini JJ (1988) Impact of PEEP on lung mechanics and work of breathing in severe airflow obstruction. J Appl Physiol 65:1488–1499
32. Tobin MJ (1988) Respiratory muscles in disease. Clin Chest Med 9:263–285
33. Tobin MJ, Lodato RF (1989) Editorial: PEEP, auto-PEEP, and waterfalls. Chest 96:449–451
34. Gurevitch MJ, Gelmont D (1989)Importance of trigger sensitivity to ventilator response delay in advanced chronic obstructive pulmonary disease with respiratory failure. Crit Care Med 17:354–359
35. Gottfried SB (1991) The role of PEEP in the mechanically ventilated COPD patient. In: Marini JJ, Roussos C (eds) Ventilatory failure. Springer, Berlin Heidelberg New York, pp 392–418
36. Scott LR, Benson MS, Pierson DJ (1986) Effect of inspiratory flow rate and circuit compressible volume on auto-PEEP during mechanical ventilation. Respir Care 31:1075–1079
37. Lodato RF, Tobin MJ (1991) Estimation of auto-PEEP. Chest 99:520–522
38. Hoffman RA, Ershowsky P, Drieger BR (1989) Determination of auto-PEEP during spontaneous and controlled ventilation by monitoring changes in end-expiratory thoracic gas volume. Chest 96:613–616
39. Petroff BJ, Legaré M, Goidberg P, Milic-Emili J, Gottfried SB (1990) Continuous positive airway pressure reduces work of breathing and dyspnea during weaning from mechanical ventilation in severe chronic obstructive pulmonary disease. Am Rev Respir Dis 141:281–289
40. Rotherman EB, Safar P, Robin ED (1964) CNS disorder during mechanical ventilation in chronic pulmonary disease. JAMA 189:993–996
41. Kilburn KH (1966) Shock, seizures, and coma with alkalosis during mechanical ventilation. Ann Intern Med 65:977–984
42. Trimble C, Smith DE, Rosenthal MH, Rosburgh RG (1971) Pathophysiologic role of hypocarbia in post-traumatic pulmonary insufficiency. Am J Surg 122:633–638
43. Gennari FJ, Kassirer JP (1982) Respiratory alkalosis. In: Cohen JL, Kassirer JP (eds) Acid-base. Little Brown, Boston, pp 349–376
44. Langer M, Mascheroni D, Marcolin R, Gattinoni L (1988) The prone position in ARDS patients: a clinical study. Chest 94:103–107
45. Glauser FL, Polatty RC, Sessler CN (1988) Worsening oxygenation in the mechanically ventilated patient: causes, mechanisms, and early detection. Am Rev Respir Dis 138:458–465
46. Argov Z, Mastaglia FL (1979) Disorders of neuromuscular transmission caused by drugs. N Engl J Med 301:409–413
47. Aitken ML, Martin TR (1987) Life-threatening theophylline toxicity is not predictable by serum levels. Chest 91:10–14
48. Pierson DJ (1990) Complications associated with mechanical ventilation. Crit Care Clin 6:711–724
49. Golden GT, Chandler JG (1975) Colonic ileus and cecal perforation in patients requiring mechanical ventilatory support. Chest 68:661–664
50. Anzueto A, Tobin MJ, Moore G, Peters JL, Seidenfeld JJ, Coalson JJ (1987) Effect of prolonged mechanical ventilation on diaphragmatic function: a preliminary study of a baboon model. Am Rev Respir Dis 135:A201
51. Marini JJ, Capps JS, Culver BH (1985) The inspiratory work of breathing during assisted mechanical ventilation. Chest 87:612–618
52. Ward ME, Corbiel C, Gibbons W, Newman S, Macklem PT (1988) Optimization of respiratory muscle relaxation during mechanical ventilation. Anesthesiology 69:29–35
53. Marini JJ, Smith TC, Lamb VJ (1988) External work output and force generation during synchronous intermittent mandatory ventilation: effect of machine assistance on breathing effort. Am Rev Respir Dis 138:1169–1179

54. Imsand C, Feihl F, Perret C, Fitting JW (1994) Regulation of inspiratory neuromuscular output during synchronized intermittent mechanical ventilation. Anesthesiology 80:13–22

55. Jubran A, van de Graaff WB, Tobin MJ (1995) Variability of patient-ventilator interaction with pressure support ventilation in patients with chronic obstructive pulmonary disease. Am J Respir Crit Care Med 152:129–136

56. Sassoon CSH, Giron AE, Ely EA, Light RW (1989) Inspiratory work of breathing on flow-by and demand-flow continuous positive airway pressure. Crit Care Med 17:1108–1114

57. Sassoon CSH, Lodia R, Rheeman CH, Kuei JH, Light RW, Mahutte CK (1992) Inspiratory muscle work of breathing during flow-by, demand-flow and continuous-flow systems in patients with chronic obstructive pulmonary disease. Am Rev Respir Dis 145:1219–1222

58. Sassoon CSH, Rosario ND, Fei R, Rheeman CH, Gruer SE, Mahutte K (1994) Influence of pressure- and flow-triggered synchronous intermittent mandatory ventilation on inspiratory muscle work. Crit Care Med 22:1933–1941

59. Sassoon CSH, Gruer SE (1995) Characteristics of the ventilator pressure- and flow-trigger variables. Intensive Care Med 21:159–168

60. Martyn J (1986) Clinical pharmacology and drug therapy in the burned patient. Anesthesiology 5:67–75

61. Hansen-Flaschen JH, Brazinsky S, Basile C, Lanken PN (1991) Use of sedating drugs and neuromuscular blocking agents in patients requiring mechanical ventilation for respiratory failure. JAMA 226:2870–2875

62. Campbell EJM, Westlake EK, Cherniack RM (1957) Simple methods of estimating oxygen consumption and efficiency of the muscles of breathing. J Appl Physiol 11:303–308

63. Cherniack RM (1959) The oxygen consumption and efficiency of the respiratory muscles in health and emphysema. J Clin Invest 38:494–499

64. Field S, Kelly SM, Macklem PT (1982) The oxygen cost of breathing in patients with cardiorespiratory disease. Am Rev Respir Dis 126:9–13

65. Aubier M, Viires N, I Syllil G, Mozes R, Roussos C (1982) Respiratory muscle contribution to lactic acidosis in low cardiac output. Am Rev Respir Dis 126:648–652

66. Coggeshall JW, Marini JJ, Newman J (1985) Improved oxygenation after muscle relaxation in adult respiratory distress syndrome. Arch Intern Med 145:1718–1720

67. Willats SM (1985) Editorial: Paralysis for ventilated patients: yes or no? Intensive Care Med 11:2–4

68. Isenstein DA, Venner DS, Duggan J (1992) Neuromuscular blockade in the intensive care unit. Chest 102:1258–1266

69. Segredo V, Caldwell JE, Matthay MA, Sharma ML, Gruenke LD, Miller RD (1992) Persistent paralysis in critically ill patents after long-term administration of vecuronium. N Engl J Med 327:524–528

70. Kupfer Y, Namba T, Kaldawi E, Tessler S (1992) Prolonged weakness after long-term infusion of vecuronium. Ann Intern Med 117:484–486

71. Hansen-Flaschen JH,: Cowen J, Raps EC (1993) Neuromuscular blockade in the ICU: more than we bargained for. Am Rev Respir Dis 147:234–236

72. Griffin D, Fairman N, Coursin D, Rawsthorne L, Grossman JE (1992) Acute myopathy during treatment of status asthmaticus with corticosteroids and steroidal muscle relaxants. Chest 102:510–514

73. Branney SW, Haenel JB, Moore FA, Tarbox BB, Schrieber RH, Moore EE (1994) Prolonged paralysis with atracurium infusion: a case report. Crit Care Med 22:1699–1701

74. Tobin MJ (1990) Respiratory monitoring during mechanical ventilation. Crit Care Clin 6:679–709

75. Tobin MJ, Jubran A (1994) Pathophysiology of failure to wean from mechanical ventilation. Schweiz Med Wochenschr 124:2139–2145

7 Critical Illness Polyneuropathy and Critical Illness Myopathy

C. Serrano-Munuera and I. Illa

Neuromuscular disorders alone can account for up to 62% of the cases of ventilatory dependency in intensive care unit (ICU) patients with no other apparent causes of failure to wean, and they may be a contributing factor in up to 86% of these patients (Spitzer et al. 1992). In addition, neuromuscular abnormalities can be detected in up to 95% of patients who stay in the ICU for a period of more than 7 days (Coakley et al. 1993). Among the neuromuscular disorders, critical illness polyneuropathy (CIP) and critical illness myopathy (CIM) have become two of the most common underlying diagnoses associated with an otherwise unexplained need for prolonged ventilatory support. Although in the earliest reports on CIP and CIM most patients had sepsis and multiple organ failure or were given neuromuscular blocking agents or high doses of corticosteroids, respectively, it is now well accepted that the spectrum of primary medical diseases in these patients is much broader than initially suspected and that the above-mentioned pharmacological precedent is not a constant feature (Berek et al. 1996; Coakley et al. 1993). In this chapter, we describe the epidemiological, clinical, electrophysiological, and pathological characteristics of both entities and summarize the relevant findings related to their pathogenesis.

7.1 Critical Illness Polyneuropathy

The occurrence of neuropathy during critical illness was described independently by American, Canadian, and French workers in the early 1980s (Bolton et al. 1984; Couturier et al. 1984; Roelofs et al. 1983). However, the clinical syndrome had been recognized decades earlier. It has classically been considered a complication of sepsis and multiple organ failure and accordingly has been called critical illness polyneuropathy (Bolton et al. 1986). In this section, the epidemiological, clinical, electrophysiological, and pathological characteristics of this syndrome will be discussed, with special emphasis on the proposed pathogenic mechanisms.

7.11 Incidence and Prevalence

Critical illness neuropathy affects both sexes equally (Witt et al. 1991) and seems to be fairly common among subjects who are in the ICU for more than 5–7 days.

In this group of patients the incidence of CIP is close to 50% (Leijten et al. 1996). Among patients with sepsis and multiple organ failure, prospective studies have shown electrophysiological evidence of neuropathy in 20%–70% (Lacomis et al. 1998; Witt et al. 1991), while clinical signs of peripheral neuropathy can be detected in only half of them. This apparent discordance could be explained by the unreliability of clinical examination in patients on endotracheal ventilation who frequently suffer from septic encephalopathy.

7.1.2 Clinical Features

The syndrome is initially suspected because of difficulties in weaning patients from the ventilator when no other apparent causes of respiratory failure are present, although CIP has been reported in isolated patients without weaning difficulties (Leijten et al. 1996). Neurological involvement usually becomes evident when the critical illness stabilizes at a median of 4.5 weeks from the onset of the acute disease (Hund et al. 1996).

The clinical picture is characterized by distal muscle weakness and wasting. Reduced or absent deep tendon reflexes are commonly found, although the presence of tendon reflexes does not exclude a diagnosis of CIP (Hund et al. 1996). In severe cases (10%), weakness may progress to tetraparesis or tetraplegia. Characteristically, the process spares the cranial nerves. There is, however, electrophysiological and morphological evidence of axonal degeneration of the phrenic nerve, supporting the idea that difficulty in weaning is due to neuropathy (Maher et al. 1995). All sensory modalities may be impaired distally in the limbs, but this clinical sign is often difficult to identify because of the limited cooperation of the patients who may suffer from encephalopathy and/or be under sedation (Berek et al. 1996). Septic encephalopathy is indeed a common feature, usually associated with abnormalities detected by electroencephalography (EEG) (Witt et al. 1991).

7.1.3 Electrophysiological Studies

Clinical examination is often unreliable and, consequently, electrophysiological studies are an essential diagnostic tool (Berek et al. 1996). Nevertheless, characteristic nerve conduction abnormalities specific to a diagnosis of CIP have not yet been established. Early electrophysiological studies (Berek et al. 1996; Bolton et al. 1986; Coakley et al. 1993; Spitzer et al. 1992) confirmed the presence of primary axonal degeneration of sensory and motor fibers with reduced sensory and compound muscle action potentials, while nerve conduction velocity, distal latencies, and F response latencies were normal or near normal. Abnormal spontaneous activity is commonly found in electromyographic studies (EMG). Although the axonal nature of this disorder seems to be well accepted and can be detected as early as 7 days after the onset of the critical illness, the electrophysiological parameters useful in the diagnosis are still being discussed. Hence, some investigators (Schwarz et al. 1997) suggested that neither reduction of the sensory nerve action potentials (SNAPs) nor reduction of the compound muscle action potentials (CMAPs) in the absence of spontaneous activity were to be considered definitive for a diagnosis of CIP. They based this assertion on findings from their short prospective study in CIP patients in whom reduction of the SNAPs did not seem to be a characteristic feature. These investigators proposed the increase in mean jitter and the spontaneous activity in EMG as the most sensitive parameters for an early diagnosis of CIP. In addition, they criticized the diagnostic value of reduction in CMAP in the absence of spontaneous activity, since such a reduction can be found in muscle wasting following inactivity and does not invariably reflect a neurogenic lesion. Further studies are needed to validate these observations. Moreover, the specificity of these findings in CIP versus CIM should be established, and the normality of SNAPs found by these investigators should be correlated with the almost constant clinical or electrophysiological sensory disturbances detected in CIP patients by other groups (Berek et al. 1996; Bolton et al. 1986; Coakley et al. 1993; Spitzer et al. 1992).

Finally, the common concomitant presence of myopathy (up to 50% of the patients with CIP may also suffer from CIM) may be difficult to assess electrophysiologically, because most of these patients are unable to cooperate in performing voluntary muscular contraction, thus preventing analysis of motor units.

7.1.4 Differential Diagnosis

Differential diagnosis must include all causes of acute neuromuscular weakness, as shown in Table 7.1. Although alternative diagnoses are numerous, most of them can easily be distinguished from CIP on clinical and electrophysiological grounds. For example, prolonged neuromuscular blockade is characterized by cranial as well as limb muscle weakness, while CIP usually spares the cranial muscles. The most difficult differential diagnosis probably concerns to the so-called axonal form of Guillain-Barré syndrome (GBS). Axonal GBS usually develops outside the ICU; it is linked to the antecedent of *Campylobacter jejuni* infections and resembles the classic form of the syndrome by cerebrospinal fluid findings and frequent bulbar involvement.

As mentioned above, concomitant CIM may be a confounding concurrent diagnosis in CIP patients. From a clinical point of view, it is not necessary to pursue the distinctive diagnosis of both conditions by performing muscle and nerve biopsies, since the prognosis will be essentially the same. However, both specimens can provide important information about the pathogenesis of both syndromes. Later in this chapter, electrophysiological tools that may help in the differential diagnosis of both entities will be discussed.

Finally, differential diagnosis in weaning difficulties should also include all other concomitant conditions that may interfere with pulmonary function, and the authors recommend being alert to alternative explanations for difficult weaning, even when CIP is present. So far, there is insufficient evidence that isolated CIP itself is responsible for weaning difficulties (Leijten et al. 1996).

Table 7.1. Causes of acute neuromuscular weakness

Neuropathies or polyneuropathies	Neuromuscular junction impairment	Muscle impairment
Onset prior to ICU admission		
Myelopathy	Botulism	Hypokalemia
Guillain-Barré syndrome	Myasthenia gravis	Hyperkalemia
Chronic inflammatory demyelinating polyneuropathy	Lambert-Eaton syndrome	Periodic paralysis
Polyneuropathy associated with: lymphoma, vasculitis, acute porphyria, diphtheria, tick bite paralysis	Hypermagnesemia	Polymyositis
Seafood poisoning, hypophosphatemia	Antibiotic-related paralysis	Rhabdomyolysis
Drugs/poisons: n-hexane, thallium, arsenic, lead, gold, lithium, vincristine, dapsone, disulfiram	Spider, scorpion, snake bite paralysis	Acid maltase deficiency
	Organophosphate poisoning	Barium poisoning
Onset during ICU admission		
Motor neuron disease	Myasthenia gravis	Acid maltase deficiency
Toxic polyneuropathies	Prolonged neuromuscular blockade	Toxic myopathy
Guillain-Barré syndrome	Anticholinesterase drug overdose	Critical illness myopathy
Critical illness polyneuropathy		

7.1.5 Pathological Findings

Morphological studies are scarce. Those published to date verify predominant axonal degeneration with loss of myelinated fibers and active Wallerian-like degeneration in most specimens (Bolton et al. 1984; Hund et al. 1996; Latronico et al. 1996; Zochodne et al. 1987). Interestingly, some degree of discordance between electrophysiological and pathological studies has been reported, with only a few patients showing abnormalities in sural biopsy compared with the high incidence of electrophysiological abnormalities reported. In an attempt to explain this discordance, it has been speculated that sepsis-related nerve failure could cause early impairment of axonal transport and transmembrane potential. This hypothesis could easily be confirmed by electrophysiological studies, but not by pathological investigations, since structural changes would take place later in the course of the disease (Latronico et al. 1996).

In addition, it should be considered that if muscle biopsy is also performed, the diagnosis of CIM as a concomitant or main diagnosis can be established in up to 65% of patients with an electrophysiological diagnosis of CIP.

7.1.6 Etiology

The etiology and pathogenesis of this syndrome remains unclear. CIP has been attributed to a variety of causes such as malnutrition (Zochodne et al. 1987), vitamin deficiencies (Bolton et al. 1984), immunological factors (Bolton et al. 1984), ischemia (Barat et al. 1987), toxin-producing bacteria (Bolton et al. 1984), gentamicin and other antibiotics (Gross et al. 1988), and the muscle relaxant pancuronium bromide (Op de Coul et al. 1985), but none has been proven so far. A statistically positive correlation has been found between the presence of neuropathy and both the number of days in ICU and serum glucose levels, while a negative correlation has been observed between CIP and serum albumin levels (Witt et al. 1991). In addition, no relationship has been proven with the cause of admission to the ICU, duration of mechanical ventilation, age, sex, number of antibiotics given, aminoglycoside blood levels, nutritional factors other than albumin serum levels, water and electrolyte disturbances, or serum muscle enzyme levels (Witt et al. 1991). Finally, the pathogenic role of the severity of organ dysfunction in terms of functional indexes and total number of impaired organs, as well as the association with aminoglycoside treatment, is still controversial (Leijten et al. 1996; Witt et al. 1991). For the last three variables, the risk of artifactual association is extremely high, since all three conditions are associated with a more severe course, are interdependent, and may represent three different ways of expressing the severity of the disease. In conclusion, these observations strongly support a major role for the septic process or multiple organ dysfunction syndrome at the beginning and probably in the maintenance of the disorder, although definitive clinical and experimental evidence is lacking.

7.1.7 Pathogenesis

Among the proposed mechanisms by which sepsis and multiple organ dysfunction may damage the peripheral nerves, the following should be taken into consideration:
- Peripheral nerve failure could be considered a nonspecific effect of sepsis in the same way as other systems become involved during sepsis (Bolton 1993; Witt et al. 1991). Endotoxin-induced cytokines, such as tumor necrosis factor, a key mediator in shock and multi-organ failure (Op de Coul et al. 1991), have been proposed as probably being involved in the pathogenesis of CIP. However, recent efforts to find an immunological factor (Verheul et al. 1994; Witt et al. 1991; Zochodne et al. 1987) and experimental treatment based on a suspected immunotoxic origin have been unsuccessful (Wijdicks and Fulgham 1994).
- The increase in serum glucose levels, probably related to the state of insulin resistance associated with sepsis, may result in increased endovascular resistance that could lead to reduced nerve flow and endoneurial hypoxia, as shown in animals with experimental diabetes. Moreover, it is now hypothesized that hypoxia of whatever origin may induce not only diabetic but also other types of neuropathy (Dyck 1989) by impairing mitochondria and, consequently, the

axonal energy-dependent transport of essential proteins (Miller and Spencer 1984). In addition, the lack of vascular autoregulation in the peripheral nerves may contribute to the generation of hypoxia during sepsis, when shunting of blood from peripheral tissues to more central tissues such as the brain, heart, liver, and kidneys takes place.

• The decrease in serum albumin levels could be related to impaired endothelial permeability and to reallocation of albumin into the endoneurial space, contributing to the creation of endoneurial edema (Fleck et al. 1985). This would be supported by susceptibility of the blood-brain barrier to the histamine-like substances that are secreted in sepsis.

7.1.8 Prognosis

CIP does not seem to worsen the long-term prognosis and, if the patient survives all other concurrent medical conditions, improvement of the neuropathy follows in 50%–70% of cases (Hund et al. 1996; Witt et al. 1991) with virtually complete recovery (44% of CIP patients become ambulatory at 4 months) (Lacomis et al. 1998). Initial reports gave a more pessimistic figure of up to 58% mortality (Zochodne et al. 1987); however, patient selection was biased towards the most severe cases and the contribution of the neuropathy to morbidity and mortality is unclear. Thus, it is extremely important to be aware of the existence of this condition to avoid an unreasonably pessimistic prognosis (Latronico et al. 1996). Although outcome is difficult to predict in terms of clinical or electrophysiological data, three parameters have been associated with poor prognosis: longer stay in the ICU, longer duration of sepsis, and greater loss of body weight (de Seze et al. 2000).

7.1.9 Treatment

There is no specific treatment for CIP, and intravenous immunoglobulin has been tried without success. Meticulous positioning is recommended in patients with CIP to prevent additional palsies caused by pressure injury, and efforts should be made to eliminate systemic infection, if present, and to prevent organ failure.

7.2 Critical Illness Myopathy

The initial identification of CIP as one of the major neuromuscular causes of ICU-acquired weakness (Bolton et al. 1984; Zochodne et al. 1994) drew attention to other neuromuscular disorders occurring in the critically ill patient and led to the identification of acute myopathy, namely critical illness myopathy (CIM) (Lacomis et al. 1993; Latronico et al. 1996; MacFarlane and Rosenthal 1977). CIM is, in the authors' experience and in agreement with other investigators (Lacomis et al. 1998), the most common and most frequently unrecognized cause of acquired muscle weakness in the ICU. However, the relative frequency of CIM and CIP is still unknown, and it varies according to the ICU population selected.

7.2.1 Clinical Features

Critical illness myopathy is clinically similar to CIP since, in the absence of other causes of respiratory failure, it is characterized by difficulties in weaning. The main difference between CIP and CIM in the bedside examination is the absence of sensory impairment in the latter, although this feature can hardly be investigated in patients under sedation or those suffering from encephalopathy, as mentioned above. Another clinical sign that may help to establish a diagnosis of the myopathic process is that deep tendon reflexes will be decreased according to the degree of weakness. Like CIP, CIM has also been reported in patients without weaning difficulties. In a few patients with the necrotic form of CIM, ophthalmoplegia or facial muscle paresis has been reported (Op de Coul et al. 1985; Ramsay et al. 1993; Zochodne et al. 1994). Therefore, the distribution of weakness may help in diagnosing this type of myopathy.

Among the ancillary examinations, the creatinine kinase (CK) serum level has limited diagnostic value due to the prevalence of ICU patients with injuries, the minor surgical procedures frequently performed during ICU admissions (i.e., tracheostomy, thoracostomy, intracranial pressure monitoring), and the fact that for most patients with CIM, serum CK levels remain within normal limits.

7.2.2 Electrophysiological Investigations

As in CIP, electrophysiological studies are an essential tool in the diagnosis of CIM. EMG studies may show an absence of spontaneous activity even in the presence of severe weakness. Mild or abundant spontaneous activity may be found in proximal and distal muscles. The latter can be misinterpreted as a sign of a neurogenic process when the patient actually has a myopathy. During contraction, the main findings are normal or early recruitment of small and polyphasic or short-duration motor unit potentials in the presence of normal sensory nerve conduction studies. However, motor unit analysis may be impossible to perform because of the difficulties in eliciting voluntary contraction in these patients. Repetitive stimulation is frequently normal, with no evidence of decremental response, but evidence of prolonged neuromuscular blockade has been found in some patients. The impairment of neuromuscular transmission may initially contribute to the development of weakness. Motor nerve conduction studies may show low or normal motor amplitudes, and sensory nerve conduction studies are characteristically normal, unless the patient has a preexisting neuropathy. Electrophysiological investigations, while an essential diagnostic tool, may not definitively establish a diagnosis of CIM. Major difficulties in establishing the diagnosis will appear in patients with low motor amplitudes, normal sensory response and no firing motor unit potentials, or a recruitment pattern that is difficult to assess due to the severity of weakness or the lack of cooperation. In these circumstances, the possibility of an axonal motor neuropathy cannot be completely excluded unless direct muscle (Rich et al. 1996; Zochodne et al. 1994) stimulation or muscle biopsy is performed. Direct muscle stimulation can be used to distinguish CIM from CIP. In both conditions the CMAP obtained by nerve stimulation can be reduced, and when the patient is severely weak or unable to cooperate, the motor unit and the recruitment pattern analysis, both commonly used to differentiate myopathy from neuropathy, cannot be performed. However, the CMAP amplitude obtained by direct muscle stimulation will differ as follows: in CIP the denervated muscle retains electrical excitability, and thus the CMAP amplitude obtained by direct muscle stimulation will be normal; in CIM, however, muscle has been found to lose electrical excitability and, consequently, the CMAP amplitude obtained by direct muscle stimulation will be reduced (Rich et al. 1997). Loss of muscle electrical excitability, however, is not a constant trait in CIM, nor is it a specific one, since it can be found in other myopathies such as periodic paralysis.

7.2.3 Pathological Findings

Three main patterns of muscle involvement with different clinical and pathological characteristics have been reported: a hypercatabolic CIM, an acute necrotizing myopathy, and a myopathy with selective loss of thick (myosin) filaments. Whether these three types of CIM represent different presentations or stages of the same pathogenic process is unclear, and some degree of all three patterns is frequently found in most muscle biopsies from CIM patients.

Hypercatabolic CIM
Pathological changes in this form of myopathy include abnormal variation in fiber size, fiber atrophy involving predominantly type II myofibers (Gutmann et al. 1996), angulated fibers, central nuclei, rimmed vacuoles, fatty degeneration, fibrosis, and single-fiber necrosis. Inflammatory infiltrates are characteristically absent (Latronico et al. 1996; Spitzer et al. 1992). The process is usually mild and the serum CK level is frequently normal, impeding identification of the myopathic process (Latronico et al. 1996). The pathogenesis of this specific form of CIM is unclear. It seems that substrate deficiency alone is insufficient to account for muscle protein degradation in critically ill patients (Clowes et al. 1983) and the pathogenic role of cytokine release is becoming more evident as the cytokine pathways in skeletal muscle metabolism are identified. Among them, the activation of the ubiquitin-proteasome pathway has recently been identified as a novel intracellular mechanism of muscle protein catabolism during sepsis (Hasselgren and Fischer 1997). In addition, glucocorticoids, interleukin-1, and tumor necrosis factor are important mediators of muscle protein breakdown during sepsis, and there is evidence that this mechanism is also operative in human beings (Gutmann et al. 1996; Tiao et al. 1997).

Necrotic Form of CIM
A predominant necrotic pattern has been reported in patients in the ICU, even in the absence of clinical weakness (Helliwell et al. 1991). The necrotic pattern has been associated with the previous use of nondepolarizing muscle-blocking agents as well as with concomitant systemic infection by legionella, influenza A and B, leptospira, *Escherichia coli*, and *Staphylococcus aureus*. The association with the use of high doses of corticosteroids remains controversial (Helliwell et al. 1991;

Ramsay et al. 1993; Zochodne et al. 1994). The most common, although not exclusive, cause for admission to the ICU in these patients is status asthmaticus.

Most of these patients, especially those who received vecuronium (Zochodne et al. 1994), have very high serum CK levels and a few patients may show myoglobin in renal tubular casts because of the progression of the disease to rhabdomyolysis.

The presence of this necrotic myopathy has been strongly associated with the total number of systems failing, to renal failure, and to patient death, and the presence of necrosis is not independently related to poor survival (Helliwell et al. 1991).

Although the medical precedents may help to distinguish this form of CIM from the other two forms, diagnosis needs to be established by pathological findings (Fig. 7.1), mainly: myonecrosis of type I and type II fibers, vacuolization and phagocytosis of muscle fibers. Lymphocytes are characteristically absent or extremely rare. Thus, muscle biopsy is the main diagnostic tool, especially during the second and third week in the ICU (Helliwell et al. 1991).

The pathogenesis of this type of CIM remains unclear. Vascular disease, poor oxygen delivery, and abnormalities of muscle biochemistry have been proposed as pathogenic mechanisms leading to muscle necrosis. The unifying hypothesis postulates that triggering factors such as neuromuscular blocking agents could act on priming factors such as corticosteroids, denervation, or sepsis to develop myonecrosis (Ramsay et al. 1993); however, experimental evidence is lacking. Recently, inflammation has also been proposed as a pathogenic mechanism, since class I major histocompatibility complex products have been identified by immunohistochemistry in the sarcolemma of muscle fibers, predominantly in perifascicular areas, of some of these patients (Bazzi et al. 1999).

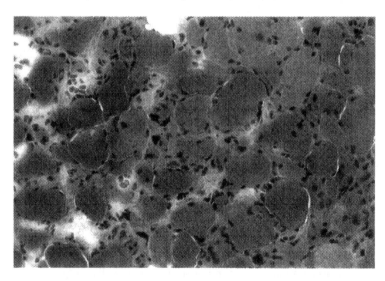

Fig. 7.1. Muscle biopsy from a patient with necrotizing myopathy. Necrotic muscle fibers are pale and are being phagocytosed by macrophages. (H&E, ×20)

Myopathy with Selective Loss of Thick (Myosin) Filaments

This form of CIM is characterized pathologically by the presence of focal regions, frequently within the center of the fibers, of negative staining with the myosin-adenosine triphosphatase reaction, with decreased amounts of skeletal muscle myosin (Fig. 7.2b) that correlate with decreased or absent myosin messenger RNA (Larsson et al. 2000). Because the pathological changes markedly influence the histochemical reactions of the muscle fibers, it is difficult to assess the fiber type. In hematoxylin and eosin staining most fibers contain centrally located light blue

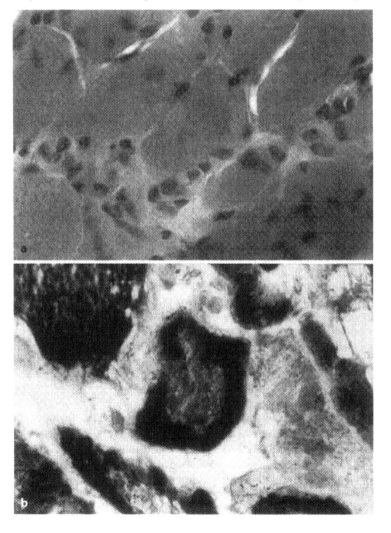

Fig. 7.2a, b. Muscle biopsy from a patient with myopathy with loss of myosin. **a** (H&E, ×60). Notice the characteristic central staining in the sarcoplasm of the muscle fibers. **b** (Myosin-ATPase, ×100). Loss of myosin-adenosine triphosphatase activity, suggesting loss of myosin filaments

or purple staining areas (Fig. 2a); in other instances, optically empty central areas are commonly found. Electron microscopy confirms the focal or even diffuse loss of thick (myosin) filaments in some of these patients, while the Z bands, thin (actin) filaments, appear unaffected. Nevertheless, it should be remembered that loss of myosin filaments is not associated exclusively with this condition, since it has occasionally been reported in dermatomyositis (Carpenter et al. 1976), thrombotic thrombocytopenic purpura (Carpenter et al. 1976), centronuclear myopathy, cytochrome *c* oxidase deficiency (Carpenter and Karpenter 1984), congenital myopathy (Yarom and Shapira 1977), and human immunodeficiency virus infection (Simpson and Bender 1988).

The most common medical precedent in these patients is fever, and causes of admission to ICU include transplantation [up to 7% of liver transplant patients may develop CIM (Campellone et al. 1998)], ketoacidotic diabetes, systemic lupus erythematosus (al-Lozi et al. 1994), and acute severe asthma (Hirano et al. 1992). This form of CIM has also been associated with the use of corticoids, either alone or in combination with high doses of neuromuscular blocking agents, but the pathological findings clearly distinguish this myopathy from the characteristic type II fiber atrophy related to corticosteroids. In terms of pathogenesis, however, the role of corticosteroids and that of neuromuscular blocking agents remain to be elucidated. Thus, there is experimental evidence that selective loss of thick filaments follows surgical denervation of muscles exposed to high doses of corticosteroids (Massa et al. 1992; Rouleau et al. 1987), and the finding that the number of corticosteroid receptors increases after surgical denervation (DuBois and Almon 1981) suggests hypersensitivity to corticosteroids as a putative mechanism. Moreover, glucocorticoids are known to augment the catabolism of skeletal muscle proteins and to decrease their synthesis (Kelly and Goldspink 1982). However, it is not known whether this action affects specifically myofibrillar proteins and, among them, predominantly myosin. Corticosteroids are known to activate at least one of the catabolic pathways in muscle, i.e., the ubiquitin-proteasome system; nevertheless, this pathway does not seem to be specifically activated in this myopathy. Increased expression of calpain, an alternative catabolic pathway, has been detected by immunohistochemistry in this entity (Showalter and Engel 1997). Corticosteroids do not increase expression of calpain in muscle. Since calpain is calcium activated, an abnormal intracellular calcium homeostasis may play a role in the pathogenesis of this disorder. Even so, activation of calpain would not explain the preferential loss of myosin because this enzyme, under certain experimental conditions, specifically removes the Z disk (actin filaments) and spares the rest of the myofibril. In conclusion, the pathogenic role of corticosteroids and of functional denervation needs to be confirmed, since some patients with this type of myopathy received neither corticosteroids nor neuromuscular blocking agents, nor did they suffer from neuropathy (Deconinck et al. 1998), suggesting that other factors play a pathogenic role. In addition, the mechanisms by which these factors generate loss of myosin need to be established.

Finally, some authors have reported impaired muscle membrane excitability in a high percentage of patients with this type of myopathy (Rich et al. 1997), and changes in the conductance of sodium and chloride channels have been associated with corticosteroid-treated denervated muscles. Moreover, tumor necrosis factor, one of the main mediators of sepsis, decreases the resting membrane potential. However, the decrease or loss of muscle membrane excitability cannot be explained by loss of myosin, and therefore, the final contribution of each of these proposed mechanisms to the development of muscle weakness requires further investigation. It has been proposed that loss of muscle excitability could be the initial cause of weakness, followed by structural changes with loss of myosin (Larsson et al. 2000).

Differential Diagnosis

Differential diagnosis of CIM includes all the conditions mentioned above under the heading of differential diagnosis in CIP. Specifically, the major differential diagnosis should be established with a pure motor axonal neuropathy acquired during ICU admission. As previously suggested, direct muscle stimulation (Rich et al. 1996) and muscle biopsy would help to elucidate whether a myopathic process is occurring. In order to avoid misinterpretations, it should be understood that response to direct muscle stimulation varies from muscle to muscle in the same patient and among patients. Finally, the second condition that should be ruled out is prolonged neuromuscular blockade. This condition may be associated with EMG findings of acute myopathy, confounding the differential diagnosis even further, and it should be suspected in patients with renal and hepatic failure.

7.2.4 Prognosis

For necrotizing myopathy, mortality is more than 70%, although the role of the myopathy in this fatal outcome has not been established (Helliwell et al. 1991). In a retrospective study, myopathy with loss of myosin filaments showed a mortality of 31%, although the cause of death was the underlying disease and not the CIM. Among surviving patients, up to 48% were ambulatory at 4 months (Lacomis et al. 1998).

7.2.5 Treatment

No specific therapy is available for CIM. The authors recommend that prolonged infusions of nondepolarizing neuromuscular blocking agents should be avoided, particularly when corticosteroids are concurrently given and when renal or hepatic failure is also present.

7.3 Conclusion

CIP and CIM are two major causes of weaning failure in ICU. Even though their etiology and pathogenesis are still unclear, physicians should be aware of the existence of both conditions in order to establish the proper diagnosis and to avoid medical actions that may worsen peripheral nerve and muscle functions.

7.4 References

al-Lozi MT, Pestronk A, Yee WC, Flaris N, Cooper J (1994) Rapidly evolving myopathy with myosin-deficient muscle fibers [see comments]. Ann Neurol 35:273–279

Barat M, Brochet B, Vital C, Mazaux J, Arne J (1987) Polyneuropathies au cours de séjours prolongés en réanimation. Rev Neurol (Paris) 143:823–831

Bazzi P, Moggio M, Prelle A, Sciacco M, Messina S, Barbieri S, Tonin P, Tomelleri G, Battistel A, Adobbati L, Checcarelli N, Veschi G, Scarlato G (1999) Critically ill patients: immunological evidence of inflammation in muscle biopsy. Clin Neuropathol 18:23–30

Berek K, Margreiter J, Willeit J, Berek A, Schmutzhard E, Mutz NJ (1996) Polyneuropathies in critically ill patients: a prospective evaluation [see comments]. Intensive Care Med 22:849–855

Bolton CF (1993) Neuromuscular complications of sepsis. Intensive Care Med 19 [Suppl 2]:S58–63

Bolton CF, Gilbert JJ, Hahn AF, Sibbald WJ (1984) Polyneuropathy in critically ill patients. J Neurol Neurosurg Psychiatry 47:1223–1231

Bolton CF, Laverty DA, Brown JD, Witt NJ, Hahn AF, Sibbald WJ (1986) Critically ill polyneuropathy: electrophysiological studies and differentiation from Guillain-Barré syndrome. J Neurol Neurosurg Psychiatry 49:563–573

Campellone JV, Lacomis D, Kramer DJ, Van Cott AC, Giuliani MJ (1998) Acute myopathy after liver transplantation [see comments]. Neurology 50:46–53

Carpenter S, Karpati G, Rothman S, Watters G (1976) The childhood type of dermatomyositis. Neurology 26:952–962

Carpenter S, Karpenter G (1984) Pathology of skeletal muscle. Churchill Livingstone, New York, pp 220–221

Clowes GH Jr, George BC, Villee CA Jr, Saravis CA (1983) Muscle proteolysis induced by a circulating peptide in patients with sepsis or trauma. N Engl J Med 308:545–552

Coakley JH, Nagendran K, Honavar M, Hinds CJ (1993) Preliminary observations on the neuromuscular abnormalities in patients with organ failure and sepsis [see comments]. Intensive Care Med 19:323–328

Couturier J, Robert D, Monier P (1984) Polynévrites compliquant des séjours prolongés en reanimation. A propos de 11 cas d'étiologie encore inconnue. Lyon Med 252:247–249

de Seze M, Petit H, Wiart L, Cardinaud JP, Gaujard E, Joseph PA, Mazaux JM, Barat M (2000) Critical illness polyneuropathy. A 2-year follow-up study in 19 severe cases. Eur Neurol 43:61–69

Deconinck N, Van Parijs V, Beckers-Bleukx G, Van den Bergh P (1998) Critical illness myopathy unrelated to corticosteroids or neuromuscular blocking agents. Neuromuscul Disord 8:186–192

DuBois DC, Almon RR (1981) A possible role for glucocorticoids in denervation atrophy. Muscle Nerve 4:370–373

Dyck PJ (1989) Hypoxic neuropathy: does hypoxia play a role in diabetic neuropathy? The 1988 Robert Wartenberg lecture. Neurology 39:111–118

Fleck A, Raines G, Hawker F, Trotter J, Wallace PI, Ledingham IM, Calman KC (1985) Increased vascular permeability: a major cause of hypoalbuminaemia in disease and injury. Lancet 1:781–784

Gross ML, Fowler CJ, Ho R, Russell RC, Harrison MJ (1988) Peripheral neuropathy complicating pancreatitis and major pancreatic surgery. J Neurol Neurosurg Psychiatry 51:1341–1344

Gutmann L, Blumenthal D, Gutmann L, Schochet SS (1996) Acute type II myofiber atrophy in critical illness [see comments]. Neurology 46:819–821

Hasselgren PO, Fischer JE (1997) The ubiquitin-proteasome pathway: review of a novel intracellular mechanism of muscle protein breakdown during sepsis and other catabolic conditions. Ann Surg 225:307–316

Helliwell TR, Coakley JH, Wagenmakers AJ, Griffiths RD, Campbell IT, Green CJ, McClelland P, Bone JM (1991) Necrotizing myopathy in critically ill patients. J Pathol 164:307–314

Hirano M, Ott BR, Raps EC, Minetti C, Lennihan L, Libbey NP, Bonilla E, Hays AP (1992) Acute quadriplegic myopathy: a complication of treatment with steroids, nondepolarizing blocking agents, or both. Neurology 42:2082–2087

Hund EF, Fogel W, Krieger D, DeGeorgia M, Hacke W (1996) Critical illness polyneuropathy: clinical findings and outcomes of a frequent cause of neuromuscular weaning failure [see comments]. Crit Care Med 24:1328–1333

Kelly FJ, Goldspink DF (1982) The differing responses of four muscle types to dexamethasone treatment in the rat. Biochem J 208:147–151

Lacomis D, Smith TW, Chad DA (1993) Acute myopathy and neuropathy in status asthmaticus: case report and literature review. Muscle Nerve 16:84–90

Lacomis D, Petrella JT, Giuliani MJ (1998) Causes of neuromuscular weakness in the intensive care unit: a study of ninety-two patients. Muscle Nerve 21:610–617

Larsson L, Li X, Edstrom L, Eriksson LI, Zackrisson H, Argentini C, Schiaffino S (2000) Acute quadriplegia and loss of muscle myosin in patients treated with nondepolarizing neuro-muscular blocking agents and corticosteroids: mechanisms at the cellular and molecular levels [see comments]. Crit Care Med 28:34–45

Latronico N, Fenzi F, Recupero D, Guarneri B, Tomelleri G, Tonin P, De Maria G, Antonini L, Riz-zuto N, Candiani A (1996) Critical illness myopathy and neuropathy. Lancet 347:1579–1582

Leijten FS, De Weerd AW, Poortvliet DC, De Ridder VA, Ulrich C, Harink-De Weerd JE (1996) Critical illness polyneuropathy in multiple organ dysfunction syndrome and weaning from the ventilator [see comments]. Intensive Care Med 22:856–861

MacFarlane IA, Rosenthal FD (1977) Severe myopathy after status asthmaticus [letter]. Lancet 2:615

Maher J, Rutledge F, Remtulla H, Parkes A, Bernardi L, Bolton CF (1995) Neuromuscular disor-ders associated with failure to wean from the ventilator. Intensive Care Med 21:737–743

Massa R, Carpenter S, Holland P, Karpati G (1992) Loss and renewal of thick myofilaments in glu-cocorticoid-treated rat soleus after denervation and reinnervation. Muscle Nerve 15:1290–1298

Miller MS, Spencer PS (1984) Single doses of acrylamide reduce retrograde transport velocity. J Neurochem 43:1401–1408

Op de Coul AA, Lambregts PC, Koeman J, van Puyenbroek MJ, Ter Laak HJ, Gabreels-Festen AA (1985) Neuromuscular complications in patients given Pavulon (pancuronium bromide) during artificial ventilation. Clin Neurol Neurosurg 87:17–22

Op de Coul AA, Verheul GA, Leyten AC, Schellens RL, Teepen JL (1991) Critical illness polyneu-romyopathy after artificial respiration. Clin Neurol Neurosurg 93:27–33

Ramsay DA, Zochodne DW, Robertson DM, Nag S, Ludwin SK (1993) A syndrome of acute severe muscle necrosis in intensive care unit patients [published erratum appears in J Neuropathol Exp Neurol (1993) 52:666]. J Neuropathol Exp Neurol 52:387–398

Rich MM, Teener JW, Raps EC, Schotland DL, Bird SJ (1996) Muscle is electrically inexcitable in acute quadriplegic myopathy [see comments]. Neurology 46:731–736

Rich MM, Bird SJ, Raps EC, McCluskey LF, Teener JW (1997) Direct muscle stimulation in acute quadriplegic myopathy. Muscle Nerve 20:665–673

Roelofs R, Serra F, Bielka N, Rosenberg L, Canton O, Delaney J (1983) Prolonged respiratory insufficiency due to acute motor neuropathy: a new syndrome? Neurology 33:240

Rouleau G, Karpati G, Carpenter S, Soza M, Prescott S, Holland P (1987) Glucocorticoid excess induces preferential depletion of myosin in denervated skeletal muscle fibers. Muscle Nerve 10:428–438

Schwarz J, Planck J, Briegel J, Straube A (1997) Single-fiber electromyography, nerve conduction studies, and conventional electromyography in patients with critical-illness polyneuropathy: evidence for a lesion of terminal motor axons. Muscle Nerve 20:696–701

Showalter CJ, Engel AG (1997) Acute quadriplegic myopathy: analysis of myosin isoforms and evidence for calpain-mediated proteolysis. Muscle Nerve :316–322

Simpson DM, Bender AN (1988) Human immunodeficiency virus-associated myopathy: analy-sis of 11 patients. Ann Neurol 24:79–84

Spitzer AR, Giancarlo T, Maher L, Rosenbuch G, Bowles A (1992) Neuromuscular causes of pro-longed ventilator dependency. Muscle Nerve 15:682–686

Tiao G, Hobler S, Wang JJ, Meyer TA, Luchette FA, Fischer JE, Hasselgren PO (1997) Sepsis is associated with increased mRNAs of the ubiquitin-proteasome proteolytic pathway in human skeletal muscle. J Clin Invest 99:163–168

Verheul GA, de Jongh-Leuvenink J, Op de Coul AA, van Landeghem AA, van Puyenbroek MJ (1994) Tumor necrosis factor and interleukin-6 in critical illness polyneuromyopathy. Clin Neurol Neurosurg 96:300–304

Wijdicks EF, Fulgham JR (1994) Failure of high dose intravenous immunoglobulins to alter the clinical course of critical illness polyneuropathy [letter]. Muscle Nerve 17:1494–1495

Witt NJ, Zochodne DW, Bolton CF, Grand'Maison F, Wells G, Young GB, Sibbald WJ (1991) Peripheral nerve function in sepsis and multiple organ failure. Chest 99:176–184

Yarom R, Shapira Y (1977) Myosin degeneration in a congenital myopathy. Arch Neurol 34:114–115

Zochodne DW, Bolton CF, Wells GA, Gilbert JJ, Hahn AF, Brown JD, Sibbald WA (1987) Critical illness polyneuropathy. A complication of sepsis and multiple organ failure. Brain 110:819–841

Zochodne DW, Ramsay DA, Saly V, Shelley S, Moffatt S (1994) Acute necrotizing myopathy of intensive care: electrophysiological studies. Muscle Nerve 17:285–292

8 Factors Associated with Mortality in Mechanically Ventilated Patients

F. Frutos Vivar, I. Alía Robledo, and A. Esteban de la Torre

Mechanical ventilation is a basic technique for the survival of a significant percentage of patients admitted to intensive care units. This percentage varies widely in the studies published, probably in relation to the type of patients included in them. If we refer to studies designed to ascertain the incidence of mechanical ventilation, where all patients requiring mechanical ventilation for more than 12 h are included, the percentage lies between 39% and 46% [1–11].

The mortality associated with mechanical ventilation has been amply described, with widely varying results. As seen in Table 8.1, mortality may be set at around 40%, although we must always remember that it will depend on different factors. These factors have been analyzed separately in a number of different studies, and on an overall basis in an international study on mechanical ventilation (ISMV) conducted at 391 intensive care units, including 5183 patients who required mechanical ventilation for more than 12 h. For their analysis a distinction was made between the factors presented by the patients at the onset of mechanical ventilation and those factors or complications that appeared during the course of ventilation.

Table 8.1. Mortality studies associated with mechanical ventilation (MV)

Author	Ref.	No. of patients	Type of patients	Mortality (%) ICU	Mortality (%) Hospital
Gillespie et al.	[3]	327	ARF with MOF	81	
Goins et al.	[4]	87	Trauma	17	
Stauffer et al.	[5]	383	Men with acute respiratory failure	39	50
Papadakis et al.	[6]	612	Medical		64
Esteban et al.	[2]	290	Medical-surgical	34	
Yaacob and Mustafa	[7]	58	Exacerbated chronic respiratory failure	60	
Lewandowski et al.	[8]	508	Acute respiratory failure		43
Vasilyev et al.	[9]	1426	Acute respiratory failure		44
Douglas et al.	[10]	57	Medical-surgical MV >5 days		44
Thompson et al.	[11]	139	Heart surgery MV >7 days		36

8.1 Factors Prior to the Onset of Mechanical Ventilation

8.1.1 Age

A number of studies have considered the influence of age on the prognosis of patients who need mechanical ventilation. In general, the results show no influence of age on prognosis, and the differences found in some of the studies are attributed to the prior functional situation and to complications during mechanical ventilation rather than to mere age in itself [12].

In a study of 365 patients (73% under 70 years of age and 27% over), Pesau et al. [13] did not find significant differences in the mortality of the two groups.

In the study by Swinburne et al. [14] there was a significant difference in the mortality by age groups: 69% in patients over 80 years old versus 56% in those under 80. When the factors associated with the increase in mortality are analyzed, however, the premorbid conditions (chronic renal failure, chronic liver disease, cancer, systemic diseases, malnutrition secondary to chronic gastrointestinal disease) have more effect than age; thus patients over 80 with these pathologies had a mortality of 93% versus 71% for younger patients, whereas the mortality was 62% and 51%, respectively, among patients who presented no prior pathology.

In the mechanical ventilation survival study conducted by Stauffer et al. [5], one of the factors associated with mortality was age; patients over 66 years of age had a relative mortality risk (RR 1.32; CI95%: 1.16–1.50) significantly higher than patients under 66.

In a study of 110 patients over 70 years of age requiring mechanical ventilation, Dardaine et al. [15] also corroborated the fact that prior functional situation and the presence of shock upon admission to the ICU were factors with a greater effect on mortality at the ICU, responsible for 38% of the deaths in their study.

We encounter a similar finding in a more recent study [16], where hospital mortality was 38% among patients over 75 years old versus 38.8% in younger patients ($p>0.2$). Cox's analysis confirms that survival does not differ between the two groups – relative risk for elderly patients is 0.82 (CI95%: 0.52–1.29).

In contrast to the above-mentioned studies is the paper published by Cohen et al.[17], where a significant correlation is found between age and mortality ($r^2=0.82$), although, due to the fact that such other factors as stay in the ICU and diagnosis also affect the prognosis, they consider that age should not be taken as the sole factor when it comes to making decisions. There is also the study by Yaacob and Mustafa [7], where increased age had an inverse correlation with survival ($r=0.96$, $p<0.05$).

In the ISMV we observe that the average age of patients who died was higher: 63 years vs. 57 years ($p<0.001$). In accordance with previously published research [16], the population was divided into two groups – those over and those under 75 years of age – and it was found that mortality was associated significantly with age [18], in that the mortality of those over 75 was 52% as compared with 37% for those under 75 – an odds ratio for the group over 75 years old of 1.4 (CI95%: 1.2–1.5).

8.1.2 Gender

As in previously published studies [1, 2], the percentage of women in the ISMV was significantly smaller (39%). As regards mortality, gender had no effect: 41% of women died versus 39% of men – an odds ratio for women of 1.03 (CI95%: 0.96–1.11). This finding is similar to that obtained in a previous study [19], where there was no difference in hospital mortality (women, 36%; men, 40.4%; $p>0.2$) and in the logistic regression analysis sex was not associated independently with mortality. It differs, however, from the results of the study by Kollef et al. [20], with 357 patients needing mechanical ventilation, where mortality was greater among women (28% vs 17.3%; $p=0.016$), female gender being an independent variable associated with mortality – an odds ratio of 2.38 (CI 95%: 1.70–3.35, $p<0.001$).

8.1.3 Reasons for Mechanical Ventilation

Following the traditional classification of reasons for respiratory failure, we will proceed to differentiate three main groups: acute exacerbation of chronic respiratory failure, coma, and acute respiratory failure.

Acute Exacerbation of Respiratory Failure

Although patients with chronic obstructive lung disease (COLD), asthma, and chronic pulmonary disease other than COLD (basically restrictive processes) may be distinguished in this group, we are going to focus our analysis on patients with COLD because of its greater incidence.

Despite the incidence of this disease there are few studies [21–34] on mortality and prognostic factors in COLD. Table 8.2 shows the studies in which the mortality of COLD patients in the ICU and/or in hospital is described. As can be seen, mortality in the ICU lies between 16% and 50% and hospital mortality overall between 32% and 50%. These differences are probably due to differences in the patients' basal situation prior to being included in the studies, since, in those that analyze the factors connected with mortality, it is observed that this situation, estimated in terms of dyspnea and degree of deterioration of the respiratory function tests, correlates significantly with mortality.

A total of 522 patients with COLD were included in the ISMV [35] and a mortality of 23% (CI95%: 19–27) was observed in the ICU, 30% (CI95%: 26–35) in the hospital. In the multivariate analysis, dyspnea at baseline was one of the independent variables connected with mortality: relative risk 2.1 (CI95%: 1.2–3.5).

Coma

The mortality of patients in the ISMV who were admitted due to coma reached a percentage (50%) considerably above the mean for the group as a whole. Since the study design did not differentiate the causes of the coma, this group may contain cases ranging from poisonings to cerebrovascular accidents, which have a very different mortality and prognosis, as we observed in a number of studies that have evaluated it. Thus, the mortality of patients with drug-induced intoxication

Table 8.2. Mortality of COLD patients requiring mechanical ventilation	Authors	Ref.	Mortality (%)	
			ICU	Hospital
	Vanderbergh et al.	[21]	50	
	Sluiter et al.	[22]	35	
	Burk and George	[23]		42
	Bone et al.	[24]		31
	Petheran and Branthwaite	[25]		44
	Gillespie et al.	[3]	25	
	Spicher and White	[26]	51	61
	Menzies et al.	[27]	21	
	Lázaro et al.	[28]	30	
	Ludwigs et al.	[29]	50	53
	Rieves et al.	[30]	43	
	Ancillo et al.	[31]	37	
	Seneff et al.	[32]	16	32
	Añón et al.	[33]	35	50
	Ely et al.	[34]		39

who need mechanical ventilation is 2% in the study by Ludwigs et al. [29], whereas the mortality of patients with cerebrovascular accidents who require mechanical ventilation, primarily due to neurological damage [36], is much higher. Burtin et al. [37] studied 199 patients with cerebral infarction who needed mechanical ventilation; 72% of the patients died during their stay in the ICU. Three variables were associated significantly with this mortality: a Glasgow coma score <10, bradycardia, and absence of brain-stem reflexes.

A recent retrospective study [36] of 230 patients with ischemic stroke or brain hemorrhage requiring mechanical ventilation showed a mortality of 57%. In this study, the prognosis was marked by signs of brain-stem dysfunction.

Acute Respiratory Failure (ARF)

The mortality of patients in need of mechanical ventilation due to acute respiratory failure has been analyzed recently by Vasilyev et al. [9] in a multicenter study conducted in 25 ICUs in the USA and Europe, where 1426 patients with acute respiratory failure of different etiologies were included. The hospital mortality of the total group was 44%, although differences were observed in mortality in relation to the cause of respiratory failure. It was lower for trauma (33%) and pneumonia (37%) and higher for sepsis-induced ARF (54%). Some of these data are similar to those found in the ISMV, where the global mortality of the ARF group was 40% (CI95%: 38–41), there being significant differences between the different ARF etiologies, with a hospital mortality of 66% (CI95%: 61–70) in sepsis patients, of 50% (CI95%: 46–54) – higher than in the aforementioned study – for pneumonia, and of 31% (CI95%: 26–37) for trauma patients.

Special mention has to be made of the high mortality among patients who needed mechanical ventilation due to cardiorespiratory arrest (61%; CI95%:

51–71), an observation already reported by Stauffer et al. [5], where cardiorespiratory arrest was associated with a significant increase in mortality risk (RR 2.88; CI95%: 1.88–4.43).

8.1.4 Severity Scores

At the present time we have a number of different systems for evaluating severity and making a prognosis for critical patients (APACHE, SAPS, MPM, etc.), but none of them has demonstrated its validity when applied solely to mechanically ventilated patients.

Thus, in the study by Portier et al. [38], carried out on 332 patients with chronic lung disease who needed mechanical ventilation for over 24 h, although the mean SAPS was higher in the group that died, it was not possible to establish a correlation between mortality and SAPS.

Something similar happens with APACHE II. In a study of 612 mechanically ventilated patients [6] the mortality observed was 1.15 times higher than that predicted by APACHE II.

In the ISMV, even though the SAPS II of the patients who died was higher than that of those who survived (51 vs 50, $p<0.001$), and having a SAPS II of more than 40 points is associated independently with hospital mortality, an odds ratio of 1.65 (CI95%: 1.25–2.18), the mortality predicted by this severity score was lower than the observed mortality (30.5 vs 39.9%).

One of the explanations for the lack of precision of these severity symptoms may be that it is determined by the changes that take place daily in the clinical situation of the patients [39]; thus in patients with a comparable Acute Physiologic Score (APS) the probability of death increases with the days of stay (Fig. 8.1). This could indicate that if the physiologic state improves or deteriorates during treat-

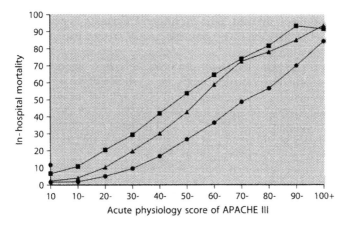

Fig. 8.1. Relation between the APACHE III Acute Physiology Score and the mortality observed for patients who are in the ICU on day 1 (*bottom line*), day 2 (*middle line*), and day 6 (*top line*). [Modified from [39]]

ment, the risk would change. It would also demonstrate that it may be necessary to calculate the APS every day in order to assess response to treatment. In other words, the admission APS is a "static" variable that needs daily correction with the next day's APS and with the increment/decrement from one day to another in order to improve its predictive capability.

8.2 Factors Subsequent to the Onset of Mechanical Ventilation

8.2.1 Method of Mechanical Ventilation

To date the only studies that have evaluated the effect of different types of mechanical ventilation on mortality have been those with ARDS patients. In a study examining all the papers published on the acute respiratory distress prognosis, Kraft et al. [40] found that the mortality was lower among patients who were treated with pressure-controlled ventilation than among patients treated with volume-controlled ventilation (35% vs 54%).

With regard to studies designed for comparing the two methods of ventilation, we find inconsistent results. Thus, in the study by Rapport et al. [41] 37 patients with ARDS were included, and similar mortality was observed in both groups (56% in the PCV group vs 64% in the CMV group), whereas in the study by Esteban et al. [42] higher mortality was observed in the CMV group (78%) than in the PCV group (51%), but this was apparently related more to a higher incidence of renal failure in the CMV group than to the method of ventilation in itself.

Apart from the above-mentioned studies, no trials including the general population of ventilated patients have been done in order to evaluate the impact of the method of mechanical ventilation on mortality.

In the ISMV the ventilation method or methods were recorded daily, and it may be observed that ventilation with CMV or with PCV was associated with an increase in mortality – the odds ratio for hospital mortality in patients ventilated with CMV was 1.45 (CI95%: 1.33–1.58), that in PCV-treated patients 1.49 (CI95%: 1.36–1.64).

Rather than a prognostic factor, however, this finding indicates that the method of mechanical ventilation might be an indicator of severity. Thus, the more severe the condition, the greater the need for ventilation support and use of total ventilation support methods instead of partial support methods, which is reflected in the comparison of the SAPS II of patients receiving each ventilation method, and it may be observed that the patients who were treated with CMV or with PCV had the most severe condition (Fig. 8.2).

This same consideration may apply for the adjuvant techniques or nonconventional methods of mechanical ventilation: inverted I:E, permissive hypercapnia, nitric oxide inhalation, prone position. The use of all these techniques entails a significant increase in mortality (Fig. 8.3). In this case too, however, if we compare the severity of the condition of patients who received any of these techniques with the patients who did not need them, the SAPS II of the former is significantly higher than the SAPS II of the latter (Fig. 8.4).

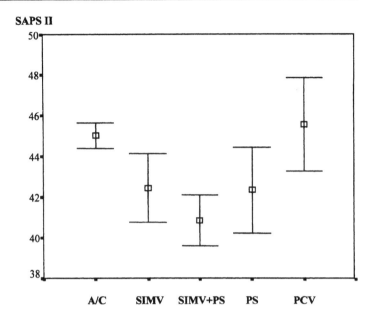

Modes of mechanical ventilation

Fig. 8.2. Comparison of the SAPS II (mean ± standard deviation) of ventilated patients with each method of mechanical ventilation: *A/C*, assisted-controlled; *SIMV*, synchronized intermittent mandatory ventilation; *PS*, pressure support ventilation; *PCV*, pressure-controlled ventilation

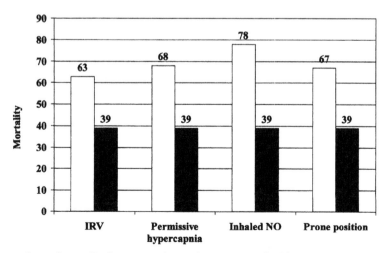

Fig. 8.3. Comparison of mortality between patients who were treated with some nonconventional method of ventilation (*light bars*) and those who did not need any of these methods (*dark bars*). *IRV*, inverted I:E ratio ventilation; *NO*, nitric oxide

SAPS II

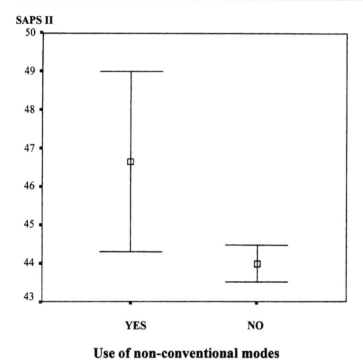

Use of non-conventional modes

Fig. 8.4. Comparison of the SAPS II (mean ± standard deviation) of patients who were treated with some nonconventional ventilation method and those who were not

8.2.2 Gasometric Variables

There are various studies where the relation of PaO_2 to prognosis has been investigated [43]. Doyle et al. [44] made a prospective analysis of 123 patients with acute lung damage. In their study no relation was found between mortality and the components of the Murray score (chest X-ray, compliance, PEEP level, PaO_2/FiO_2 ratio) determined during the first 3 days of hospitalization. Taking a PaO_2/FiO_2 ratio of 300 as the cutoff point, they divided the patients into two groups, but they found no differences in mortality.

Other authors have reported similar results. Thus, in a study of 188 consecutive admissions to a respiratory ICU, no relation was found between PaO_2 and mortality [45]. Another two studies with 63 and 134 patients with respiratory failure secondary to pneumonia [46, 47] show an absence of correlation in the multivariate analysis between the worst PaO_2/FiO_2 ratio in the first 24 h of hospitalization and mortality. In the studies by Jiménez et al. [45] and Potgeiter and Hammond [46] the factors associated with mortality were severity of the patient's condition (measured in the former by the SAPS and in the latter by APACHE II) and the number of organs that failed, which suggests that nonpulmonary dysfunction is the determinant of mortality.

Another standpoint from which we may analyze the possible relationship between hypoxemia and mortality is the one we are offered by calculating some of the gravity scores (SAPS, APACHE, MPM). The three scores include an oxygenation-related variable, which suggests that hospital mortality is related to PaO_2 on admission. An in-depth analysis of the scores, however, does not allow us to draw that conclusion. The oxygenation variable in SAPS II is defined as the lowest PaO_2/FiO_2 ratio value in the first 24 h after admission, in ventilated patients or in those with a pulmonary artery catheter. Thus, what could be associated with mortality is FiO_2, the need for mechanical ventilation, the presence of a pulmonary artery catheter or PaO_2, but the isolated effect of the latter cannot be determined. Something similar happens with APACHE II, where the oxygenation-related variable is the O_2 alveoloarterial gradient, which does not allow the relation between oxygenation and mortality to be evaluated separately either.

In spite of this, there does seem to be an association between the PaO_2/FiO_2 ratio and mortality. We find this association in the analysis of the ISMV data. Figure 8.5 shows the mortality associated with three different cutoff points (<300, <200, <150) of the value of the PaO_2/FiO_2 ratio on two consecutive days during the period mechanical ventilation was maintained. We also find it in the study by Vasilyev et al. [9], where the higher the PaO_2/FiO_2 ratio determined upon admission, the longer the survival: 19.1% for a PaO_2/FiO_2 ratio <100 and 70.4% for a PaO_2/FiO_2 ratio >225.

This may be due to the fact that it would be the FiO_2 rather than the PaO_2 which is associated with mortality. We find a fact supporting this theory in the information obtained from the British Intensive Care Society's APACHE II data base,

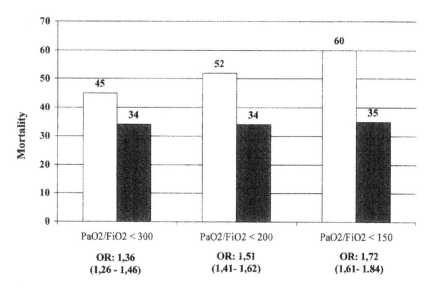

Fig. 8.5. Comparison of the mortality at three different levels of PaO_2/FiO_2 ratio. The *light bars* correspond to patients who had the PaO_2/FiO_2 shown and the *dark bars* to the patients whose PaO_2/FiO_2 ratio remained above the value shown. *OR*, odds ratio; the 95% confidence interval is stated in brackets

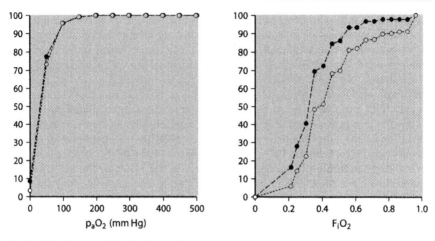

Fig. 8.6. Distribution of deaths (*dotted line*) and survivals (*continuous line*) for the lowest PaO₂ and the highest FiO₂ in the first 24-h stay in the ICU. [Taken from [48]]

which contains data on 7136 patients admitted to 26 units [48]. In Fig. 8.6 we see that there are no differences in the PaO_2 between patients who died and those who survived, while FiO_2 tends to be higher in those who died.

On the other hand, not only in the Vasilyev et al. study [9] but also in the ISMV data it may be observed that both PaO_2 and FiO_2 correlate significantly with mortality. Thus, in the former study [9] a lower rate of survival (<30%) is observed both for patients who present a PaO_2 lower than 60 mmHg at admission and for those needing an FiO_2 above 0.8. In the case of the ISMV, where the mortality associated with having a PaO_2 of less than 60 mmHg and needing an FiO_2 of more than 0.8 for at least two consecutive days during mechanical ventilation was analyzed, both variables were associated in the multivariate analysis, with increased mortality, with greater significance for FiO_2: odds ratio for $FiO_2 \geq 0.8$, 2.90 (CI95%: 2.23–3.78) versus an odds ratio for PaO_2 <60 mmHg, 1.69 (CI95%: 1.01–2.81), while FiO_2 remains as an independent variable associated with mortality in the multivariate analysis.

As regards $PaCO_2$, the presence of hypercapnia at the time of starting mechanical ventilation is not associated with increased mortality in the Vasilyev study [9] and in the ISMV, even though the patients who maintained a $PaCO_2$ above 55 mmHg for 2 days running during the period of mechanical ventilation did exhibit higher mortality (48.4 vs 39.1, $p<0.001$) in the ISVM.

8.2.3 Pulmonary Mechanics Variables

One of the first studies to relate a lung mechanics parameter, specifically static pulmonary compliance, to the mortality of ventilated patients was that conducted by Mancebo et al. [49]. In their study of 55 patients with acute respiratory failure needing mechanical ventilation, they developed a mortality predictive model in which compliance was included as an independent variable. Although no discriminating cutoff point was offered, it was observed that the lower the compliance, the higher the probability of death.

The studies published since then have fixed their attention on pressures in the airway. In the study by Vasilyev et al. [9], a pressure peak at the onset of mechanical ventilation above 50 cmH_2O was associated with a survival of less than 20%, whereas a peak pressure below 30 cmH_2O was associated with a survival of 60%. We find similar data in the ISMV, where the patients who have a peak pressure above 50 cmH_2O for two consecutive days have a mortality of 77%, an odds ratio for hospital mortality of 1.32 (CI95%: 1.17–1.48).

Since, physiologically speaking, the most important estimator of alveolar pressure at the end of inspiration is plateau pressure, this parameter has been the target of the studies published in the past few years. On the basis of the fact that in a person with normal lungs a pressure plateau of 35–40 cmH_2O is sufficient to achieve total pulmonary capacity, this is the maximum safety limit which was adopted at the Consensus Conference on mechanical ventilation of the American College of Chest Physicians [50]. However, in the five randomized clinical trials on tidal volume modification, where plateau pressure differences seem to be a decisive factor in determining the effect of the treatment, the plateau pressure level, which appears to be a predictor of high death risk in patients with ARDS, is 32 cmH_2O [51].

The ISMV analyzed the relation of the two plateau pressure levels proposed – 32 cmH_2O and 35 cmH_2O – to hospital mortality. It was observed that the existence of a plateau pressure above those levels over two consecutive days, at any time during the mechanical ventilation period, is accompanied by a significant increase in mortality. A plateau pressure higher than 32 cmH_2O had a mortality of 70%, an odds ratio of 1.81 (CI95%: 1.63–2.02), and a plateau pressure higher than 35 cmH_2O carried a mortality of 76.5%, an odds ratio of 1.96 (CI95%: 1.75–2.20).

8.2.4 Complications Appearing During Mechanical Ventilation

Barotrauma

There are few studies that examine the relation between the appearance of barotrauma and the mortality of patients receiving mechanical ventilation. In a study of 100 patients with acute lung damage, Schnapp et al. [52] found an incidence of barotrauma of 13% and, although the mortality of patients with barotrauma is not different from that of patients without (76% vs 64%), barotrauma was an independent mortality indicator when adjusted for other predictors, odds ratio 6.15 (CI95%: 1.11–33.9).

In a more recent study [53], conducted on a selected group of subjects (patients with ARDS secondary to sepsis) who had an incidence of pneumothorax and other air leaks of 10.6%, Weg et al. found no relation between the presence of barotrauma and a significant increase in mortality.

In ISVM [54] the incidence of barotrauma – defined as the presence, at any time during the mechanical ventilation period, of any of the following processes connected directly with mechanical ventilation: pneumothorax, subcutaneous emphysema, interstitial emphysema, pneumomediastinum or pneumoperitoneum – was 3%. The patients who presented barotrauma had a higher mortality (60%) than those who did not, odds ratio of 1.5 (CI95%: 1.32–1.76).

Acute Respiratory Distress Syndrome

The majority of studies have described mortality in acute lung injury and in ARDS as being 40%–60% [44, 55–57]. Although a few have suggested that this mortality may be decreasing [58–60], there are one or two recent studies where a mortality similar to the rates in previous decades is described [40, 61]. This observation was confirmed in the ISVM, where the appearance of ARDS – defined as a PaO_2/FiO_2 ratio <200 – had a hospital mortality of 71% [62].

These differences could be determined by the heterogeneity of the populations included in each study, as mortality may depend on various factors: time when the ARDS is diagnosed (the mortality of ARDS as a reason for mechanical ventilation is not the same as when it is a complication after mechanical ventilation has started); failure of organs other than the lungs; prior chronic diseases, especially cirrhosis; sepsis as a risk factor for ARDS; age; and an extrapulmonary cause of ARDS [44, 55, 60–63]. Surprisingly enough, in the studies published to date, the traditional indices of oxygenation and ventilation, including PaO_2/FiO_2 ratio and lung injury score, are not prognostic. In various studies the mortality among patients with an initial PaO_2/FiO_2 ≤300 was similar to that of patients with a ratio of ≤200 [44, 55, 60]. However, the absence of improvement in gas exchange during the first few days of mechanical ventilation is a factor that is related negatively to prognosis [64]. Furthermore, in the past few years special interest has been placed in the prognostic value of the so-called oxygenation rate $[(P_{mean\ of\ the\ airway} \times FiO_2 \times 100)/PaO_2]$. In their study of 229 patients, Monchi et al. [61] found that the oxygenation index was a variable associated with mortality. For their part, in 117 ARDS patients, Meyer et al. [65] compared the mortality predictive capability of the oxygenation index with that of the PaO_2/FiO_2 ratio. In the multivariate analysis, the oxygenation index was predictive of hospital mortality at day 3, odds ratio of 3.5 (CI95%: 1.5–8.6) and also at day 7, odds ratio of 5.9 (CI95%: 1.6–23.3). The PaO_2/FiO_2 ratio was not a predictor of mortality at any time during the clinical course.

Nosocomial Pneumonia

Mortality attributable to ventilator-associated pneumonia (VAP) has been the subject of numerous studies and continues to be a controversial matter. The studies that compared mortality between patients with and those without VAP have reached contradictory conclusions. Other studies, using univariate analysis, have suggested that VAP is associated with increased mortality, but this association is not so evident when a multivariate analysis is carried out. However, the use of logistic regression to control the effect of confounding variables has shown that VAP significantly increases the risk of death in the ICU.

In the ISMV, nosocomial pneumonia was associated with a significant increase in mortality in the univariate analysis: odds ratio of 1.19 (CI95%: 1.08–1.31) but this association was not confirmed in the logistic regression analysis.

In an attempt to clarify this question, in a cohort study with control cases, Heyland et al. [66] compared 177 patients diagnosed as suffering from VAP with the same number of patients without pneumonia. Although there were no significant differences in mortality between patients with and those without VAP (23.7% vs 17.7%, $p=0.16$), the authors reached the conclusion that pneumonia could increase the risk of death by 33% (an absolute risk increase of 5%).

Sepsis

Sepsis continues to show a high mortality despite the improvement in support measures, advances in the knowledge of the inflammatory processes involved in sepsis, and the availability of new and more powerful antibiotics.

A mortality of 56% [67] was observed in a recent review of severe sepsis at French units. During the first 3 days after diagnosis of severe sepsis, shock and acidosis were predictive of mortality. After the first 3 days, the factors associated with mortality were the development of thrombocytopenia, hypothermia, and the presence of various foci of infection.

In a series of 153 patients with clinical evidence of sepsis, Sasse et al. [68] found a hospital mortality of 51%. Likewise, on evaluating the impact of sepsis associated with positive hemocultures in a cohort of 5457 patients admitted to a surgical ICU, Pittet et al. [69] found that the death risk was five times higher for patients with sepsis.

In the ISMV, during the ventilation support period, 567 patients (12%) presented sepsis criteria with a hospital mortality of 62%, and in the univariate analysis sepsis correlated with mortality: odds ratio 1.70 (CI95%: 1.58–1.83).

Multiorgan Failure

If we define multiorgan failure (MOF) as severe acquired dysfunction of at least two organs which is maintained for at least 24–48 h, there are two relevant facts: on the one hand, 15% of the patients admitted to an ICU present with MOF; on the other hand, this is the primary cause of death [70]. We should mention that the incidence of MOF does not appear to have declined in the past few years. The incidence of 48% of MOF in a series of 17,440 patients observed by Zimmerman et al. from 1988 to 1990 was similar to the rate of 44% recorded between 1979 and 1982 [71]. In the ISMV, 28% of the patients who required mechanical ventilation presented with failure of at least one organ.

Various studies have evaluated mortality associated with MOF (Table 8.3). In the ISMV the global mortality of patients with organ failure was 68% and a significant correlation was observed between the number of failed organs and mortality. Thus, patients who presented with failure of one or two organs had a relative death risk of 1.80 (CI95%: 1.68–1.92) and those who presented with failure of more than three organs had a relative risk of death of 2.52 (CI95%: 2.39–2.65). Mortality depends not only on the number of organs that fail, but also on which organ fails. In a 617-patient study Kollef and Sherman [75] evaluated the appearance of MOF and the relative importance presented by each dysfunction: pulmonary, 23.6%; gastrointestinal, 25%; hepatic, 42.4%; hematologic, 47.9%; cardiac, 54%; renal, 54.8% and neurological, 65.9%. Apart from the number of organs that failed and the APACHE II, in the logistic regression analysis the variables that were associated with mortality were cardiac dysfunction, odds ratio of 3.96 (CI95%: 2.63–5.99), and neurological dysfunction, odds ratio of 3.20 (CI95%:

Table 8.3. Incidence and mortality of multiorgan failure

Authors	Ref.	Type of patient	No.	Incidence (%)	Mortality by number of failed organs (%)		
					1	2	3
Bell et al.	[72]	Severe acute respiratory failure	84	47	40	54	80–100
Knauss et al.	[73]	Medical-surgical	5815	15	40	60	100
Spanier et al.	[74]	Liver transplant	113	27	20	20	80–100
Zimmerman et al.	[71]	Medical-surgical	17,440	14	30–60	20–80	80–100

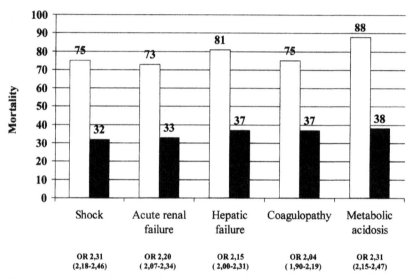

Fig. 8.7. Comparison of mortality between patients who presented with the organ dysfunction shown (*light bars*) and those who did not (*dark bars*). *OR*, odds ratio; the 95% confidence interval is stated in brackets

1.95–5.25). It is seen in Fig. 8.7 that in the ISMV the mortality also depended on the organ that failed during the period of mechanical ventilation.

8.2.5 Mechanical Ventilation Days

A number of authors have found a significant correlation between mechanical ventilation and mortality. In a study in which they analyzed the factors associated with the survival of 383 men with acute respiratory failure who needed mechanical ventilation, Stauffer et al. [5] found that the duration of the mechanical ventilation period had no significant effect on ICU mortality but did reduce hospital survival: Each 5-day increase in the length of the mechanical ventilation period increased the probability of dying in hospital by 1.65 (CI95%: 1.19–2.28).

In the multicenter study conducted by Vasilyev et al. [9], the duration of ventilation support also has a negative impact on survival, so a short period of mechanical ventilation was associated with a longer hospital survival. The patients who received mechanical ventilation for at least 48 h had a survival of 38% versus 30% among those who had mechanical ventilation for more than 2 weeks. Figure 8.8 shows the relation of mechanical ventilation time to mortality observed in the ISMV.

8.3 Conclusion

In the light of the studies published we conclude that the mortality of patients requiring mechanical ventilation due to respiratory failure of any etiology is in the region of 40%, and that this mortality will depend on various factors that we may differentiate into two groups: First, factors connected with the patient's characteristics – age, for instance; with the pathological process, giving rise to the need for mechanical ventilation, e.g., increased mortality in the case of coma, sepsis or community-acquired pneumonia; and with the severity of the patient's condition at the onset of ventilation support. Second, factors which, we could say, will

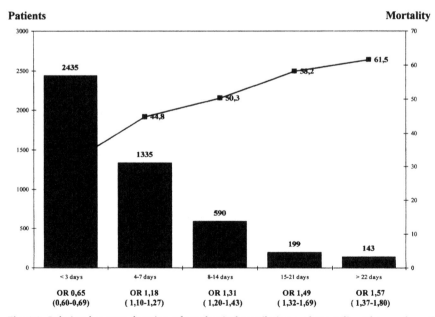

Fig. 8.8. Relation between duration of mechanical ventilation and mortality. The number of patients in each interval of time is shown in *bars* and the mortality in *lines*. *OR*, odds ratio; the 95% confidence interval is shown in brackets

modify with their presence the a priori prognosis presented by a patient, and which appear during the course of the mechanical ventilation period, organ dysfunction being the most important cause of death in this cohort of patients.

8.4 References

1. Esteban A, Anzueto A, Alía I, et al for the Mechanical Ventilation International Study Group (2000) How is mechanical ventilation employed in the intensive care unit? An international utilization review. Am J Respir Crit Care Med 161:1450–1458
2. Esteban A, Alía I, Ibañez J, Benito S, Tobin MJ and the Spanish Lung Failure Collaborative Group (1994) Modes of mechanical ventilation and weaning. A National Survey of Spanish Hospitals. Chest 106:1188–1193
3. Gillespie DJ, Marsh HM, Divertie MB, Meadows JA (1986) Clinical outcome of respiratory failure in patients requiring (>24 hours) mechanical ventilation. Chest 90:364–369
4. Goins WA, Reynolds HN, Wyansom D, Dunham CM (1991) Outcome following prolonged intensive care unit stay in multiple trauma patients. Crit Care Med 19:339–345
5. Stauffer JL, Fayter NA, Graves B, Cromb M, Lynch JC, Goebel P (1993) Survival following mechanical ventilation for acute respiratory failure in adult men. Chest 104:1222–1229
6. Papadakis MA, Lee KK, Browner WS, et al (1993) Prognosis of mechanically ventilated patients. West J Med 159:659–664
7. Yaacob I, Mustafa M (1994) The immediate outcome of ventilation for pulmonary diseases. Singapore Med J 35:512–514
8. Lewandowski K, Metz J, Deutschmann C, et al (1995) Incidence, severity, and mortality of acute respiratory failure in Berlin, Germany. Am J Respir Crit Care Med 151:1121–1125
9. Vasilyev S, Schaap RN, Mortensen JD (1995) Hospital survival rates of patients with acute respiratory failure in modern respiratory intensive care units. An international, multicenter, prospective survey. Chest 107:1083–1088
10. Douglas SL, Daly BJ, Brennan PF, Harris S, Nochomovitz M, Dyer MA (1997) Outcomes of long-term ventilator patients: a descriptive study. Am J Crit Care 6:99–105
11. Thompson MJ, Elton RA, Mankad PA, et al (1997) Prediction of requirement for, and outcome of, prolonged mechanical ventilation following cardiac surgery. Cardiovasc Surg 5:376–381
12. Meinders AJ, van der Hoeven JG, Meinders AE (1996) The outcome of prolonged mechanical ventilation in elderly patients: are the efforts worthwhile? Age Ageing 25:353–356
13. Pesau B, Falger S, Berger E, et al (1992) Influence of age on outcome of mechanically ventilated patients in an intensive care unit. Crit Care Med 20:489–492
14. Swinburne AJ, Fedullo AJ, Bixby K, Lee DK, Wahl GW (1993) Respiratory failure in the elderly. Analysis of outcome after treatment with mechanical ventilation. Arch Intern Med 153:1657–1662
15. Dardaine V, Constans T, Lasfargues G, Perrotin D, Ginies G (1995) Outcome of elderly patients requiring ventilatory support in intensive care. Aging (Milano) 7:221–227
16. Ely EW, Evans GW, Haponik EF (1999) Mechanical ventilation in a cohort of elderly patients admitted to an intensive care unit. Ann Intern Med 131:96–104
17. Cohen IL, Lambrinos J (1995) Investigating the impact of age on outcome of mechanical ventilation using a population of 41,848 patients from a statewide database. Chest 107: 1673–1680
18. Esteban A, Anzueto A, Alía I, et al for the International Mechanical Ventilation Study Group (2000) Indications for, complications from, and outcome of mechanical ventilation: effect of age. Am J Respir Crit Care Med 161:A385
19. Epstein SK, Vuong V (1999) Lack of influence of gender on outcomes of mechanically ventilated medical ICU patients. Chest 116:732–739
20. Kollef MH, Brien JD, Silver P (1997) The impact of gender on outcome from mechanical ventilation. Chest 111:434–441

21. Vandenbergh E, van de Woestijne KP, Gyselin A (1968) Conservative treatment of acute respiratory failure in patients with chronic obstructive lung disease. Am Rev Respir Dis 98:60–69
22. Sluiter HJ, Blokzjil EJ, van Dijl W, van Haeringen JR, Hilvering C, Steenhuis EJ (1972) Conservative and respirator treatment of acute respiratory insufficiency in patients with chronic obstructive lung disease: a reappraisal. Am Rev Respir Dis 105:932–943
23. Burk RH, George RB (1973) Acute respiratory failure in chronic obstructive pulmonary disease: immediate and long-term prognosis. Arch Intern Med 132:865–868
24. Bone RC, Pierce AK, Johnson RL (1978) Controlled oxygen administration in acute respiratory failure in chronic obstructive pulmonary disease: a reappraisal. Am J Med 65:896–902
25. Petheram IS, Branthwaite MA (1980) Mechanical ventilation for pulmonary disease. Anaesthesia 35:467–473
26. Spicher JE, White DP (1987) Outcome and function following prolonged mechanical ventilation. Arch Intern Med 147:421–425
27. Menzies R, Gibbons W, Goldberg P (1989) Determinants of weaning and survival among patients with COPD who require mechanical ventilation for acute respiratory failure. Chest 95:398–405
28. Lázaro A, López-Mesa J, Aragón C, Fernández A, Cerdá E (1990) Evolución a corto y largo plazo de 100 enfermos con EPOC tratados con ventilación mecánica. Med Intensiva 14:245–248
29. Ludwigs UG, Baehrendtz S, Wanecek M, Matell G (1991) Mechanical ventilation in medical and neurologic disease: 11 years of experience. J Intern Med 229:117–124
30. Rieves RD, Bass D, Carter RR, Griffith JE, Norman JR (1993) Severe COPD and acute respiratory failure. Correlates for survival at the time of tracheal intubation. Chest 104:854–860
31. Ancillo P, Cortina JJ, Moreno J, Campos JM, López MJ, Macías S (1994) EPOC y ventilación mecánica en UCI. Med Intensiva 18:18–21
32. Seneff MG, Wagner DP, Wagner RP, Zimmerman JE, Knaus WA (1995) Hospital and 1-year survival of patients admitted to intensive care units with acute exacerbation of chronic pulmonary disease. JAMA 274:1852–1857
33. Añón JM, García de Lorenzo A, Zarazaga A, Gómez-Tello V, Garrido G (1999) Mechanical ventilation of patients on long-term oxygen therapy with acute exacerbations of chronic obstructive pulmonary disease: prognosis and cost-utility analysis. Intensive Care Med 25:452–457
34. Ely WE, Baker AM, Evans GW, Haponik EF (2000) The distribution of costs of care in mechanically ventilated patients with chronic obstructive pulmonary disease. Crit Care Med 28:408–413
35. Alía I, Frutos F, Esteban A, Anzueto A, Benito S for the International Mechanical Ventilation Study Group (2000) Pronóstico de los pacientes BNCO agudizados que reciben ventilación mecánica en la UCI. Med Intensiva 24 [Suppl 1]:58 (abstract)
36. Gujjar AR, Deibert E, Manno EM, Duff S, Diringer MN (1998) Mechanical ventilation for ischemic stroke and intracerebral hemorrhage: indications, timing, and outcome. Neurology 51:447–451
37. Burtin P, Bollaert PE, Feldmann L, et al (1994) Prognosis of stroke patients undergoing mechanical ventilation. Intensive Care Med 20:32–36
38. Portier F, Defouilloy C, Muir JF, and the French Task Group for Acute Respiratory Failure in Chronic Respiratory Insufficiency (1992) Determinants of immediate survival among chronic respiratory insufficiency patients admitted to an intensive care unit for acute respiratory failure. Chest 101:204–210
39. Wagner DP, Knaus WA, Harrell FE, Zimmerman JE, Watts C (1994) Daily prognostic estimates for critically ill adults in intensive care units: results from a prospective, multicenter, inception cohort analysis. Crit Care Med 22:1359–1372
40. Krafft P, Fridrich P, Pernerstorfer T, et al (1996) The acute respiratory distress syndrome: definitions, severity and clinical outcome. An analysis of 101 clinical investigations. Intensive Care Med 22:519–529

41. Rappaport SH, Shpiner R, Yoshihara G, Wright J, Chang P, Abraham E (1994) Randomized, prospective trial of pressure-limited versus volume-controlled ventilation in severe respiratory failure. Crit Care Med 22:22–32

42. Esteban A, Alía I, Gordo F, et al for the Spanish Lung Failure Collaborative Group (2000) Prospective randomized trial comparing pressure-controlled ventilation and volume-controlled ventilation in ARDS. Chest 117:1690–1686

43. Young JD (2000) Hypoxemia and mortality in the ICU. In: Vincent JL (ed) Yearbook of intensive care and emergency medicine. Springer, Berlin Heidelberg New York, pp 239–246

44. Doyle RL, Szaflarski N, Modin GW, Wiener-Kronish JP, Matthay MA (1995) Identification of patients with acute lung injury. Predictors of mortality. Am J Respir Crit Care 152:1818–1824

45. Jimenez P, Torres A, Roca J, Cobos A, Rodriguez-Roisin R (1994) Arterial oxygenation does not predict the outcome of patients with acute respiratory failure needing mechanical ventilation. Eur Respir J 7:730–735

46. Georges H, Leroy O, Vandenbussche C (1999) Epidemiological features and prognosis of severe community-acquired pneumococcal pneumonia. Intensive Care Med 25:198–206

47. Potgieter PD, Hammond JM (1996) The intensive care management, mortality and prognostic indicators in severe community-acquired pneumococcal pneumonia. Intensive Care Med 22:1301–1306

48. Rowan KM, Kerr JH, Major E, McPherson K, Short A, Vessey MP (1993) Intensive Care Society's APACHE II study in Britain and Ireland. I: Variations in case mix of adult admissions to general intensive care units and impact on outcome. Br Med J 307:972–977

49. Mancebo J, Benito S, Martin M, Net A (1988) Value of static pulmonary compliance in predicting mortality in patients with acute respiratory failure. Intensive Care Med 14:110–114

50. Slutsky AS (1993) Mechanical ventilation: American College Of Chest Physicians' Consensus Conference. Chest 104:1833–1859

51. Tobin MJ (2000) Culmination of an era in research on the acute respiratory distress syndrome. N Engl J Med 342:1360–1361

52. Schnapp LM, Chin DP, Szaflarski, Matthay MA (1995) Frequency and importance of barotrauma in 100 patients with acute lung injury. Crit Care Med 23:272–278

53. Weg JG, Anzueto A, Balk RA, et al (1998) The relation of pneumothorax and other air leaks to mortality in the acute respiratory distress syndrome. N Engl J Med 338:341–346

54. Esteban A, Anzueto A, Frutos F, Alía I, Benito S for the International Mechanical Ventilation Group (2000) Barotrauma en los pacientes que reciben ventilación mecánica. Med Intensiva 24 [Suppl 1]:86 (abstract)

55. Zilberberg MD, Epstein SK (1998) Acute lung injury in the medical ICU: comorbid conditions, age, etiology, and hospital outcome. Am J Respir Crit Care Med 157:1159–1164

56. Sloane PJ, Gee MH, Gottlieb JE, et al (1992) A multicenter registry of patients with acute respiratory distress syndrome: physiology and outcome. Am Rev Respir Dis 146:419–426

57. Suchyta MR, Clemmer TP, Elliot CG, Orme JF jr, Weaver LK (1992) The adult respiratory distress syndrome: a report of survival and modifying factors. Chest 101:1074–1079

58. Milberg JA, Davis DR, Steinberg KP, Hudson LD (1995) Improved survival of patients with acute respiratory distress syndrome (ARDS): 1983–1993. JAMA 273:306–309

59. Abel SJC, Finney SJ, Brett SJ, Keogh BF, Morgan CJ, Evans TW (1998) Reduced mortality in association with the acute respiratory distress syndrome (ARDS). Thorax 53:292–294

60. Luhr OR, Antonsen K, Karlsson M, et al (1999) Incidence and mortality after acute respiratory failure and acute respiratory distress syndrome in Sweden, Denmark, and Iceland. The ARF Study Group. Am J Respir Crit Care Med 159:1849–1861

61. Monchi M, Bellenfant F, Cariou A, et al (1998) Early predictive factors of survival in the acute respiratory distress syndrome. A multivariate analysis. Am J Respir Crit Care Med 158:1076–1081

62. Anzueto A, Esteban A, Alía I, et al for the International Mechanical Ventilation Study Group (2000) ARDS before and after mechanical ventilation. Am J Respir Crit Care Med 161:A382

63. Viellard-Baron A, Girou E, Valente E, et al (2000) Predictors of mortality in acute respiratory distress syndrome. Focus on the role of right heart catheterization. Am J Respir Crit Care Med 161:1597–1601

64. Heffner JE, Brown LK, Barbieri CA, Harpel KS, DeLeo J (1995) Prospective validation of an acute respiratory distress syndrome predictive score. Am J Respir Crit Care Med 152:1518–1526
65. Meyer J, Wong DT, Yacoub A, Wong G, Bohn D, Kavanagh BP (2000) Oxygenation index vs PaO_2/FiO_2 ratio to predict outcome in ARDS. Am J Respir Crit Care Med 161:A210
66. Heyland DK, Cook DJ, Griffith L, Keenan SP, Brun-Buisson C, for the Canadian Critical Care Trials Group (1999) The attributable morbidity and mortality of ventilator-associated pneumonia in the critically ill patient. Am J Respir Crit Care 159:1249–1256
67. Brun-Buisson C, Doyon F, Carlet J, et al for the French ICU Group for severe sepsis (1995) Incidence, risks factors, and outcome of severe sepsis and septic shock in adults: a multicenter prospective study in intensive care units. JAMA 274:968–974
68. Sasse KC, Nauenberg E, Long A, et al (1995) Long-term survival after intensive care unit admission with sepsis. Crit Care Med 23:1040–1047
69. Pittet D, Thievent B, Wenzel RP, et al (1996) Bedside prediction of mortality from bacteremic sepsis: a dynamic analysis of ICU patients. Am J Respir Crit Care Med 153:684–693
70. Matuschak GM (1998) Multiple organ system failure: clinical expression, pathogenesis, and therapy. In: Hall JB, Schmidt GA, Wood LDH (eds) Principles of critical care, 2nd edn. McGraw-Hill, New York, pp 221–248
71. Zimmerman JE, Knaus WA, Wagner DP, Sun X, Hakim RB, Nystrom PO (1996) A comparison of risks and outcomes for patients with organ system failure: 1982–1990. Crit Care Med 24:1633–1641
72. Bell RC, Coalson JL, Smith JD, Johanson WG (1983) Multiple organ system failure and infection in adult respiratory distress syndrome. Ann Intern Med 99:293–298
73. Knaus WA, Draper EA, Wagner DP, Zimmerman JE (1985) APACHE II: a severity of disease classification system. Crit Care Med 13:818–829
74. Spanier TB, Klein RD, Nasraway SA, et al (1995) Multiple organ failure after liver transplantation. Crit Care Med 23:466–473
75. Kollef MH, Sherman G (1999) Acquired organ system derangements and hospital mortality: are all organ systems created equally? Am J Crit Care 8:180–183

9 Pathophysiology of Weaning-Associated Respiratory Failure

C.S.H. Sassoon, A. Manka, and K.G. Chetty

Supported by the Department
of Veterans Affairs Medical Research Service

9.1 Introduction

Weaning of a small proportion of patients receiving mechanical ventilatory support from mechanical ventilation poses a challenge to the clinician in charge of their care. In general, the etiology of unsuccessful weaning is related to the incomplete resolution of the underlying illness that dictates the need for ventilatory support, the development of ventilator-associated complications, or new problems. The cause of weaning failure is multi-factorial (Jubran and Tobin 1997; Vassilakopoulos et al. 1998), and an isolated factor can rarely be defined. Regardless of the etiologies, the fundamental derangement underlying weaning-associated respiratory failure is a decrease in respiratory neuromuscular capacity (Table 9.1) and

Table 9.1. Decreased respiratory neuromuscular capacity. (Adapted from Tobin et al. 1998)

1. Decreased respiratory center drive
2. Phrenic nerve dysfunction
3. Decreased neuromuscular transmission
4. Decreased respiratory muscle strength and/or endurance
   a) Hyperinflation
   b) Sepsis
   c) Decreased oxygen supply
   d) Hypoxemia
   e) Cardiovascular dysfunction
   f) Organ dysfunction with "stealing effect"
   g) Malnutrition
   h) Mineral and electrolyte abnormalities
   i) Acid-base disorder
   j) Endocrine disorder
   k) Drug-induced neuro/myopathy
   l) Respiratory muscle fatigue
   m) Disuse muscle atrophy or muscle injury

Table 9.2. Excessive load to the respiratory muscles. (Adapted from Tobin et al. 1998)

1. Increased ventilatory demand
   a) Increased CO_2 production
   b) Increased dead-space ventilation
   c) Inappropriate increased respiratory drive (e.g., anxiety)
2. Increased mechanical workload
   a) Increased resistive load
   b) Increased lung and/or chest wall elastic load
   c) Elevated intrinsic positive end-expiratory pressure (PEEPi)

an excessive load to the respiratory system (Table 9.2), particularly the respiratory muscles (Tobin et al. 1998). The pattern of breathing in these patients is generally rapid and shallow (Jubran and Tobin 1997). The best method for determining the interplay among the factors involved in weaning failure is an experimental design, with the patients acting as their own control during both failed and successful trials. The two most recent studies which have met the above criterion (Vassilakopoulos et al. 1998, Capdevila et al. 1998) will be the basis of this review article.

9.2 Imbalance Between Respiratory Neuromuscular Capacity and Respiratory Muscle Load

In the first study, Vassilakopoulos and co-workers (1998) studied 30 patients with chronic obstructive pulmonary disease (COPD; $n=10$), adult respiratory distress syndrome (ARDS; $n=10$) and other categories such as trauma and pneumonia ($n=10$). The patients had mechanical ventilatory support for 14–20 days prior to the study, and the average interval between failed and successful weaning trial was 9 days. During the failed trial, the patients had a markedly elevated load to the respiratory muscles, which decreased significantly during the subsequent successful weaning trial. The elevated respiratory muscle load was reflected by the increased intrinsic positive end-expiratory pressure (PEEPi), maximum respiratory system resistance (Rmax), and the ratio of mean to maximum inspiratory airway pressure (PI/PImax) (Table 9.3). At the same time, the ability to generate maximum inspiratory pressure (PImax) was reduced during the failed weaning trial and improved during the successful trial. Dynamic hyperinflation was also present, altering the coupling of the diaphragm and rib-cage expansion and producing inadequate tidal volume (VT) (Grassino et al. 1994). Indeed, the breathing pattern of these patients was more rapid and shallow during the failed weaning trial than during the successful weaning trial (Table 9.3). The imbalance between respiratory muscle load and neuromuscular capacity resulted in increased energy demand, estimated as the tension-time index (TTI) of the global respiratory muscles. TTI during the failed trial fell within the critical threshold (0.15–0.18) above which respiratory muscle fatigue will occur (Bellemare and Grassino 1982) (Fig. 1, panel A). Using multiple logistic regression analysis, these investigators demonstrated that the TTI and f/VT ratio were the main pathophysiological determinants of weaning failure.

Table 9.3. Respiratory muscle load and frequency-to-tidal volume ratio during failed and successful weaning trials

		Vassilakopoulos et al. (1998) $n=30$	Capdevila et al (1998) $n=11$
PEEPi (cmH$_2$O)	Failure	6.1±2.5	na
	Success	3.9±2.7	na
Rmax (cmH$_2$O/l/s)	Failure	14.1±4.9	na
	Success	11.2±4.0	na
PI (cmH$_2$O)	Failure	22.3±1.3	28.1±9.1
	Success	17.9±1.5	19.7±5.5
PImax (cmH$_2$O)	Failure	48.4±13.3	47.7±13.7
	Success	57.6±14.6	54.0±15.4
PI/PImax (cmH$_2$O)	Failure	0.46±0.1	0.59±0.7
	Success	0.31±0.1	0.36±0.4
TTI (PI/PImax	Failure	0.16±0.03	0.34±0.20
× Ti/Ttot)	Success	0.10±0.02	0.10±0.10
f/VT (min/l)	Failure	98±38	93±30
	Success	62±21	56±21

PEEPi, intrinsic positive end-expiratory pressure; *Rmax*, maximum respiratory system resistance; *PI*, mean airway pressure; *PImax*, maximum inspiratory airway pressure; *PI/PImax*, ratio of mean airway pressure to maximum airway pressure; *TTI*, tension-time index; *f/VT*, ratio of respiratory frequency to tidal volume. *na*, not available. Values are mean ±SD.

In the second study, Capdevila et al. (1998) determined respiratory muscle load and capacity in 17 difficult-to-wean patients who had been on prolonged mechanical ventilation for an average of 20 days and had undergone tracheotomies. Eleven of the patients who had initially failed the trial were eventually able to sustain spontaneous breathing, with an average interval of 19 days between trials. Six of the patients continued to require mechanical ventilation. This study allows intra- and intergroup comparisons of respiratory muscle load and function. In the group of those who eventually weaned successfully, the initial mean PI was elevated but decreased significantly during the successful trial (Table 9.3). Similarly, the initial average TTI of 0.34, a value which falls within their predetermined critical threshold for respiratory muscle fatigue (TTI of 0.27–0.43), decreased to 0.10 during the successful weaning trial (Table 9.3, Fig. 1, panel B). In this study, mean PI (for the calculation of TTI) was derived from the measurement of airway occlusion pressure (P0.1) in which PI=5 P0.1 × inspiratory time (TI) (Ramonatxo et al. 1995). In the group of those who subsequently weaned successfully, the P0.1 decreased from a mean of 7.2 cmH$_2$O to 3.6 cmH$_2$O. In contrast, in the group who remained ventilator dependent, indices of respiratory muscle load (PI), energy demand (TTI), and P0.1 remained elevated. The breathing pattern was also more rapid and shallow during the failed weaning trial than when they weaned successfully (Table 9.3).

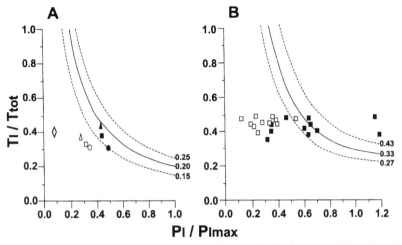

Fig. 9.1 A,B. Tension-time index of patients who initially failed weaning (*closed symbols*) and who eventually weaned successfully (*open symbols*). All patients served as their own control. A presents data from Vassilakopoulos et al. 1998 (with permission). The data are mean values of three groups (ten patients in each group) consisting of patients with COPD (*circle*), ARDS (*triangle*) and other categories (*square*). During the failed weaning trial, TTI fell at or above the critical threshold value of respiratory muscle fatigue of 0.15. At the time of successful weaning, TTI fell below its critical threshold value. For comparison, the TTI of a healthy subject is indicated by the *diamond* symbol. B presents data from Capdevila et al. 1998 (with permission). Only the data of patients who initially failed and subsequently weaned successfully are displayed. Initially, seven of 11 such patients had TTI greater than 0.27, according to the modified calculation of TTI (see text for explanation). During the successful weaning trial, all but one had TTI below 0.27

9.2.1 Respiratory Muscle Load

Both of the above studies (Vassilakopoulos et al. 1998, Capdevila et al. 1998) have clearly demonstrated that the major determinants of weaning failure are the excessive load to the respiratory muscles, together with a decrease in their capacity. A decrease in the load imposed on the respiratory muscles with a concomitant increase in capacity, reduced energy demand, and a more efficient breathing pattern resulted in a successful weaning outcome. In patients with COPD who failed a weaning trial, a large proportion of inspiratory muscle effort was expended to overcome both PEEPi and resistive load (20% and 42%, respectively), and to a lesser extent non-PEEPi elastic load (Jubran and Tobin 1997). However, at the end of the trial, the increase in inspiratory effort to overcome these respiratory loads was 111%, 42%, and 33%, respectively (Fig. 9.2). Similarly, in patients with ARDS, PEEPi and resistive load contributed 19% and 55% of the total inspiratory muscle work, respectively (Vassilakopoulos et al. 1998). Elevated airflow resistance in patients with ARDS has already been shown (Pelosi et al. 1995). The increased resistance is most likely due to a reduced lung volume and possibly to a reduced amount of ventilated lung, rather than to anatomic airway narrowing (Pelosi et al. 1995).

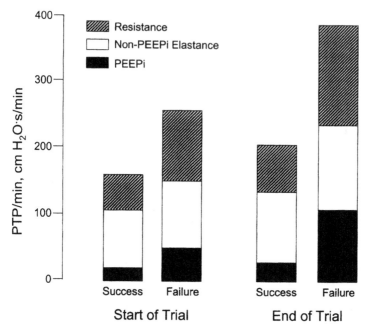

Fig. 9.2. Partitioning of pressure-time product during weaning trial of patients with COPD into resistive (*hatched rectangles*), nonintrinsic positive-end expiratory pressure elastic (*non-PEEPi*) and PEEPi components at the start and end of the trial in the success (*n=14*) and failure (*n=17*) groups. At the end of the trial, the increase in PTP/min in the failure group was due to increases in the PEEPi component by 111%, in the nonPEEPi elastic component by 33%, and in the resistive component by 42%. The increase in PTP/min at the end of the trial in the success group resulted primarily from the increase in non-PEEPi elastic and resistive components, but not from the PEEPi component. (From Jubran and Tobin 1997, with permission)

9.2.2 Respiratory Muscle Capacity

Does a decrease in central neuromuscular drive contribute to the decreased neuromuscular capacity? In Jubran and Tobin's study of 17 patients with COPD (1997), inspiratory excursions of the esophageal pressure (Pes) increased at the end of the weaning trial, in comparison to those at the beginning of the trial, suggesting that central neuromuscular drive was not depressed. Using P0.1 as a measure of neuromuscular drive, Capdevila and co-workers (1998) found similar results. In 11 of the patients who were eventually weaned, P0.1 was elevated during the failed weaning trial and decreased as the patients weaned successfully. In fact, in the patients who were ventilator dependent, P0.1 remained elevated throughout the study trials (8.9 and 9.8 cmH$_2$O). It appears that for the majority of patients who fail weaning, the reduced respiratory muscle capacity does not result from depressed central neuromuscular drive.

Does phrenic nerve dysfunction contribute to the decreased neuromuscular capacity? Critical illness polyneuropathy (CIP) has been implicated as a cause of weaning difficulty (Leijten et al. 1995). CIP is defined as a predominantly axonal polyneuropathy with acute onset in a setting of systemic inflammatory response with multiple organ dysfunction. However, it has not been determined how *diaphragmatic denervation* with and without CIP contributes to weaning failure. In a recent retrospective study, 44 of 102 patients met the electrodiagnostic criteria for CIP. Twenty-four (54%) of these patients had diaphragmatic denervation; however, the clinical history of the majority of them suggested that the diaphragmatic denervation was caused by mechanisms other than CIP, such as cardioplegia, high cervical trauma, and mediastinal pathology (Sander et al. 1999). Of the patients who did not meet the electrodiagnostic criteria for CIP, 13 (22%) had diaphragmatic denervation that could be explained by the clinical presentation. Similarly, a prospective study by Leijten et al. (1996) found no convincing association between CIP and weaning failure. These studies suggest that it is unlikely that the decreased respiratory muscle capacity is related to phrenic nerve dysfunction.

Does the increase in TTI to its critical threshold value indicate inspiratory muscle fatigue? Respiratory muscle fatigue is defined as a condition in which the muscle is incapable of developing force and/or velocity as a result of activity under load which is reversible by rest (NHLBI Workshop Summary 1990). Two types of contractile fatigue have been described, according to the force generated at different discharge frequencies of the motor nerves. High-frequency fatigue is the reduced contractile force of a muscle at stimulation frequency of 50–100 Hz, and occurs soon after exposure to a very high load. After removal of the load, the muscle's force-generating capacity recovers rapidly (Aubier et al. 1981). High-frequency fatigue is thought to result from accumulation of intracellular hydrogen ions, inorganic phosphates, altered calcium concentrations in the sarcoplasmic reticulum, or T-tubules which may interfere with action potential propagation (Grassino et al. 1994). High discharge frequencies occur in human beings only when they are exposed to a very heavy load that can be sustained very briefly (Bigland-Ritchie 1984). During regular breathing, the discharge frequency of the parasternal intercostal and scalene motor nerve is 7–14 Hz in healthy subjects and 8–19 Hz in patients with COPD (Gandevia et al. 1996). Similarly, the discharge frequency of phrenic motoneurons is 9–12 Hz in healthy subjects and 14–22 Hz in patients with COPD (De Troyer et al. 1997). The decreased contractile force at this stimulation frequency is called low-frequency fatigue. In contrast to high-frequency contractile fatigue, the development of low-frequency contractile fatigue requires a prolonged period of loading, as well as a longer period of recovery, i.e., more than 24 h (Laghi et al 1995). This form of fatigue is thought to result from load-induced injury (Reid et al. 1994), which in turn may be mediated by the production of oxygen-free radicals (Anzueto et al. 1994). Load-induced injury may also be mediated by mechanical disruption of the sarcolemma and/or sarcoplasmic reticulum, with consequent entry of calcium into the cytoplasm, activating lipolytic and proteolytic enzymes to degrade membrane phospholipid and myofilament proteins (Armstrong et al. 1991). The load-induced injury appears in the form of myofibril disruption with loss of distinct A and I bands and development of Z-band streaming. Irrespective of the mechanisms, even modest respiratory muscle loads, comparable to those endured by patients with severe obstructive pulmonary disease, can induce substantial muscle damage (Zhu et al. 1997). Although it is tempting to speculate that load-induced injury occurs in the human diaphragm and is associated with weaning difficulty, such evidence is still lacking.

In animal experiments, the ventilator mode itself appears to be responsible for the decrease in force generation of the diaphragm (Bourdelles et al. 1994; Anzueto et al. 1997). Two days of controlled mechanical ventilation were sufficient to result in a decrease of 42% in the diaphragm force-generating capacity compared with that of the control animals (Bourdelles et al. 1994). In the study of Anzueto and co-workers (1997), transdiaphragmatic pressure (Pdi) decreased 38% from the initial Pdi after 11 days of controlled mechanical ventilation. Preliminary observation from our laboratory seems to support earlier findings of other investigators (Bourdelles et al. 1994; Anzueto et al. 1997). Sarcomere disruption was observed in the animals that were placed on mechanical ventilation for 3 days, but not in animals breathing spontaneously (Sassoon et al. 1996). If a similar condition in human beings can be inferred, controlled mechanical ventilation may contribute to the diminished respiratory muscle capacity.

Bellemare and Grassino (1982) proposed the tension-time index (TTI) as an alternative to pressure-time product for quantifying the magnitude and duration of muscle contractions. They found that during inspiratory resistive loading, at a diaphragm TTI of less than 0.15, breathing could be sustained indefinitely. On the other hand, above this critical threshold value, endurance time was limited. Capdevila et al. (1998) used the modified TTI as described by Ramonatxo et al. (1995), in which the calculation of mean PI was based on measurement of P0.1 (PI=5 P0.1 × TI). With this method, the critical threshold value equivalent to the diaphragm TTI was 0.33. Although in the studies of both Vassilakopoulos et al. (1998) and Capdevila et al. (1998) the average TTI during the failure trial exceeded the critical threshold value, this was not observed in the study of Jubran and Tobin (1997). Only five of the 17 patients who failed the weaning trial had a TTI of greater than 0.15 at the end of the trial. One of the limitations of measurement with TTI is an underestimation of the maximum force generation included in the calculation of TTI. This is due to the dynamic hyperinflation which commonly develops in the critically ill patients and which reduces the force-generating capacity of the inspiratory muscles. Although a TTI above the critical threshold value indicates respiratory muscle fatigue, a recent study by Laghi et al. (1998) shows that in healthy subjects breathing against inspiratory resistive loading, progressive diaphragm muscle fatigue occurs even before the development of task failure. Diaphragm muscle fatigue was assessed as the decline in twitch Pdi produced with magnetic stimulation of the phrenic nerves. Hence, respiratory muscle fatigue of the low-frequency contractile type may develop and may be responsible for the decreased neuromuscular capacity in the patients who failed weaning.

9.3 Pattern of Breathing During Weaning Failure

The majority of patients who fail weaning demonstrate a rapid shallow breathing pattern (Jubran and Tobin 1997; Vassilakopoulos et al. 1998; Capdevila et al. 1998), and in fact, the frequency to tidal volume ratio (f/VT) has been used as the most simple index for predicting the outcome of weaning (Yang and Tobin 1991). Some investigators have attributed its development to respiratory muscle fatigue (Cohen et al. 1982). However, if a rapid shallow breathing pattern were an effective strategy for avoiding respiratory muscle fatigue, a significant correlation between the degree of rapid shallow breathing pattern and a measure of respiratory muscle fatigue would be expected. Jubran and Tobin (1997) demonstrated a poor correlation between f/VT and TTI ($r=0.08$) in the 17 patients who failed weaning. Vassilakopoulos et al. (1998) also showed a lack of relationship between f/VT and TTI in their 30 patients who failed weaning trial ($r=0.16$). The pathophysiological mechanism(s) responsible for the rapid shallow breathing pattern is unknown and may be the result of increased mechanical load, chemoreceptor stimulation, operating lung volume, reflexes originating from the lungs and respiratory muscles, altered respiratory motoneuron discharge patterns, sense of effort, and cortical influences (Jubran and Tobin 1997).

In summary, the mechanism of weaning-associated respiratory failure is the imbalance between respiratory muscle load and respiratory neuromuscular capacity. The reduced respiratory muscle capacity may be due to respiratory muscle fatigue. A practical and reliable method for detecting respiratory muscle fatigue in critically ill patients would be a welcome addition to our understanding of the pathophysiology of weaning-associated respiratory failure. With the availability of magnetic stimulation to the phrenic nerve, the realization of such a method may not be too far off.

9.4 References

Anzueto A, Supinski GS, Levine SM, Jenkinson SG (1994) Mechanisms of disease: are oxygen-derived free radicals involved in diaphragmatic dysfunction? Am J Respir Crit Care Med 149:1048–1052

Anzueto A, Peters JI, Tobin MJ, De Los Santos R, Seidenfeld JJ, Moore G, Cox WJ, Coalson JJ (1997) Effects of prolonged controlled mechanical ventilation on diaphragmatic function in healthy adult baboons. Crit Care Med 25:1106–1107

Armstrong RB, Warren GL, Warren JA (1991) Mechanisms of exercise-induced muscle fiber injury. Sports Med 12:349–356

Aubier M, Farkas G, De Troyer A, Mozes R, Roussos C (1981) Detection of diaphragmatic fatigue in man by phrenic stimulation. J Appl Physiol 50:538–544

Bellemare F, Grassino A (1982) Effect of pressure and timing of contraction of human diaphragm fatigue. J Appl Physiol 53: 1190–1195

Bigland-Ritchie B (1984) Muscle fatigue and the influence of changing neural drive. Clin Chest Med 5:21–34

Bourdelles GL, Viires N, Boczkowski J, Seta N, Pavlovic D, Aubier M (1994) Effects of mechanical ventilation on diaphragmatic contractile properties in rats. Am J Respir Crit Care Med 149: 1539–1544

Capdevila X, Perrigault PF, Ramonatxo M, Roustan JP, Peray P, d'Athis F, Prefaut C (1998) Changes in breathing pattern and respiratory muscle performance parameters during difficult weaning. Crit Care Med 26:79–87

Cohen CA, Zagelbaum G, Gross D, Roussos C, Macklem PT (1982) Clinical manifestations of inspiratory muscle fatigue. Am J Med 73:308–316

De Troyer A, Leeper JB, McKenzie DK, Gandevia SC (1997) Neural drive to the diaphragm in patients with severe COPD. Am J Respir Crit Care Med 155:1335–1340

Gandevia C, Leeper JB, McKenzie DK, De Troyer A (1996) Discharge frequencies of parasternal intercostal and scalene motor units during breathing in normal and COPD subjects. Am J Respir Crit Care Med 153: 622–628

Grassino A, Comtois N, Galdiz HJ, Sinderby C (1994) The unweanable patient. Monaldi Arch Chest Dis 49:522–526

Jubran A, Tobin MJ (1997) Pathophysiologic basis of acute respiratory distress in patients who fail a trial of weaning from mechanical ventilation. Am J Respir Crit Care Med 155:906–915

Laghi F, D'Alfonso N, Tobin MJ (1995) Pattern of recovery from diaphragm fatigue over 24 hours. J Appl Physiol 79:539–546

Laghi F, Topeli A, Tobin MJ (1998) Does resistive loading decrease diaphragmatic contractility before task failure? J Appl Physiol 85:1103–1112

Leijten FSS, Harinck-De Weerd JE, Poortvliet DCJ, De Weerd AW (1995) The role of polyneuropathy in motor convalescence after prolonged mechanical ventilation. JAMA 274: 1221–1225

Leijten FSS, De Weerd AW, Poortvliet DCJ, De Ridder VA, Ulrich C, Harinck-De Weerd JE (1996) Critical illness polyneuropathy in multiple organ dysfunction syndrome and weaning from the ventilator. Intensive Care Med 22: 856–861

NHLBI Workshop Summary (1990) Respiratory muscle fatigue: report of the respiratory muscle fatigue workshop group. Am Rev Respir Dis 142:474–480

Pelosi P, Cereda M, Foti G, Giacomini M, Pesenti A (1995) Alterations of lung and chest wall mechanics in patients with acute lung injury: effects of positive end-expiratory pressure. Am J Respir Crit Care Med 152:531–537

Ramonatxo M, Boulard P, Prefaut C (1995) Validation of a noninvasive tension-time index of inspiratory muscles. J Appl Physiol 78:646–653

Reid WD, Huang J, Bryson S, Walker DC, Belcastro AN (1994) Diaphragm injury and myofibrillar structure induced by resistive loading. J Appl Physiol 76:176–184

Sander HW, Saadeh PB, Chandswang N, Greenbaum D, Chokroverty S (1999) Diaphragmatic denervation in intensive care unit patients. Electromyogr Clin Neurophysiol 39:3–5

Sassoon CSH, Yeam I, Gruer SE, Wuerker RB, Caiozzo VJ, Sieck GC. Effect of controlled mechanical ventilation on diaphragm contractile properties (1996) Am J Respir Crit Care Med 153:A372

Tobin MJ, Laghi F, Jubran A (1998) Respiratory muscle dysfunction in mechanically ventilated patients. Mol Cell Biochem 179:87–98

Vassilakopoulos T, Zakynthinos S, Roussos C (1998) The tension-time index and the frequency/tidal volume ratio are the major pathophysiologic determinants of weaning failure and success. Am J Respir Crit Care Med 158:378–85

Yang K, Tobin MJ (1991) A prospective study of predicting outcome of trials of weaning from mechanical ventilation. N Engl J Med 324: 1445–1450

Zhu E, Petrof BJ, Gea J, Comtois N, Grassino AE (1997) Diaphragm muscle fiber injury after inspiratory resistive breathing. Am J Respir Crit Care Med 155:1110–1116

10 Rapid Shallow Breathing: Causes and Consequences

A. Jubran

A patient failing a weaning trial often shows physical signs of respiratory distress, such as increased usage of accessory muscles, retraction of intercostal spaces, paradoxical motion of the abdomen, and cyanosis. A common finding on physical exam in a weaning failure patient is tachypnea – one of the earliest signs of impending respiratory disaster.

When breathing pattern was studied systematically during weaning, patients who fail a weaning trial developed an increase in respiratory frequency and a fall in tidal volume (V_T) immediately upon discontinuation of mechanical ventilation [1] (Fig. 10.1). It was reasoned that measuring these changes might be useful in predicting weaning outcome. Subsequently, Yang and Tobin [2] measured fre-

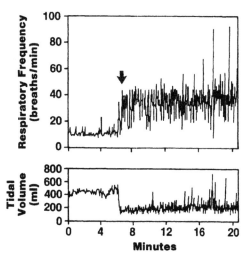

Fig. 10.1. A time-series, breath-by-breath plot of respiratory frequency and tidal volume in a patient who failed a weaning trial. The *arrow* indicates the point of resuming spontaneous breathing following discontinuation of ventilator support. Rapid shallow breathing developed almost immediately, suggesting the prompt establishment of a new steady state. Although it has been considered that rapid shallow breathing may reflect the presence of respiratory muscle fatigue, its almost instantaneous development without subsequent progression is difficult to reconcile with the development of respiratory muscle fatigue. (From [1], with permission)

quency and V_T over 1 min using a simple hand-held spirometer. These measurements were made while the patient was disconnected from the ventilator and breathing room air. Then they combined these measurements into an index of rapid shallow breathing, the frequency-to-tidal volume ratio (f/V_T ratio), and evaluated its usefulness as a predictor of weaning. In an initial "training data set", an f/V_T ratio of 105 breaths/min/l provided the best separation between patients who were successfully weaned and those in whom weaning failed. This threshold was then prospectively evaluated in 64 patients. The index had a positive predictive value of 0.78 and a negative predictive value of 0.95. Analyzing the data with receiver operating characteristic (ROC) curves, the area under the curve for the f/V_T was the highest of ten weaning predictors.

The pathophysiological basis for the development of rapid shallow breathing is unknown. A shortened inspiratory time (T_I) with a consequent decrease in tidal volume indicates that a resetting of the inspiratory cutoff point is a major problem in weaning failure patients [1]. So the failure patients appear to have a reduction not in overall motor output but rather in the distribution of volume and time components.

Patients with COPD commonly display tachypnea, which is a maladaptive response, since the accompanying reductions in T_I and expiratory time (T_E) decrease end-inspiratory and increase end-expiratory lung volume, respectively. This truncation in V_T volume from below and above may be sufficient to offset any increase in minute ventilation resulting from tachypnea. Moreover, a decrease in tidal volume leads to an increase in dead-space ventilation (V_D/V_T) and hypercapnia. Furthermore, since expiratory muscle recruitment is ineffective in patients with airflow limitation, these patients are unable to lower end-expiratory lung volume and they become dependent on inspiratory pressure activity – a response pattern that is energetically inefficient because of the nonlinear relationship between pressure generation and ventilation [3–5].

10.1 Causes of Rapid Shallow Breathing

Several factors might be responsible for the development of rapid shallow breathing. These include chemoreceptor stimulation, increased lung volume, reflexes originating in the lungs and respiratory muscles, altered motoneuron discharge patterns, sense of effort, and cortical influences [6–9]. These factors are interdependent, making the mechanism of a net response pattern extremely difficult to decipher.

It has been suggested that alterations in loading might be an important factor in the development of rapid shallow breathing. To address this issue, passive mechanics were measured in weaning-failure and weaning-success patients right before they were taken off the ventilator prior to the T-piece trial [10]. Respiratory system resistance was not different between the two group of patients. When resistance was partitioned into the ohmic component, reflecting airway resistance, and the component arising from stress inhomogeneities in the system secondary to pendelluft and viscoelastic properties, no differences were observed between the two groups. Likewise, dynamic elastance of the respiratory system ($E_{dyn,rs}$) was found to be similar between the groups before the trial. Dynamic elastance ($E_{dyn,L}$) was significantly higher in the failure group than in the success group (Fig. 10.2), but the individual values showed a considerable overlap among the patients in the two groups, thus limiting its usefulness in signaling a patient's ability to sustain spontaneous ventilation. That the respiratory mechanics were similar in the two groups before the start of the weaning trial suggests that an increase in loading is likely not to be an important underlying mechanism of rapid shallow breathing.

During spontaneous breathing, however, changes in lung mechanics were observed between weaning-success and weaning-failure patients [6]. Dynamic elastance was higher in the failure than in the success group at 2 min into the trial of spontaneous breathing, and it increased more in the failure than in the success group throughout the trial. Inspiratory resistance was similar in the two groups at 2 min of the trial of spontaneous breathing. At the end of the trial, resistance increased in the failure group whereas it remained unchanged in the successfully weaned patients.

At the start of the trial, intrinsic positive end-expiratory pressure (PEEPi) was higher in the failure than in the success group, and this variable was higher in the failures throughout the course of the trial. The increase in PEEPi at the start of the trial is most likely due to high respiratory rate. The associated decease in expiratory time does not allow sufficient time for emptying of lung units with long time constants, and therefore, end-expiratory lung volume or FRC increases. Tidal volume, frequency, and inspiratory resistance accounted

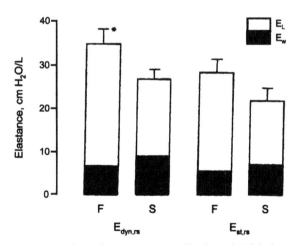

Fig. 10.2. Dynamic ($E_{dyn,rs}$, overall column height) and static ($E_{st,rs}$, overall column height) elastance of the respiratory system in the weaning-failure (F) and weaning-success (S) groups during passive ventilation; the *white* portions of the columns represent lung elastance while the *shaded* portions represent chest wall elastance. $E_{dyn,L}$ was higher in the failure group than in the success group ($p<0.01$), and $E_{dyn,rs}$ tended to be higher in the failure group ($p=0.07$); $E_{dyn,w}$ was not different between the two groups. $E_{st,L}$ tended to be higher in the failure group than in the success group ($p=0.07$), while $E_{st,rs}$ and $E_{st,w}$ were not significantly different between the two groups. *Upward-directed bars* represent ±SE of lung elastance (E_L), while *downward-directed bars* represent ±SE of chest wall elastance (E_w). (From [10], with permission)

for 85% of the variance in PEEPi, highlighting the importance of rapid shallow breathing as a cause of PEEPi.

During the weaning trial, patient effort was quantitated using pressure-time product (PTP), which is the time integral difference between esophageal pressure and chest wall recoil pressure [6, 11]. Both an upper and a lower bound PTP were calculated to include the entire possible range of patient effort. Upper bound PTP assumes that the decrease in esophageal pressure is due to dynamic hyperinflation, whereas lower bound PTP assumes that it is due to cessation of expiratory effort. At the beginning of the trial, upper and lower bound PTP were not different between the two groups. Between the beginning and the end of the trial of spontaneous breathing, both indices of PTP increased in the failure and the success groups. Over the course of the trial, the failure group had higher values of both upper bound and lower bound PTP than the success patients.

An increase in the energy expenditure of the respiratory muscles can place these patients at an increased risk for fatigue. To determine whether fatigue is likely in these patients, the tension-time index of the inspiratory muscles was measured at the start and at the end of the trial. Five of 17 failure patients had values above 0.15 – a value that has been shown to be associated with respiratory muscle fatigue in normal subjects. This observation suggests that diaphragmatic fatigue does occur in some weaning-failure patients. Of course, the tension-time index has limitations and cannot be accepted as definitive proof of fatigue.

10.2 Consequences of Rapid Shallow Breathing

Patients who fail a trial of spontaneous breathing develop an increase in arterial carbon dioxide tension ($PaCO_2$). The $PaCO_2$ is determined by the relationship between the metabolic production of CO_2 and alveolar ventilation. In turn, a reduction in alveolar ventilation could be due to a decrease either in overall minute ventilation or in ratio of physiological dead space to V_T [12]. The minute ventilation in itself is not a significant determinant of CO_2 retention, as it is similar in weaning-failure and weaning-success patients [1]. Instead, the increase in $PaCO_2$ is due to differences in frequency and V_T (Fig. 10.3), and these two variables account for 80% of the variance in $PaCO_2$. Thus one of the consequences of rapid shallow breathing is an increase in $PaCO_2$ with an inevitable increase in dead-space ventilation.

The failure group developed an increase not only in $PaCO_2$ but also in PTP. Normally, as one increases effort, PCO_2 should fall; that is PCO_2 is inversely proportional to PTP. On rearranging this equation, the product of PCO_2 and PTP is equivalent to a constant, k. The more efficient the respiratory muscle pump, the lower the value of k and vice versa. So the $PCO_2 \times PTP$ product can be used as an index of the efficiency of the respiratory muscle pump.

At the end of the trial of spontaneous breathing, the $PTP \times PCO_2$ product was found to be twice as high in the failure group as in the success group [6]. Using a threshold of 13, all but one of the failure patients had a value above it and all but three of the successes had a value below it. When the f/VT ratio was added to this product, the separation between the two groups is complete except for one patient in each group (Fig. 10.4).

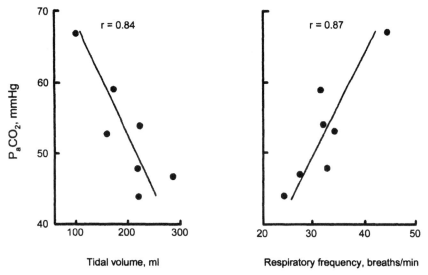

Fig. 10.3. Relationship between tidal volume (V_T) and respiratory frequency with carbon dioxide tension ($PaCO_2$) in seven patients who failed a spontaneous breathing trial. $PaCO_2$ was significantly correlated with VT ($r=0.84$, $p<0.025$) and frequency ($r=0.87$, $p<0.025$); 81% of the variance in $PaCO_2$ could be explained by the changes in these two variables (From [1], with permission)

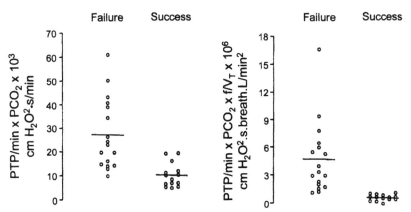

Fig. 10.4. *Left panel*: PTP/min $\times$ PCO_2 product, an index of the inefficiency of the respiratory pump in clearing CO_2, was higher in the failure group than in the success group at the end of the trial of spontaneous breathing ($p<0.0005$). *Right panel*: PTP/min $\times$ PCO_2 $\times$ f/V_T product was higher in the failure than in the success group at the end of the trial of spontaneous breathing ($p<0.0001$). *Bar* indicates group mean value. (From [6], with permission)

It has been suggested that the development of rapid shallow breathing in patient's being weaned from mechanical ventilation is a helpful indication of respiratory muscle fatigue. In a study of 12 patients who were having weaning difficulty, Cohen and co-workers [13] observed that seven developed a fall in high/low ratio of the power spectrum of the diaphragmatic electromyogram (EMG), which they considered indicative of diaphragmatic fatigue. These initial changes in the EMGs were followed by an increase in respiratory rate and rapid shallow breathing and abdominal paradox. The investigators concluded that rapid shallow breathing was a manifestation of fatigue. Several limitations of the study exist. First, all patients, including those without EMG changes and an abnormal breathing pattern, were returned to mechanical ventilation within 40 min, thus limiting the clinical significance of these findings. Also, a shift in the power spectrum of the EMG has not been shown to bear a relationship to the form of fatigue that is physiologically important, i.e., low-frequency fatigue. In addition, no attempt was made to separate the effect of the work of breathing from fatigue in these patients.

Cohen et al. [13] concluded that abdominal paradox was a reliable sign of respiratory muscle fatigue. Tobin et al. [14] found that asynchrony and paradox of the rib cage and abdomen were more severe in patients who failed weaning than in those who were successfully weaned. However, there was considerable overlap among individual patients in the two groups, indicating that spontaneous ventilation can be sustained despite the presence of abdominal paradox.

To determine the pathophysiological basis of abnormal rig cage-abdominal motion, healthy volunteers were studied while breathing against resistive loads [15]. Paradoxical volumes increased during the first minute of loaded breathing, did not progress during the loaded breathing run, and returned to baseline immediately following discontinuation of the load. So it is clear that respiratory muscle fatigue is neither a sufficient nor a necessary condition for the development of rib cage-abdominal asynchrony or paradox, and that the abnormal motion is determined primarily by load rather than by fatigue.

The importance of fatigue as a mechanism of rapid shallow breathing was studied during CO_2 rebreathing before and after the induction of fatigue in healthy subjects using Hey plot analysis (Fig. 10.5) [16]. The slope of V_T and minute ventilation was decreased following the induction of diaphragmatic fatigue, indicating that the breathing pattern became slower and deeper. These data suggest that it is unlikely that rapid shallow breathing is a manifestation of fatigue.

A small V_T decreases work per breath and sense of effort/dyspnea [17]. Accordingly, shallow breathing has been considered a useful strategy to avoid fatigue [18, 19]. In disease states, however, a low V_T is almost always accompanied by an increase in frequency, so that energy expenditure per unit increases, especially with the simultaneous development of dynamic hyperinflation and hypercapnia. Respiratory muscle work is least with a normal breathing pattern – that is, frequency of 17 breath/min, V_T of 400 ml, and f/V_T 43 b/min/l. Employing the model of Otis and colleagues [20], an increase in f/V_T will result in an exponential increase in work of breathing: $work=40356e^{(0.0017 \times f/V_T)}$, $r=0.90$. Although admittedly crude, tension-time index appears to be the best available framework for considering the risk of fatigue. Data on patients who failed a trial of spontaneous breathing indicate that rapid shallow breathing was not a useful strategy for

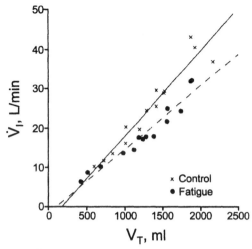

Fig. 10.5. The minute ventilation: tidal volume ($\dot{V}_I : V_T$) relationship before (*crossed symbols, continuous line*) and following induction of diaphragmatic fatigue (*closed symbols, interrupted line*) in a representative subject. The slope of the ($\dot{V}_I : V_T$) relationship was significantly reduced with fatigue, indicating that the breathing pattern became relatively slower and deeper. (Based on data from [16])

avoiding fatiguing contractions; to serve as a compensatory strategy, f/V_T should have a negative correlation with tension-time index, whereas r was 0.08 [6].

In summary, the cause of rapid shallow breathing is unknown and is likely to involve several different mechanisms, including increased chemoreceptor and mechanoreceptor stimulation, increased mechanical load, increased operating lung volume reflexes, sense of effort, and cortical influences. This is the aspect of rapid shallow breathing that we know the least.

The consequences of rapid shallow breathing are the following: The decrease in tidal volume will cause an increase in physiological dead space, leading to an increase in $PaCO_2$. The increase in frequency is associated with a decrease in expiratory time, which, in turn, leaves insufficient time for lung emptying; as a result, hyperinflation and PEEPi develop. The rapid shallow breathing and PEEPi both can lead to an increase in the work of breathing. Whether or not this leads to fatigue needs to be further studied.

10.3 References

1. Tobin MJ, Guenther SM, Perez W, Mador MJ, Semmens BJ, Allen SJ, et al (1986) The pattern of breathing during successful and unsuccessful trials of weaning from mechanical ventilation. Am Rev Respir Dis 134:1111–1118
2. Yang K, Tobin MJ (1991) A prospective study of indexes predicting outcome of trials of weaning from mechanical ventilation. N Engl J Med 324:1445–1450
3. Dodd DS, Brancastisano T, Engel LA (1984) Chest wall mechanics during exercise in patients with severe chronic air-flow obstruction. Am Rev Respir Dis 129:33–38

4. Younes M (1993) Mechanisms of ventilatory failure. Current pulmonology. Mosby-Year Book, St. Louis, pp 243–292
5. O'Donnell DE, Webb KA (1993) Exertional breathlessness in patients with chronic airflow limitation: the role of hyperinflation. Am Rev Respir Dis 148:1351–1357
6. Jubran A, Tobin MJ (1997) Pathophysiological basis of acute respiratory distress in patients who fail a trial of weaning from mechanical ventilation. Am J Respir Crit Care Med 155:906–915
7. Tobin MJ (1998) Noninvasive monitoring of ventilation. In: Tobin MJ (ed) Principles and practice of intensive care monitoring. McGraw-Hill, New York, pp 465–495
8. Winning AJ, Widdicombe JG (1976) The effect of lung reflexes on the pattern of breathing in cats. Respir Physiol 27:253–266
9. Tallarida G, Baldoni F, Peruzzi G, Raimondi G, Massaro M, Abate A, et al (1983) Different patterns of respiratory reflexes originating in exercising muscle. J Appl Physiol 55:84–91
10. Jubran A, Tobin MJ (1997) Passive mechanics of lung and chest wall in patients who failed and succeeded in trials of weaning. Am J Respir Crit Care Med 155:916–921
11. Jubran A, Van de Graaff WB, Tobin MJ (1995) Variability of patient-ventilator interaction with pressure- support ventilation in patients with COPD. Am J Respir Crit Care Med 152:129–136
12. Sorli J, Grassino A, Lorange G, Milic-Emili J (1978) Control of breathing in patients with chronic obstructive pulmonary disease. Clin Sci Mol Med 54:295–304
13. Cohen C, Zagelbaum G, Gross D, Roussos C, Macklem PT (1982) Clinical manifestations of inspiratory muscle fatigue. Am J Med 73:308–316
14. Tobin MJ, Guenther SM, Perez W, Lodato RF, Mador MJ, Allen SJ, et al (1987) Konno-Mead analysis of ribcage-abdominal motion during successful and unsuccessful trials of weaning from mechanical ventilation. Am Rev Respir Dis 135:1320–1328
15. Tobin MJ, Perez W, Guenther SM, Lodato RF, Dantzker DR (1987) Does ribcage-abdominal paradox signify respiratory muscle fatigue? J Appl Physiol 63:851–860
16. Mador MJ, Tobin MJ (1992) The effect of inspiratory muscle fatigue on breathing pattern and ventilatory response to CO_2. J Physiol (Lond) 445:17–32
17. Jones GL, Killian KJ, Summers E, Jones NL (1985) Inspiratory muscle forces and endurance in maximum resistive loading. J Appl Physiol 58:1608–1615
18. Roussos C, Moxham J, Bellemare F (1995) Respiratory muscle fatigue. In: Roussos C (ed) The thorax. Dekker, New York, pp 1405–1461
19. Yan S, Sliwinski P, Gauthier AP, Lichros I, Zakynthinos S, Macklem PT (1993) Effect of global inspiratory muscle fatigue on ventilatory and respiratory muscle responses to CO_2. J Appl Physiol 75:1371–1377
20. Otis AB, Fenn WO, Rahn H (1950) The mechanics of breathing in man. J Appl Physiol 2:592–607

11 Cardiopulmonary Interactions and Gas Exchange During Weaning from Mechanical Ventilation

M. Ferrer, J. Roca, and R. Rodriguez-Roisin

Supported by the Comissionat per a Universitats i Recerca,
Generalitat de Catalunya (1999 SGR 00228)

11.1 Introduction

The major function of the lung is to exchange physiological (respiratory) gases, namely, oxygen (O_2) and carbon dioxide (CO_2). In normal conditions, an equilibrium between oxygen uptake (VO_2) and carbon dioxide elimination (VCO_2) in the lungs, and the metabolic demands regarding oxygen consumption and carbon dioxide production, must be attained with whatever partial pressures of both gases in arterial blood are necessary to achieve this equilibrium. Only when the lungs fail as a gas exchanger do arterial hypoxemia and hypercapnia or both appear, and respiratory failure ensues. Arterial oxygen (PaO_2) and carbon dioxide ($PaCO_2$) tensions are the directly measurable end-point variables used routinely by clinicians to properly manage patients with acute respiratory failure. When this is severe, mechanical ventilation is then considered the best strategy for treating patients. Traditionally, the mechanisms of hypoxemia are alveolar hypoventilation, limitation of alveolar to end-capillary O_2 diffusion, shunt, and ventilation-perfusion (V_A/Q) mismatching; major causes of hypercapnia are alveolar hypoventilation and V_A/Q inequalities [1].

Ideally, it would be of great interest to clinicians to direct therapy toward blood gas measurements only, including their most common calculated indices, i.e., alveolar-arterial PO_2 difference (A-aO_2), venous admixture ratio (Q_S/Q_T), and physiologic dead space (V_D/V_T), as a general functional marker of the overall status of the lung. Thus impaired or improved results of all these variables, the principal merits of which are their simplicity and the relative ease of access to measurement, could correspond to impaired or improved pulmonary gas exchange, respectively. Unfortunately, all these variables reflect not only the state of the lung, i.e., V_A/Q inequality, shunt, and limitation of O_2 diffusion, but also the conditions under which the lung is operating. These conditions, which uniquely determine the PO_2 and PCO_2 in any single gas exchange unit of the lung, are the V_A/Q ratio, the composition of the inspired gas, and the composition of the mixed venous blood [2]. It is important to appreciate the key role played by these three factors governing the respiratory gases in any single gas-exchange unit.

Weaning from mechanical ventilation is a critical period in the evolution of patients admitted to intensive care units (ICUs). The resolution of two important factors regarding the behavior of pulmonary function is involved in weaning success. First, a higher activity of the respiratory muscles is needed at the beginning of spontaneous breathing, thus increasing the metabolic demands of the organism (increased O_2 consumption and CO_2 production), which must be compensated with an increased efficacy of the lung as gas exchanger. Second, the ventilatory and hemodynamic changes accompanying the switch from mechanical to spontaneous ventilation give way to a profound remodeling of the interactions between the intra- and extrapulmonary factors determining the arterial blood partial pressure of respiratory gases.

11.2 Factors Determining PaO$_2$

In contrast to more traditional views, the mechanisms of hypoxemia are currently classified as intrapulmonary and extrapulmonary (Table 11.1). Assessment of the intrapulmonary factors of abnormal gas exchange using the multiple inert gas elimination technique (MIGET) represents a major conceptual breakthrough in our understanding of the pathophysiology of pulmonary disease states [3, 4]. The basic principles and technical details of MIGET have been addressed extensively in other publications [5]. The MIGET has three major advantages: (a) It estimates the pattern of pulmonary blood flow and alveolar ventilation and calculates the mismatch of V_A/Q relationships; (b) it partitions the alveolar-arterial PO_2 difference into components of shunt, V_A/Q inequality, and limitation of diffusion of O_2; and (c) it apportions and unravels arterial oxygenation into intrapulmonary and extrapulmonary components. Of great importance is the ability to perform measurements at any level of inspired fraction of O_2 (F_IO_2) without perturbing the vascular and bronchial wall tone, since the level of F_IO_2 need not be altered.

Table 11.1. Factors determining arterial hypoxemia

Intrapulmonary	Extrapulmonary	
V_A/Q mismatch	Major:	↓ alveolar ventilation
Shunt		↓ cardiac output
O_2 diffusion limitation		↓ PiO$_2$
		↑ O_2 consumption
	Secondary:	↓ P_{50}
		↓ [Hb]
		↑ pH

V_A/Q, ventilation-perfusion; *[Hb]*, hemoglobin concentration; P_{50}, PO_2 corresponding to 50% of oxyhemoglobin saturation.

11.2.1 Intrapulmonary Factors

Heterogeneity of V_A/Q relationships is, undoubtedly, the most important cause of hypoxemia in the vast majority of patients during weaning from mechanical ventilation. In fact, V_A/Q mismatch is the principal mechanism of hypoxemia in patients with respiratory failure secondary to exacerbations of chronic airflow limitation – e.g., chronic obstructive pulmonary disease (COPD), asthma – throughout the period of exacerbation [6, 7]. The presence of increased intrapulmonary shunt (perfusion of unventilated alveolar units, i.e., V_A/Q ratios equal to zero) [8] plays a minor secondary role as a mechanism of hypoxemia during early stages of exacerbation of COPD, due to obstruction of peripheral airways caused by mucus retention and plugging, with insufficient compensation by collateral ventilation, never exceeding 10% of cardiac output. Other factors causing hypoxemia, such as limitation of alveolar to end-capillary O_2 diffusion [9], are negligible. It has occasionally been reported that reopening of the *foramen ovale* associated with abrupt increases in chronic pulmonary hypertension can cause hypoxemia secondary to shunt during the early stages of acute exacerbation of the disease, but this is infrequent during weaning. Even in diseases such as the acute respiratory distress syndrome (ARDS) [10], where increased intrapulmonary shunt is the major mechanism of arterial hypoxemia, this mechanism does not play a vital role during weaning from mechanical ventilation.

Arterial PO_2 and PCO_2 of each alveolar unit, and thus, PO_2 and PCO_2 at the end of the pulmonary capillary (if limitation of alveolar to end-capillary O_2 diffusion is not present), are essentially determined by (a) the composition of inspired gas; (b) the partial pressures of these gases in mixed venous blood; and, (c) the ventilation-to-perfusion (V/Q) ratio. The V/Q ratio can range from nonventilated but perfused alveolar units (V/Q = 0 or intrapulmonary shunt) to ventilated but nonperfused alveolar units (V/Q equal to infinite or physiologic dead space). Alveolar units with very low V/Q ratios, near to zero, behave similar to shunt alveolar units, in that their PO_2 and PCO_2 values are similar to those from mixed venous blood. When room air is breathed (F_IO_2) = 0.21, as V/Q ratios increase, increases in alveolar PO_2 (PAO_2) and decreases in alveolar PCO_2 ($PACO_2$) occur. Oxyhemoglobin is nearly completely saturated at the end of the pulmonary capillary in alveolar units with V/Q ratios higher than 0.1. In alveolar units with V/Q ratios = 1 at F_IO_2 0.21, values of PAO_2 and $PACO_2$ are approximately 100 and 40 mmHg, respectively. When V/Q ratio increases, PAO_2 and $PACO_2$ become similar to those of inspired gas. In an alveolar unit with V/Q equal to infinite, PAO_2 is approximately 150 mmHg and $PACO_2$ is nearly 0 mmHg. However, due to the sigmoid shape of the dissociation curve of oxyhemoglobin, the presence of alveolar units with high V_A/Q rations is not associated with a significant increase of the arterial oxygen content.

Figure 11.1 illustrates V_A/Q distributions in a healthy young individual breathing room air at rest, obtained with MIGET. Each data point represents a particular amount of blood flow or alveolar ventilation, while overall pulmonary perfusion and total ventilation correspond to the sum of the data points (the lines have been drawn for clarity only). These quantities (distributions) are plotted against a large range of 50 V_A/Q ratios from zero (shunt) to infinity (dead space) on a log scale. The unimodal profile of each distribution has three main components: symmetry,

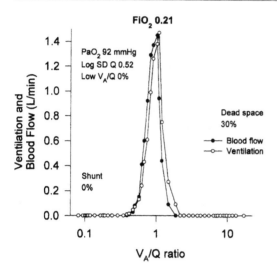

Fig. 11.1. Distributions of alveolar ventilation and pulmonary blood flow plotted versus V_A/Q ratio

location around a V_A/Q ratio of 1.0, and narrowness (i.e., very little dispersion). Note that there is no inert gas shunt (compared with the concept of venous admixture ratio) since the tracer nature of inert gases used for MIGET is insensitive to the presence of postpulmonary shunt (i.e., the bronchial and thebesian circulations). Inert gas physiologic dead space is also slightly lower than Bohr's dead space (approximately 30% of alveolar ventilation) because it does not include the alveolar units which have an alveolar PCO_2 that is lower than arterial blood.

The patterns of disordered V_A/Q distributions characteristic of different diseases have been extensively described in the literature [6, 10–19]. In the analysis of the V_A/Q distributions we are considering the following aspects: the shape (unimodal or bimodal) and dispersion (or second moment) of the perfusion (log SD Q) and ventilation (log SD V) distributions; the position of these distributions (first moment of both distributions, mean Q and V, respectively); and the magnitude of the two extreme compartments (shunt and dead space). Intrapulmonary shunt has been previously defined as the percent of perfusion directed to non-ventilated alveolar units (V_A/Q ratios <0.005), and dead space is the percent of ventilation to nonperfused alveolar units (V_A/Q ratios >100).

11.2.2 Extrapulmonary Factors

Alveolar ventilation (V_A), the fraction of inspired O_2, cardiac output (Q_T) and O_2 consumption (VO_2) are considered the most relevant extrapulmonary factors influencing arterial oxygenation (Table 11.1). Other factors playing a secondary role are blood pH, hemoglobin concentration, and the affinity of the dissociation curve of oxyhemoglobin (P_{50}). Alveolar ventilation is considered an extrapulmonary factor because it is determined by the tidal volume, the physiologic dead space, and the respiratory frequency, modulated in part by the mechanisms of the control of ventilation.

Increases of F_IO_2 have a great impact on PaO_2 and the arterial O_2 content (CaO_2) in disorders of the V_A/Q distributions characterized by an increase in the perfusion to areas with V/Q ratios lower than the unit (between 0.01 and 1.0). When V_A/Q distributions are normal, the increase in F_IO_2 is associated with an increase in PaO_2 but, due to the shape of the oxyhemoglobin dissociation curve, the impact on the CaO_2 is minimal. By contrast, as stated above, when arterial hypoxemia is caused by an increase of intrapulmonary shunt, as occurs in ARDS, increases in F_IO_2 are not associated with significant increases in PaO_2.

The effects of alveolar ventilation on arterial respiratory blood gases have been documented extensively [20]. When V_A/Q distributions are normal, increases of ventilation are effective in increasing PaO_2 and decreasing $PaCO_2$ without causing significant changes in CaO_2, due to the shape of the oxyhemoglobin dissociation curve. However, when V_A/Q relationships are severely impaired, the increase in alveolar ventilation is more effective in reducing $PaCO_2$ than in increasing PaO_2.

Cardiac output can influence arterial oxygenation via three mechanisms [21]. The most important is due to the relation between Q_T and mixed venous O_2 content (C_VO_2), according to the Fick principle ($VO_2 = Q_T \cdot (CaO_2 - C_VO_2)$). If metabolic requirements remain constant, a decrease in Q_T will go along with an increase in the peripheral O_2 extraction to keep VO_2 constant; thus, C_VO_2 and mixed venous PO_2 (P_VO_2) will decrease. As stated above, P_VO_2 is an important determinant of arterial oxygenation. A second mechanism influencing arterial oxygenation can occur in those clinical conditions (emphysema, pulmonary fibrosis) in which the increase of Q_T (i.e., during exercise) is not accompanied by an effective recruitment of pulmonary capillaries. Under these circumstances, the transit time of erythrocytes through the pulmonary capillary will decrease, thus facilitating, in an impaired lung parenchyma, hypoxemia due to limitation of alveolar to end-capillary O_2 diffusion [19]. The third mechanism by which Q_T influences gas exchange is intrapulmonary redistribution of blood flow, in the well-known association between increases in Q_T and intrapulmonary shunting [22, 23], whose underlying mechanism is poorly known.

Changes in VO_2 can modulate PaO_2 through the above-described relation between C_VO_2 and P_VO_2 (Fick principle). Arterial PO_2 is less sensitive to changes in VO_2 in conditions causing predominantly increased intrapulmonary shunt (i.e., ARDS) than in conditions causing V_A/Q mismatching and increased perfusion to alveolar units with low V_A/Q ratios (i.e., COPD).

11.3 Factors Determining PaCO$_2$

Factors influencing CO_2 retention can be of either intrapulmonary origin, such as V_A/Q mismatching, as extensively described above [1], or extrapulmonary origin, including (a) decrease of effective alveolar ventilation; (b) changes in acid-base equilibrium; and (c) increases of CO_2 production (VCO_2) [24].

Regarding decreases of alveolar ventilation, disorders of ventilatory mechanics leading to respiratory muscle fatigue must be considered. Chest wall deformities, neuromuscular disorders, and disorders of the control of ventilation associated with changes of the breathing pattern are the most important extrapulmonary factors, potentially causing decreases of effective alveolar ventilation and, consequently, development of hypercapnia.

Metabolic alkalosis can cause depression of the respiratory drive even in subjects with normal lungs. Finally, increases in VCO_2 during exercise, fever, parenteral nutrition with high carbohydrate intake, or laparoscopic surgery with pneumoperitoneum using CO_2 can be factors facilitating the development of hypercapnia, especially in patients with underlying lungs diseases unable to appropriately increase effective alveolar ventilation.

11.4 Summary of Physiologic Concepts

In summary, there are several determinants governing PaO_2 and $PaCO_2$ in critically ill patients [25]. The most important intrapulmonary factors are V_A/Q mismatching and increased intrapulmonary shunt; in contrast, diffusion limitation of O_2 plays a minor role. Among extrapulmonary factors, inspired PO_2, overall ventilation, cardiac output, and O_2 uptake are the most influential. Note that the three intrapulmonary factors plus one of the extrapulmonary determinants, O_2 consumption, are not under the direct control of the physician, although the remaining extrapulmonary factors are. By manipulating mechanical ventilation, clinicians may easily control inspired PO_2, the amount and pattern of total ventilation, and cardiac output, particularly when positive endexpiratory pressure (PEEP) is applied or the patient exhibits significant intrinsic PEEP (PEEPi). Cardiac output also may be influenced directly by the use of pharmacological agents. Arterial PO_2 may fall due to decreases in inspired PO_2, overall ventilation, and/or cardiac output, and/or an increase in O_2 consumption, even though the intrapulmonary factors remain unaltered. Conversely, increases in inspired PO_2, ventilation, and/or cardiac output and/or a decrease in O_2 consumption may produce an increase in PaO_2, irrespective of changes in the intrapulmonary factors. Note also that the three intrapulmonary factors in combination with total ventilation represent the four classic mechanisms of hypoxemia and hypercapnia [1]. Finally, changes in the minor factors influencing the oxyhemoglobin dissociation curve also may determine PaO_2, although minimally, just as changes in acid-base status and/or in CO_2 production may significantly influence the level of $PaCO_2$.

This is why PaO_2 and $PaCO_2$ become the end-point variables of the interaction of all these intrapulmonary and extrapulmonary determinants of gas exchange. This represents a more appealing approach to proper interpretation of arterial blood gas abnormalities at the bedside and is important to an understanding of the gas exchange response to mechanical ventilation.

11.5 Nature of Gas Exchange in Disease States

From the clinical standpoint, the three principal mechanisms of altered arterial respiratory gases during spontaneous breathing in any pulmonary disease state are V_A/Q mismatching, increased intrapulmonary shunt, and alveolar hypoventilation. The role of diffusion limitation to O_2 is modest and plays only a small role in patients with pulmonary fibrosis [19] and in healthy individuals under very extreme conditions such as strenuous exercise [26]. During mechanical ventilation, however, alveolar hypoventilation is under control in such a way that $PaCO_2$ does not represent a problem by itself, except when clinical conditions concur to increase $PaCO_2$ in order to protect the lung from barotrauma or volutrauma. V_A/Q inequality plays a pivotal role in those disorders essentially characterized by chronic lung disease ("dry lung"), namely COPD and bronchial asthma, which have in common expiratory airflow limitation, large pulmonary volumes, and intrinsic PEEP, whereas increased intrapulmonary shunt is a key determinant of hypoxemia in conditions characterized by acute lung injury ("wet lung"), such as acute respiratory distress syndrome (ARDS) and severe life-threatening pneumonia, having in common small lung volumes [27].

11.5.1 Acute Lung Injury ("Wet Lung")

Although it may occasionally be difficult to differentiate ARDS from other causes of acute lung injury (after all, ARDS is a constellation of many entities, among which pneumonia, trauma, and cardiac surgery are common causes), it is clear that from the viewpoint of gas exchange, functional findings are different. Furthermore, the response to high inspired O_2 concentrations differs substantially among these disorders.

Gas exchange in patients with acute lung injury behaves differently according to the underlying disorder. Patients with ARDS show moderate to severe increases in intrapulmonary shunt as the major cause of hypoxemia, although approximately half of these patients have some degree of V_A/Q inequality (blood flow distributed to areas with low V_A/Q ratios) [28]. The application of PEEP induces a reduction of shunt and an increase of dead space, whereas V_A/Q distributions remain essentially unaltered. Figure 11.2 represents two patterns of V_A/Q distributions in patients with ARDS with and without PEEP. Patients with severe life-threatening pneumonia have both moderate to severe increases in intrapulmonary shunt and a moderate degree of low V_A/Q regions (greater than in patients with ARDS) [18, 29]. Figure 11.3 represents the pattern of V_A/Q distributions in a patient with pneumonia under mechanical ventilation. While breathing 100% O_2, patients with ARDS increase shunt, but the dispersion of blood flow remains essentially unchanged, suggesting the development of reabsorption atelectasis without release of hypoxic pulmonary vasoconstriction [30]; moreover, arterial oxygenation will not increase substantially, due to refractory hypoxemia. In contrast, in patients with severe pneumonia, intrapulmonary shunt remains unaltered, while the dispersion of pulmonary perfusion increases significantly, suggesting that hypoxic pulmonary vasoconstriction is released [18]. Increases in PaO_2 are higher in the latter than in ARDS patients. Diffusion limitation for O_2, as an additional mechanism of hypoxemia, is never present (Table 11.2). Gas-exchange characteristics in patients with head trauma or following cardiac surgery do not differ significantly from those in patients with severe pneumonia.

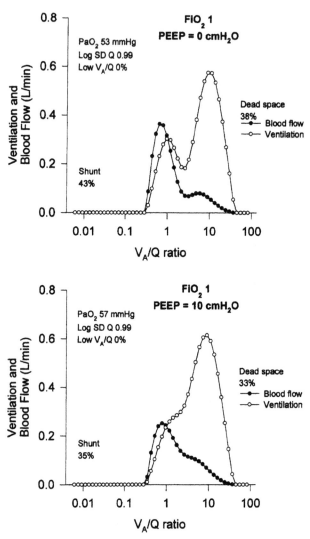

Fig. 11.2. Two patterns of V_A/Q distribution in a patient with ARDS, without (*upper panel*) and with PEEP (*lower panel*). Note that intrapulmonary shunt and dead space are considerably increased, and that PEEP markedly reduced the amount of shunt

11.5.2 Chronic Airflow Limitation

Although both COPD and bronchial asthma have a common functional hallmark, namely chronic airflow obstruction with or without associated reversibility, they also show several pathophysiologic differences. A contrasting feature between pulmonary gas exchange in patients with "dry lung" and in those with "wet lung"

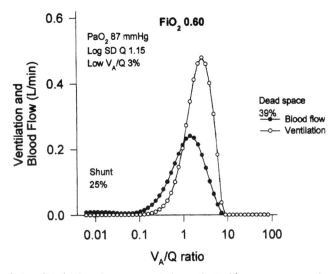

Fig. 11.3. Ventilation-perfusion distributions in a representative patient with severe pneumonia requiring mechanical ventilation. Note that shunt and dead space are moderately elevated; likewise, a considerable amount of blood flow is distributed to lung units with low V_A/Q ratios (below 0.1)

Table 11.2. Characteristics of pulmonary gas exchange in acute lung injury

	ARDS	Pneumonia
Principal mechanisms		
Shunt	Severe	Severe
V_A/Q mismatch	Absent/mild	Mild/moderate
O_2 diffusion limitation	Absent	Absent
Effects of 100% O_2		
Increase in PaO_2	Mild/moderate ($\leq$300 mmHg)	Marked ($\geq$400 mmHg)
Increase in shunt	Mild/moderate	Absent
Hypoxic vascular response	Absent	Increased

V_A/Q, ventilation-perfusion.

is that the functional findings observed during acute conditions can be better interpreted in light of the findings shown during the stable chronic state.

While the severity of V_A/Q mismatch at baseline is similar in patients with COPD and in those with bronchial asthma, increased intrapulmonary shunting is modestly present in the former but negligible in the latter. Yet, the profiles of V_A/Q abnormalities need not to be the same in the two entities. Patients with COPD may show up to four different patterns of V_A/Q inequality during acute exacerbations (Fig. 11.4) [25]: (a) increased blood flow diverted to lung units with low V_A/Q ratios; (b) increased alveolar ventilation to lung units with high V_A/Q ratios; (c) both increased perfusion to units with low V_A/Q ratios and ven-

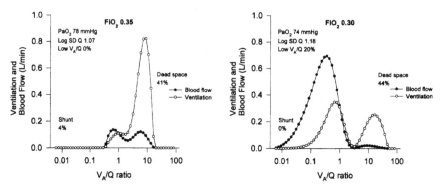

Fig. 11.4. Two patterns of V_A/Q distribution in patients with COPD. The typical bimodal pattern of the blood flow distribution is presented in the *left panel*, while the bimodal pattern of the ventilation distribution is shown in the *right panel*. Note that intrapulmonary shunt is modestly present only in the patient represented in the left panel

tilation to lung units with high V_A/Q ratios; and (d) two broadly unimodal patterns. In mechanically ventilated COPD patients during exacerbations, the decrease of PEEPi by means of reducing minute ventilation and changing ventilatory pattern decreases PaO_2 and increases $PaCO_2$. However, the fall in PaO_2 is partially offset, because mixed venous PO_2 increases due to increased cardiac output which, in turn, increases systemic oxygen delivery [31]. Most patients with acute severe asthma show considerable alterations of pulmonary blood flow dispersion with a marked bimodal blood flow profile, which may include 50% or more of cardiac output [12, 32]. In adult asthma, nevertheless, high V_A/Q ratios are rarely seen. Moreover, while breathing 100% O_2 ablates hypoxic pulmonary vasoconstriction in COPD patients [13, 30], shunt modestly increases (less than 10% of cardiac output) only in patients with status asthmaticus [12], suggesting the development of reabsorption atelectasis and/or redistribution of pulmonary blood flow to preexisting small shunts. Limitation of alveolar to end-capillary O_2 diffusion is absent (Table 11.3).

11.6 Gas Exchange During Discontinuation of Mechanical Ventilation

Most changes of gas exchange and hemodynamics induced by positive pressure ventilation are reversed during weaning from mechanical ventilation. Our group [13] studied V_A/Q abnormalities in mechanically ventilated COPD patients ready for weaning during mechanical ventilation and spontaneous breathing. No major differences in pulmonary and systemic hemodynamics were shown between mechanical ventilation and spontaneous breathing, but cardiac output increased significantly when patients were removed from the ventilator. There were no significant changes in PaO_2, alveolar-arterial O_2 gradient, or venous admixture ratio between the two conditions, but mixed venous PO_2 and O_2 delivery increased sig-

Table 11.3. Characteristics of pulmonary gas exchange in chronic airflow limitation

	COPD	Asthma
Principal mechanisms		
Shunt	Mild	Absent
V_A/Q mismatch	Severe (nonuniform pattern)	Severe (uniform pattern)
O_2 diffusion limitation	Absent	Absent
Effects of 100% O_2		
Increase in PaO_2	Marked ($\geq$400 mmHg)	Marked ($\geq$400 mmHg)
Increase in shunt	Absent	Mild/moderate
Hypoxic vascular response	Increased	Increased

V_A/Q, ventilation-perfusion.

nificantly when patients were weaned from mechanical ventilation. Oxygen consumption (calculated according to the Fick principle) did not change. Another important finding during spontaneous breathing was that minute ventilation remained essentially unchanged, while respiratory frequency increased and tidal volume fell significantly, i.e., a rapid and shallow breathing developed. This inefficient pattern of breathing caused an increase in $PaCO_2$ and a decrease in arterial pH. A considerable increase in the percentage of blood flow to low V_A/Q areas was observed during spontaneous breathing. Moreover, both the dispersion of ventilation and the overall V_A/Q heterogeneity increased (worsened) significantly. In contrast, intrapulmonary shunt, the dispersion of blood flow, and dead space remained essentially unchanged. Therefore, there was further V_A/Q worsening during spontaneous ventilation after removal of ventilatory support. This worsening can be explained by alterations in the breathing pattern and also by changes in cardiac output. Yet, neither the PaO_2 nor the alveolar-to-arterial PO_2 difference underwent major changes, indicating that arterial blood gases were not sufficiently sensitive to detect V_A/Q changes, because other factors, such as minute ventilation and cardiac output, were modulating pulmonary gas exchange in this clinical setting. Indeed, cardiac output increased substantially after cessation of mechanical ventilation because of a simultaneous abrupt increase in venous return. Similarly, there were increases in mixed venous PO_2 and systemic O_2 delivery due to the increased cardiac output. Nevertheless, the resulting beneficial effect of the increased cardiac output on PaO_2 was counterbalanced by the simultaneous decrease in overall V_A/Q ratio, induced in turn by the less efficient breathing pattern and an increased overall blood flow.

More recently, our group [33] studied the V_A/Q abnormalities during discontinuation from mechanical ventilation in mechanically ventilated COPD patients during exacerbations, comparing assist-control ventilation (ACV) with both spontaneous breathing and pressure-support ventilation (PSV). Compared with both ventilatory modalities, and as in the study alluded to above [13], patients developed a more rapid and shallow pattern of spontaneous breathing with no changes in minute ventilation, which in turn caused a significant increase in both dead space and $PaCO_2$. Arterial oxygenation remained unchanged throughout the study. A trend to worsening of V_A/Q distributions during spontaneous breathing, compared with both ventilatory modalities, was shown, although none of these changes were significant. Cardiac output, as well as mixed venous PO_2 and systemic oxygen delivery, increased during spontaneous breathing, which explained why PaO_2 did not fall. No changes were observed during PSV compared with ACV, indicating that increased cardiac output prevented an arterial oxygenation drop during spontaneous breathing, and that pulmonary gas exchange essentially did not change during PSV compared with ACV. All patients were successfully weaned within 24 h of the measurements in both studies [13, 33].

Inert gas and lung isotopic scanning measurements have been assessed simultaneously in a similar group of patients with COPD after more than 5 days of attempted weaning from the ventilator [34]. It was suggested that the abnormal ventilatory pattern shown during spontaneous breathing was the major determinant of V_A/Q mismatch, preferentially located at the basal zones of the lung. An impaired diaphragmatic function, unable to support the weight of the abdominal content, was postulated as a plausible explanation for the development of low basal V_A/Q areas. This gas exchange response was insensitive to the use of inspiratory pressure support at a level of 10 cmH_2O.

The key role played by hemodynamic changes during unsuccessful weaning was stressed in patients with severe advanced COPD and cardiovascular disease who were recovering from acute cardiopulmonary decompensation [35]. Although inert gas exchange data were not measured, there was significant impairment of both PaO_2 and $PaCO_2$, together with an increase in cardiac output and significant deterioration in hemodynamics with marked increase of the transmural pulmonary artery occlusion pressure (PAOP). Oxygen uptake also increased significantly. The increased demands in these patients could have further negatively influenced the final PaO_2, thus offsetting the positive effects of the increased cardiac output on mixed venous oxygen content. Patients were treated with diuretics, resulting in a reduction of blood volume, and 60% of them were then weaned successfully from mechanical ventilation with unchanged PAOP. Additional factors contributing to weaning failure included preexisting cardiovascular disease, which may be aggravated by dramatic changes in venous return. An increase of gastric pressure during spontaneous ventilation with subsequent increased splanchnic blood flow could be an additional mechanism [36].

Other investigators [37] have shown that discontinuation of mechanical ventilation, in the form of both continuous positive-pressure ventilation and pressure-support ventilation, resulted in increased O_2 consumption and decreased minute ventilation, with consequent marked increments in $PaCO_2$ and no change in PaO_2. Conceivably, the simultaneous increase in cardiac output (not measured) prevented a fall in PaO_2.

The large variability in cardiac output measurements obtained with the thermodilution technique may explain the absence of an increase in O_2 consumption (calculated according to the Fick equation) in our previous study [13]. Oxygen consumption measures can be underestimated because both bronchial and thebesian veins empty into the systemic circulation, such that the O_2 consumed by parts of the lung and the heart may not necessarily be reflected in the Fick measurement [38]. It is considered that oxygen consumption measured from the mixed expired samples at the mouth is more accurate than that calculated from the Fick equation. It also has been shown that the correlation between the two measurements of O_2 consumption is relatively weak [39].

The increased consumption of oxygen by the respiratory muscles during discontinuation of mechanical ventilation may cause changes in the regional blood flow distribution, thus reducing the splanchnic circulation and causing gastric mucosal acidosis, as assessed by gastric tonometry. Several reports suggested that more profound changes in gastric intramucosal pH (pHi) might occur in patients who are later unsuccessfully weaned from the ventilator compared with those weaned successfully [40, 41]. Mohsenifar and co-workers [40] found significant differences for only 20 min within the pressure-support weaning period but not during mechanical ventilation. In this study, the authors estimated pHi from intraluminal pH measurements, which may be inaccurate in patients receiving drugs that alter intraluminal pH (e.g., histamine-2-receptor blockers). In another study, Bouachour and co-workers [41] observed patients with weaning failure to have lower pHi before the weaning period, while the patients were still on ventilatory support. In the latter study tonometry with an intragastric latex balloon filled with saline solution was employed, hence circumventing some of the problems associated with direct measurements of pHi. Yet the long equilibrium time of around 60 min needed to ensure the measurements in saline solution precludes the use of this technique in a clinical setting with short-time changes in the physiologic conditions, such as discontinuation from mechanical ventilation. In addition, both studies looked at pHi either before mechanical ventilation was stopped or very early during weaning in order to use measurements of pHi as a predictor of weaning outcome. Our group [42] has recently studied pHi measurements during weaning and after ventilatory support was withdrawn to verify that the differences observed are attributable to the weaning process. This study was done using capnometric recirculation gas tonometry, a recently developed technique based in the analysis of CO_2 tension in an intragastric latex balloon filled with gas [43], whose major advantage in weaning is that only 5 min are required as the equilibrium time to perform measurements. Despite the fact that values of pHi during spontaneous breathing were significantly lower in patients who failed the weaning trial compared with those successfully extubated, differences between patients with weaning success and failure were small and capnometric recirculation gas tonometry did not replace or improve the predictive power of the rapid and shallow breathing index for weaning outcome prediction.

In summary, cardiopulmonary interactions determining gas exchange and oxygen transport are complex. The switch from mechanical ventilation to spontaneous breathing is associated with the development of a rapid and shallow breathing pattern and an increase in oxygen consumption and systemic venous return. An appropriate cardiovascular response to these increased demands, avoiding both left ventricular failure and increasing mixed venous oxygen content, will further determine the success of weaning from mechanical ventilation.

11.7 References

1. West JB (1971) Causes of carbon dioxide retention in lung disease. N Engl J Med 284:1232–1236
2. West JB (1977) Ventilation-perfusion relationships. Am Rev Respir Dis 116:919–943
3. Wagner P, West JB, West (1974) Measurements of continuous distributions of ventilation-perfusion ratios: theory. J Appl Physiol 36:588–599
4. Evans J, Wagner P (1977) Limits on V_A/Q distributions from analysis of experimental inert gas elimination. J Appl Physiol 42:600–605
5. Roca J, Wagner P (1994) Contribution of multiple inert gas elimination technique to pulmonary medicine. I: Principles and information content of the multiple inert gas elimination technique. Thorax 49:815–824
6. Wagner PD, Dantzker DR, Dueck R, Clausen JL, West JB (1977) Ventilation-perfusion inequality in chronic obstructive pulmonary disease. J Clin Invest 59:203–216
7. Dantzker DR (1984) Gas exchange. In: Montenegro H (ed) Chronic obstructive pulmonary disease. Churchill Livingstone, Edinburgh, pp 141–160
8. Glauser F, Pollaty R, Sessler C (1988) Worsening oxygenation in the mechanically ventilated patient. Causes, mechanisms, and early detection. Am Rev Respir Dis 138:458–465
9. Agusti A, Barbera JA, Roca J, Wagner P, Guitart R, Rodriguez-Roisin R (1990) Hypoxic pulmonary vasoconstriction and gas exchange in chronic obstructive pulmonary disease. Chest 97:268–275
10. Dantzker DR (1987) Ventilation-perfusion inequality in lung disease. Chest 91:749–754
11. Roca J, Ramis L, Rodriguez-Roisin R, Ballester E, Montserrat J, Wagner P (1989) Serial relationships between VA/Q inequality and spirometry in acute severe asthma requiring hospitalization. Am Rev Respir Dis 139:732–739
12. Rodriguez-Roisin R, Ballester E, Roca J, Torres A, Wagner PD (1989) Mechanisms of hypoxemia in patients with status asthmaticus requiring mechanical ventilation. Am Rev Respir Dis 139:732–739
13. Torres A, Reyes A, Roca J, Wagner PD, Rodriguez-Roisin R (1989) Ventilation-perfusion mismatching in chronic obstructive pulmonary disease during ventilator weaning. Am Rev Respir Dis 140:1246–1250
14. Barbera JA, Ramirez J, Roca J, Wagner PD, Sanchez-Loret J, Rodriguez-Roisin R (1990) Lung structure and gas exchange in mild chronic obstructive pulmonary disease. Am Rev Respir Dis 141:895–901
15. Ringstedt C, Eliasen K, Andersen J, Heslet L, Qvist J (1989) Ventilation-perfusion distributions and central hemodynamics in chronic obstructive pulmonary disease. Chest 96:976–983
16. Melot C, Hallemans R, Naeije R, Mols P, Lejeune P (1984) Deleterious effect of nifedipine on pulmonary gas exchange in chronic obstructive pulmonary disease. Am Rev Respir Dis 130:612–616
17. Ballester E, Reyes A, Roca J, Guitart R, Wagner P, Rodriguez-Roisin R (1989) Ventilation-perfusion mismatching in acute severe asthma: effects of salbutamol and 100% oxygen. Thorax 44:258–267
18. Gea J, Roca J, Torres A, Agusti A, Wagner P, Rodriguez-Roisin R (1991) Mechanisms of abnormal gas exchange in patients with pneumonia. Anesthesiology 75:782–789
19. Agusti A, Roca J, Gea J, Wagner PD, Xaubet A, Rodriguez-Roisin R (1991) Mechanisms of gas exchange impairment in idiopathic pulmonary fibrosis. Am Rev Respir Dis 143:219–225
20. West JB (1985) Ventilation/blood flow and gas exchange. Blackwell Scientific Publications, Oxford
21. Dantzker DR (1983) The influence of cardiovascular function on gas exchange. Clin Chest Med 4:149–159
22. Lynch JP, Mhyre J, Dantzker DR (1979) Influence of cardiac output on intrapulmonary shunt. J Appl Physiol 46:315–321
23. Breen P, Schumacker P, Hedenstierna G, Ali J, Wagner P, Wood LDH (1982) How does increased cardiac output increase shunt in pulmonary edema? J Appl Physiol 53:1487–1495
24. Weinberger S, Schwartzstein R, Weiss J (1989) Hypercapnia. N Engl J Med 321:1223–1231

25. Rodriguez-Roisin R, Roca J (1994) Pulmonary gas exchange. In: Calverley P, Pride N (eds) Chronic obstructive pulmonary disease. Chapman & Hall, London, pp 161–184
26. Torre-Bueno J, Wagner P, Saltzman G (1985) Diffusion limitation in normal humans during exercise at sea level and simulated altitude. J Appl Physiol 58:989–995
27. Wagner P, Rodriguez-Roisin R (1991) Clinical advances in pulmonary gas exchange. Am Rev Respir Dis 143:883–888
28. Dantzker DR, Brook C, Dehart P, et al (1979) Ventilation-perfusion distribution in the adult respiratory distress syndrome. Am Rev Respir Dis 120:1039–1052
29. Lampron, Lemaire F, Teisserie B, Harf A, Palot M, Matamis D, Lorino A (1985) Mechanical ventilation with 100% oxygen does not increase intrapulmonary shunt in patients with severe bacterial pneumonia. Am Rev Respir Dis 131:409–413
30. Santos C, Ferrer M, Roca J, Torres A, Hernández C, Rodriguez-Roisin R (2000) Pulmonary gas exchange response to oxygen breathing in acute lung injury. Am J Respir Crit Care Med 161:26–31
31. Rossi A, Santos C, Roca J, Torres A, Felez MA, Rodriguez-Roisin R (1994) Effects of PEEP on V_A/Q mismatching in ventilated patients with chronic airflow obstruction. Am J Respir Crit Care Med 149:1077–1084
32. Ferrer A, Roca J, Wagner PD, Lopez F, Rodriguez-Roisin R (1993) Airway obstruction and ventilation-perfusion relationships in acute severe asthma. Am Rev Respir Dis 147:579–584
33. Ferrer M, Roca J, Hernandez C, Iglesia R, Gomez F, Rodriguez-Roisin R (1997) Pulmonary gas exchange and hemodynamics during weaning from mechanical ventilation in COPD patients. Eur Respir J 10:22s (Abstract)
34. Beydon L, Cinotti L, Rekik N, et al (1991) Changes in the distribution of ventilation and perfusion associated with separation from mechanical ventilation in patients with obstructive pulmonary disease. Anesthesiology 75:730–738
35. Lemaire F, Teboul J, Cinotti L, Giotto G, Abrouk F, Steg G, Macquin-Mavier I, Zapol W (1988) Acute left ventricular dysfunction during unsuccessful weaning from mechanical ventilation. Anesthesiology 69:171–179
36. Permutt S (1988) Circulatory effects of weaning from mechanical ventilation: the importance of transdiaphragmatic pressure. Anesthesiology 69:157–160
37. Annat GJ, Viale JP, Dereymez CP, Bouffard YM, Delafosse BX, Motin JP (1990) Oxygen cost of breathing and diaphragmatic pressure-time index: measurement in patients with COPD during weaning with pressure support ventilation. Chest 98:411–414
38. Light R (1988) Intrapulmonary oxygen consumption in experimental pneumococcal pneumonia. J Appl Physiol 64:2490–2495
39. Hubmayr RD, Loosbrock L, Gillespie DJ, Rodarte JR (1988) Oxygen uptake during weaning from mechanical ventilation. Chest 94:1148–1155
40. Mohsenifar Z, Hay A, Hay J, Lewis MI, Koerner SK (1993) Intramural pH as a predictor of success or failure in weaning patients from mechanical ventilation. Ann Intern Med 119:794–798
41. Bouachour G, Guiraud MP, Gouello JP, Roy PM, Alquier P (1996) Gastric Intramucosal pH: an indicator of weaning outcome from mechanical ventilation in COPD patients. Eur Respir J 9:1868–1873
42. Maldonado A, Bauer TT, Ferrer M, Hernández C, Arancibia F, Rodriguez-Roisin R, Torres A (2000) Capnometric recirculation gas tonometry and weaning from mechanical ventilation. Am J Respir Crit Care Med 161:171–176
43. Guzman JA, Kruse JA (1996) Development and validation of a technique for continuous monitoring of gastric intramucosal pH. Am J Respir Crit Care Med 153:694–700

12 Weaning-Induced Cardiac Failure

A. Jubran

The most common cause of unsuccessful weaning from mechanical ventilation is thought to be the failure of the respiratory muscle pump. The alterations in lung volume and intrathoracic pressure that occur during weaning can have detrimental effects on cardiovascular performance and lead to a decreased supply of oxygen to the overworked respiratory muscles. Thus, the complex interactions between the heart and the lung during spontaneous breathing can determine whether the patient can be weaned successfully.

The most characteristic finding in patients who fail a weaning trial is that they develop rapid shallow breathing immediately upon discontinuation of mechanical ventilation [1]. Compared with successes, patients who fail weaning have a higher respiratory rate and lower tidal volume throughout the weaning trial. The increase in frequency is commonly associated with dynamic hyperinflation, as reflected by the presence of intrinsic positive end-expiratory pressure (PEEPi). During a trial of spontaneous breathing, dynamic PEEPi was higher in the failure patients than in the success patients. From the start to the end of the trial, dynamic PEEPi increased progressively in weaning-failure patients, suggesting the development of dynamic hyperinflation; however, expiratory muscle contraction may have also contributed [2].

Hyperinflation has numerous adverse effects on respiratory muscle function. The increase in lung volume causes the inspiratory muscles to shorten, with a consequent decrease in their force of contraction. Flattening of the diaphragm is associated with an increase in its radius of curvature, which, according to the law of Laplace, causes a decrease in the efficiency of transdiaphragmatic pressure generation. The medial rather than axial orientation of the muscle fibers may cause diaphragmatic contraction to produce rib-cage deflation rather than expansion. The zone of apposition between the diaphragm and the rib cage is decreased by hyperinflation, which also decreases the efficiency of chest wall expansion. Likewise, the horizontal (rather than the normal oblique bucket-handle) orientation of the ribs makes it more difficult for the respiratory muscles to expand the rib cage [3]. In addition, hyperinflation forces the patient to breathe on the upper, less-compliant portion of the pressure-volume curve, so that the inspiratory pressure requirement for a given tidal volume is increased. Because tidal volume is incompletely exhaled, alveolar pressure remains positive at the end of expiration. Thus, when the patient begins to inspire, he has to first generate a negative inspiratory pressure equal in magnitude to the level of PEEPi, which results in a marked increase in the work of inspiration.

An increase in lung volume can also have detrimental effect on pulmonary vascular resistance. Indeed, lung volume is one of the major determinants of pulmonary blood flow. The pulmonary vasculature can be divided into alveolar and extra-alveolar vessels. Alveolar vessels are located within the alveolar walls and are surrounded by alveolar pressure. As lung volume increases from residual volume to total lung capacity, resistance of the alveolar vessels increases secondary to compression and the associated increase in transpulmonary pressure. The extra-alveolar vessels are surrounded by lung interstitial pressure, which is similar to intrathoracic pressure. As lung volume increases, interstitial pressure decreases as a result of the increased elastic recoil of the lung. These opposing forces induce a complex relation between lung volume, pulmonary vascular resistance, and pulmonary vascular capacitance. However, the net effect of increasing lung volume is to increase pulmonary vascular resistance, which, in turn, will cause a decrease in cardiac index [4].

The second major alteration in breathing that can affect cardiovascular function during weaning is changes in intrathoracic pressure that occur upon switching from mechanical ventilation to spontaneous breathing (Fig. 12.1).

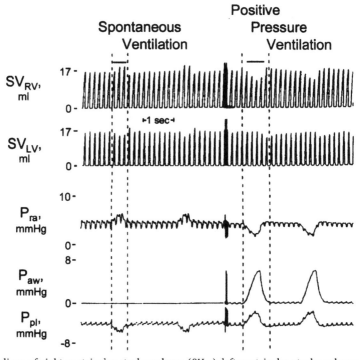

Fig. 12.1. Recordings of right ventricular stroke volume (SV_{RV}), left ventricular stroke volume (SV_{LV}), transmural right atrial pressure (P_{ra}), airway pressure (P_{aw}) and pleural pressure (P_{pl}) during spontaneous ventilation (*left*) and positive-pressure ventilation (*right*) in an intact, closed-chested canine model. The *vertical dotted lines* are reference points for the start and end of a breath for each condition. See text for details. (Modified from [4], with permission)

During a spontaneous breath, as pleural pressure becomes more negative, systemic venous return to the right side of the heart is augmented and transmural right atrial pressure, a measure of right ventricular preload, increases; this, in turn, increases the right ventricular stroke volume. But the decrease in pleural pressure causes a corresponding increase in left ventricular afterload, and therefore the stroke volume of the left ventricle decreases. Conversely, during the positive pressure breath, as pleural pressure rises, the gradient for venous return decreases. This decreases right atrial transmural pressure (or right ventricular preload), leading to a decrease in right ventricular stroke volume. But the increase of pleural pressure during positive breathing will cause a decrease in left ventricular afterload, which in turn causes an increase in the stroke volume of the left ventricle (Fig. 12.1).

During a trial of spontaneous breathing, swings in esophageal pressure were much greater in patients who failed the trial than in those who were successfully extubated (Fig. 12.2) [2]. Moreover, these swings in esophageal pressure increased from the beginning to the end of the trial. These alterations in intrathoracic pressure can have a detrimental impact on cardiac function.

In a very influential study, Lemaire et al. [5] considered the hemodynamic changes in 15 patients with chronic obstructive pulmonary disease (COPD) and

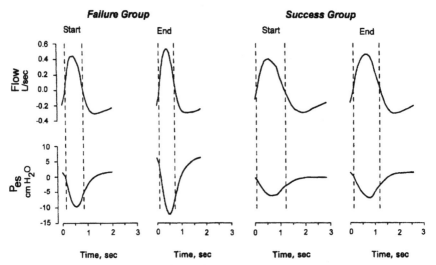

Fig. 12.2. Ensemble average plots of flow and esophageal pressure (P_{es}) at the start and end of a trial of spontaneous breathing in 17 ventilator-dependent patients who failed the trial and 14 patients who tolerated the trial and were successfully extubated. At the start of the trial, the inspiratory excursion in P_{es} was greater in the failure group, and it showed a further increase by the end of the trial. To generate these plots, flow and P_{es} tracings were divided into 25 equal time intervals over a single respiratory cycle for each of the five breaths for each patient in the two groups. For a given patient, the five breaths from the start of the trial were then superimposed and aligned with respect to time, and the average at each time point was calculated. The group mean tracings were then generated by ensemble averaging of the individual mean from each patient. The same procedure was performed for breaths at the end of the trial. (From [2], with permission)

cardiovascular disease who failed a weaning trial. After 10 min of spontaneous breathing, patients developed large swings in esophageal pressure resulting in an increase in left-ventricular afterload, which in turn caused an increase in pulmonary artery occlusion pressure. Some patients developed a large increase in left ventricular end-diastolic volume, which may further elevate the pulmonary artery occlusion pressure by placing the left ventricular end-diastolic pressure on the ascending portion of the left ventricular pressure-volume relationship curve. The authors attributed the increase in left ventricular end-diastolic volume to an increase in venous return – due to low pleural pressure during spontaneous breathing and central translocation of blood volume secondary to peripheral vasoconstriction and an increase in transdiaphragmatic pressure.

To extend Lemaire's observation, Jubran et al. [6] obtained detailed measurements of mixed venous oxygen saturation (S_vO_2) and other hemodynamic variables in a group of ventilator-supported patients during a trial of spontaneous breathing. No difference in S_vO_2 was observed between the group of patients who failed a weaning trial and those who were successfully extubated (Fig. 12.3). On discontinuation of the ventilator, S_vO_2 did not change in the successes, whereas it fell progressively in the failure group.

Arterial oxygen saturation (S_aO_2) was lower in the failures than in the successes during mechanical ventilation and throughout the course of the weaning trial, and this may have contributed to the decrease in S_vO_2. The low S_aO_2 is due partly to the higher venous admixture (Q_{va}/Q_t) in the failure group,

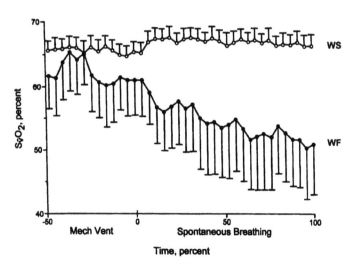

Fig. 12.3. Ensemble averages of the interpolated values of mixed venous oxygen saturation (S_vO_2) during mechanical ventilation and a trial of spontaneous breathing in the success group (*open symbols*) and failure group (*closed symbols*). During mechanical ventilation, S_vO_2 was similar in the two groups ($p=0.28$). Between the onset and the end of the trial, S_vO_2 decreased in the failure group ($p<0.01$), whereas it remained unchanged in the success group ($p=0.48$). Over the course of the trial, S_vO_2 was lower in the failure group than in the success group ($p<0.02$). (*Bars* represent SE). (From [6], with permission)

which increased with spontaneous breathing. The increase in Q_{va}/Q_t with resumption of spontaneous breathing in weaning-failure patients is probably due to derecruitment of lung units secondary to withdrawal of positive-pressure ventilation [7].

To determine the reason for the fall in S_vO_2, it is important to examine the factors that determine the S_vO_2-O_2 transport, O_2 consumption, and O_2 extraction ratio. By the end of the trial, O_2 consumption was virtually identical in the two groups, but the manner by which this O_2 demand was met differed between the two groups. The successes met the demand by significantly increasing O_2 transport from mechanical ventilation to the onset and end of the trial. The failures showed little change in transport – if anything, it went in the opposite direction to the successes. Instead, they significantly increased O_2 extraction between the beginning and end of the trial. That is, the failures increased O_2 extraction by the tissues – presumably largely by the respiratory muscles – which, together with the decrease in O_2 transport, resulted in a fall in S_vO_2. Parenthetically, SvO_2 in the failure group was significantly correlated with O_2 transport ($r=0.80$) and with the O_2 extraction ratio ($r=-0.83$).

Extraction ratio is normally 0.2–0.3 [8], and it increases to greater than 0.8 during maximal exercise. When the O_2 extraction ratio is less than 0.60, increased metabolic demand appears to be met aerobically, whereas energy requirements are met via the anaerobic pathway when the O_2 extraction exceeds 0.60 [9]. In patients who failed a weaning trial, the O_2 extraction ratio at the end of a weaning trial (0.37) did not reach the ratio reported to signify the onset of anaerobic metabolism. Furthermore, the respiratory origin of the acidosis in weaning-failure patients suggests that energy requirements were met solely via aerobic pathways.

The ability of weaning-failure patients to deal with respiratory muscle energy demands through aerobic pathways is probably due to the capacity of the diaphragm to achieve higher blood flow than most other skeletal muscles [10, 11]. The diaphragm is extremely resistant to hypoxic stress, and animals can maintain a ventilation that is sufficient to avoid hypercapnia until phrenic vein PO_2 falls to 12 mmHg [10]. Similarly, studies indicate that a PO_2 of ~10 mmHg in the phrenic vein is the threshold associated with the onset of lactate production by the diaphragm [12] and the development of fatigue [13]. The lowest mixed venous PO_2 in weaning-failure patients was 26 mmHg, which is above the threshold for onset of diaphragmatic lactate production. This association needs to be interpreted with caution, however, since mixed venous blood contains effluents from many tissue beds other than the diaphragm.

The opposing changes in O_2 transport between weaning-success and weaning-failure patients are due mostly to changes in cardiac index. The success group increased O_2 transport by increasing cardiac index. An increase in the cardiac index is the expected response to discontinuation of mechanical ventilation in patients with normal cardiovascular function, and it is mediated largely by an increase in preload [4] (Fig. 12.4).

The relative decrease in cardiac index in patients who fail weaning is the result of several mechanisms. Cardiac index can decrease in response to an impairment of cardiac contractility secondary to the hypoxemia and respiratory acidosis that

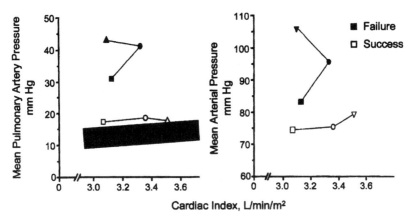

Fig. 12.4. Mean pulmonary artery pressure (P_{pa}) and mean arterial pressure (P_a) versus cardiac index (CI) during mechanical ventilation (*squares*) and at the onset (*circles*) and end (*triangles*) of a spontaneous breathing trial in the success (*open symbols*) and failure group (*closed symbols*). The shaded area represents the normal range of increase in mean P_{pa} with CI. In the success group, CI increased between mechanical ventilation and the end of the trial, mean P_{pa} remained slightly above the normal range, and mean P_a remained unchanged. In contrast, in the failure group, CI was similar during mechanical ventilation and at the end of the weaning trial, but mean P_{pa} and mean P_a were higher by the end of the trial ($p<0.025$ and $p<0.05$, respectively). The increases in mean P_{pa} and mean P_a, together with the lack of change in CI, strongly suggest increases in right- and left-ventricular afterload in the failure group. (From [6], with permission)

develop in weaning-failure patients [14, 15]. An impairment of cardiac contractility can also result from the myocardial ischemia that has been documented during weaning [16,17]; however, impairment of left ventricular contractility owing to the development of myocardial ischemia during weaning appears to be confined largely to patients with documented coronary artery disease [18]. Finally, the decrease in cardiac index could occur as a result of the increase in left ventricular afterload, because of the more negative swings in intrathoracic pressure [2, 6, 19].

The decrease in O_2 transport in weaning-failure patients can also affect respiratory muscle function. In critically ill patients, the O_2 cost of breathing was more than 20% of the total body oxygen consumption [20]. It is extremely difficult to measure the O_2 consumption by the respiratory muscles, i.e., the O_2 cost of breathing. Instead, investigators tend to measure work of breathing. However, mechanical work can substantially underestimate oxygen consumption by the respiratory muscles. In particular, measurement of mechanical work is totally insensitive to energy expenditure during an isometric contraction.

Pressure-time product (PTP) avoids these problems, and several investigators have shown that measurements of magnitude and duration of pressure generation – namely, PTP – is more closely related to respiratory muscle oxygen consumption than is mechanical work [21]. In healthy volunteers breathing through resistors, oxygen consumption of respiratory muscles was better correlated with tension-time index than with mechanical work.

In weaning-failure patients, inspiratory PTP at the end of a T-tube trial is markedly increased, indicating an increase in energy consumption. If the O_2 transport is not adequate, it may not meet the high demands placed on the respiratory muscles and will cause them to fatigue.

Tension-time index (TTI), which quantifies the magnitude and duration of inspiratory muscle contraction, appears to be the best available framework for considering the risk of respiratory muscle fatigue. Jubran and Tobin [2] measured the TTI in 17 patients with COPD who failed a trial of weaning from mechanical ventilation and in 14 patients who tolerated such a trial and were extubated (Fig. 12.5). At the onset of the trial, TTI was not different in the two groups. However, while it increased over the course of the trial in the weaning-failure group, it remained unchanged in the success group. Five of the failure patients developed a TTI greater than 0.15 – a value that has been shown to be associated with respiratory muscle fatigue. These results suggest that respiratory muscle fatigue may be responsible for some instances of weaning failure in patients with COPD.

A problem with fatigue is that it can cause severe muscle destruction. The only way to recover from this type of fatigue is by resting the respiratory muscles. In healthy volunteers, diaphragmatic fatigue was induced by having subjects breathe through a resistor to the limits of tolerance [22]. Fatigue was measured as the transdiaphragmatic pressure response to phrenic nerve stimulation. Fatigue caused a decrease in the twitch pressures of each subject, and, importantly, the reduction in twitch pressure was still evident after 24 h. This observation indicates that a considerable period of rest is needed to recover from fatigue.

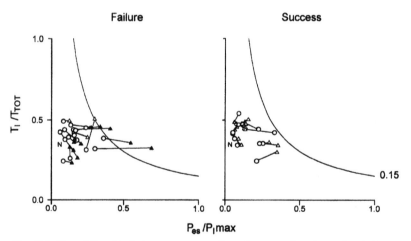

Fig. 12.5. The relationship between mean esophageal pressure/maximum inspiratory pressure ratio (P_{es}/P_Imax) and duty cycle (T_I/T_{TOT}) in ventilator-supported patients with COPD who failed a trial of spontaneous breathing and patients who tolerated the trial. *Circles* and *triangles* represent values at the start and end of the trial, respectively; *closed symbols* indicate patients who developed an increase in P_aCO_2 during the trial. Five of the 17 patients in the failure group developed a tension time index of >0.15 (indicated by the *isopleth*), suggesting respiratory muscle fatigue. *N* represents value in a normal subject. (From [2], with permission)

In summary, the major reason why patients fail a trial of spontaneous breathing is because of the enormous workload that they face in being weaned from mechanical ventilation. Such increases in workload lead to an increase in left-ventricular afterload and a relative decrease in oxygen transport. Thus, the inability to increase oxygen delivery to the tissues, including the respiratory muscles, during a period of increased O_2 demand can place the patient at considerable risk for the development of diaphragmatic fatigue.

12.1 References

1. Tobin MJ, Guenther SM, Perez W, Mador MJ, Semmens BJ, Allen SJ, et al (1986) The pattern of breathing during successful and unsuccessful trials of weaning from mechanical ventilation. Am Rev Respir Dis 134:1111–1118
2. Jubran A, Tobin MJ (1997) Pathophysiological basis of acute respiratory distress in patients who fail a trial of weaning from mechanical ventilation. Am J Respir Crit Care Med 155:906–915
3. Tobin MJ (1988) Respiratory muscles in disease. Clin Chest Med 9:263–266
4. Miro AM, Pinsky MR (1994) Heart-lung interaction. In: Tobin MJ (ed) Principles and practice of mechanical ventilation. McGraw-Hill, New York, pp 647–671
5. Lemaire F (1988) Weaning from mechanical ventilation. In: Ledingham IM (ed) Recent advances in critical care medicine. Churchill Livingstone, New York, pp 15–30
6. Jubran A, Mathru M, Dries D, Tobin MJ (1998) Continuous recordings of mixed venous oxygen saturation during weaning from mechanical ventilation and the ramifications thereof. Am J Respir Crit Care Med 158:1763–1769
7. Gattinoni L, Pesenti A, Bombino M, Baglioni S, Rivolta M, Rossi F, et al (1988) Relationship between lung computed tomography density gas exchange, and PEEP in acute respiratory failure. Anesthesiology 69:824–832
8. Russell JA, Phang PT (1994) The oxygen delivery/consumption controversy. Approaches to management of the critically ill. Am J Respir Crit Care Med 149:533–537
9. Weber KT, Kinasewitz GT, Janicki JS, Fishman AP (1982) Oxygen utilization and ventilation during exercise in patients with chronic cardiac failure. Circulation 65:1213–1223
10. Reid MB, Johnson RL jr (1983) Efficiency, maximal blood flow, and aerobic work capacity of canine diaphragm. J Appl Physiol 54:763–772
11. Rochester DF, Bettini G (1976) Diaphragmatic blood flow and energy expenditure in the dog. Effects of inspiratory airflow resistance and hypercapnia. J Clin Invest 57:661–672
12. Rochester DF, Briscoe AM (1979) Metabolism of the working diaphragm. Am Rev Respir Dis 119:101–106
13. Bark H, Supinski G, Bundy R, Kelsen S (1988) Effect of hypoxia on diaphragm blood flow, oxygen uptake, and contractility. Am Rev Respir Dis 138:1535–1541
14. Walley KR, Lewis TH, Wood LD (1990) Acute respiratory acidosis decreases left ventricular contractility but increases cardiac output in dogs. Circ Res 67:628–635
15. Walley KR, Becker CJ, Hogan RA, Teplinsky K, Wood LD (1988) Progressive hypoxemia limits left ventricular oxygen consumption and contractility. Circ Res 63:849–859
16. Hurford WE, Lynch KE, Strauss HW, Lowenstein E, Zapol WM (1991) Myocardial perfusion as assessed by thallium-201 scintigraphy during the discontinuation of mechanical ventilation in ventilator-dependent patients. Anesthesiology 74:1007–1016
17. Chatila W, Jacob B, Guaglionone D, Manthous CA (1996) The unassisted respiratory rate-tidal volume ratio accurately predicts weaning outcome. Am J Med 101:61–67
18. Richard C, Teboul JL, Archambaud F, Hebert JL, Michaut P, Auzepy P (1994) Left ventricular function during weaning of patients with chronic obstructive pulmonary disease [see comments]. Intensive Care Med 20:181–186
19. Buda AJ, Pinsky MR, Ingels NB jr, Daughters GT, Stinson EB, Alderman EL (1979) Effect of intrathoracic pressure on left ventricular performance. N Engl J Med 301:453–459

20. Field S, Kelly SM, Macklem PT (1982) The oxygen cost of breathing in patients with cardiorespiratory disease. Am Rev Respir Dis 126:9–13
21. Field S, Sanci S, Grassino A (1984) Respiratory muscle oxygen consumption estimated by the diaphragm pressure-time index. J Appl Physiol 57:44–51
22. Laghi F, D'Alfonso N, Tobin MJ (1995) Pattern of recovery from diaphragmatic fatigue over 24 hours. J Appl Physiol 79:539–546

13 Physiopathological Determinants of Patient-Ventilator Interaction and Dyssynchrony During Weaning

C.S.H. Sassoon, T.S. Gallacher, and A. Manka

*Supported by the Department
of Veterans Affairs Medical Research Service*

13.1 Introduction

During weaning from mechanical ventilation, the patient assumes a greater proportion of the work of breathing as ventilatory assistance is gradually withdrawn. The gradual withdrawal of ventilator assistance can be accomplished by the application of pressure-support ventilation (PSV) (Brochard et al. 1994; Esteban et al. 1995), synchronous intermittent mandatory ventilation (SIMV) (Brochard et al. 1994; Esteban et al. 1995), proportional assist ventilation (PAV) (Georgopoulos 1998), bi-level continuous positive airway pressure ventilation (Bi-level CPAP) or airway pressure release ventilation, mandatory minute ventilation (Davis et al. 1989), adaptive lung ventilation (Linton et al. 1994), or continuous positive airway pressure (CPAP) with or without automatic tube compensation (Stocker et al. 1997). Sometimes short intervals of T-piece trials (Esteban et al. 1995) are interspersed between high levels of ventilatory assistance or prolonged T-piece trials are applied (Esteban et al. 1997). Among the available methods of weaning, only PSV, SIMV, and T-piece have been studied prospectively (Brochard et al.1994, Esteban et al.1995; Esteban et al.1997). With PSV or SIMV the patient receives partial ventilatory support, whereas with T-piece the patient assumes full spontaneous breathing effort. In one prospective study (Esteban et al. 1994), the prevalence of weaning with either PSV, SIMV, or a combination of both PSV and SIMV with or without T-piece in succession was 75%. Thus, the majority of weaning was accomplished with the application of partial ventilatory support. In this regard, it is imperative that the ventilator be properly adjusted so as to avoid respiratory system reloading that would exceed the patient's respiratory muscle capacity. Respiratory muscle reloading may develop as a result of premature removal of ventilatory support in a patient with unremitting elevated load to the respiratory system (if the underlying disease has not recovered), inappropriate ventilator settings, or high ventilator circuit resistance including the endotracheal tube. All of these may result in ineffective triggering or wasted efforts. This review will discuss the prevalence of improper interaction between the patient and the ventilator, or patient-ventilator dyssynchrony, the pathophysiological determinants of this dyssynchrony during weaning from mechanical ventilation, and ways of possibly improving patient-ventilator interaction. Patient-ventilator dyssynchrony is defined as the mismatch between patient- and ventilator-triggered breaths.

13.2 Prevalence and Significance of Patient-Ventilator Dyssynchrony During Weaning

To our knowledge, there is only one study addressing the prevalence of patient-ventilator dyssynchrony during weaning from mechanical ventilation. Chao and co-workers (1997) studied 174 patients admitted to a regional weaning center. The patients had been on mechanical ventilation for a median of 29 days prior to transfer to the facility. Ineffective triggering efforts were quantified by bedside physical examination for a minimum of 2 min. Nineteen of the patients (11%) demonstrated patient-ventilator dyssynchrony while they were receiving assist-control mechanical ventilation (AMV) with a mean tidal volume (VT) of 576 ml, a peak inspiratory flow of 82 l/min, and an effective respiratory rate (f) of 15 breaths/min. Ineffective triggering efforts consisted of 45% of total inspiratory efforts. Patients with ineffective triggering efforts had significantly lower maximum inspiratory pressure (PI_{max}) compared with the group without patient-ventilator dyssynchrony (15.9 vs 29.2 cmH_2O, respectively). Eighty-four percent of the patients with dyssynchrony suffered from chronic obstructive pulmonary disease (COPD). In contrast, 40% of the patients without patient-ventilator dyssynchrony had COPD. The patients with ineffective triggering efforts also had an unfavorable weaning outcome. Only three (16%) of the 19 patients with ineffective triggering efforts, compared with 88 (57%) of the 155 patients without ineffective triggering efforts, were successfully weaned from mechanical ventilation. Although this study suggests that patient-ventilator dyssynchrony results in a poor outcome, the underlying disease with associated inspiratory muscle weakness itself may have been responsible for the adverse outcome (Vallverdu et al. 1998). Furthermore, there has been no study evaluating the accuracy of ineffective triggering efforts using bedside physical examination in comparison to, for example, diaphragm electrical activity (EMGd).

13.3 Pathophysiological Determinants of Patient-Ventilator Dyssynchrony

During partial ventilatory support, the patient pulls while the ventilator pushes gas flow. Alterations in patient respiratory center drive, timing, and/or respiratory system mechanics will affect the interaction between the patient and the ventilator. Since PSV is an effective weaning method (Brochard et al. 1994), our discussion will focus on PSV as the ventilator-related factor. With PSV, the trigger variable, the inspiratory pressure, the pressure rate of rise, and the inspiratory cycle-off or expiratory sensitivity, individually or in combination, can all influence patient-ventilator interaction. During PSV, the pressure applied to overcome the impedance of the respiratory system is the sum of the pressure provided by the ventilator (P_{vent}) and the respiratory muscles (P_{mus}) according to the equation of motion:

$$P_{vent}+P_{mus}=(VT{\cdot}E_{rs})+(airflow{\cdot}R_{rs})+PEEPi, \tag{1}$$

in which E_{rs} is the elastance of the respiratory system, VT is tidal volume, R_{rs} is the respiratory system resistance, and PEEPi is the intrinsic positive end-expiratory pressure. In this section we will discuss both the patient- and the ventilator-related factors that may contribute to patient-ventilator dyssynchrony.

13.3.1 Respiratory Center Drive and Timing

A decrease in neuromuscular drive during weaning may result in ineffective triggering of the ventilator, particularly when the set trigger variable is insufficiently sensitive. In addition, ineffective triggering effort increases with high levels of PSV as the result of an accompanying decrease in drive (Leung et al. 1997). An augmented neuromuscular drive during weaning suggests elevated inspiratory muscle work of breathing. With PSV, in the presence of high neuromuscular drive, inspiratory flow demand increases, but because the set inspiratory pressure is fixed, this is achieved at the expense of increasing P_{mus} (see equation 1).

The underlying mechanism of ineffective triggering efforts is the mismatch between patient and ventilator inspiratory time (TI_{neural} vs TI_{mech}, respectively). When TI_{neural} is longer than TI_{mech}, double cycling may occur since the patient's ventilatory demand has not been fully satisfied. On the other hand, when TI_{neural} is shorter than TI_{mech}, ineffective efforts may develop since the ventilator continues to deliver gas flow, encroaching on neural expiratory time (TE_{neural}) and leaving less time for exhalation. The next inspiratory effort occurs at a high lung volume and is insufficient to overcome the high elastic recoil of the respiratory system. Consequently, inspiratory effort is wasted and the ventilator fails to deliver fresh gas flow. Hence, at a moderate or high level of PSV, a shortened TI_{neural} increases the likelihood of TI_{neural}-mechanical mismatching with ensuing patient-ventilator dyssynchrony.

Could TI_{neural} shorten, e.g., with elevated $PaCO_2$, or could it be that the shortening of TI_{neural} is closely linked to the ventilator setting? Under anesthesia the duration of TI_{neural} during spontaneous breathing is determined by the attainment of volume threshold via the Herring-Breuer reflex (Younes and Remmers 1981). Yet in conscious subjects the increase in tidal volume induced by hypercapnia is associated with little or no change in TI_{neural} (Clark and von Euler 1972). In healthy conscious subjects receiving assist-control mechanical ventilation, however, TI_{neural} is sensitive to set inspiratory flow; that is, TI_{neural} becomes shorter as flow delivery increases (Fernandez et al. 1999). Although the relationship between TI_{neural} and flow during PSV has not been determined, a high set inspiratory pressure is associated with a high flow delivery. This high flow delivery may induce a flow-terminating reflex and shorten TI_{neural}. The shortened TI_{neural}, combined with a prolonged TI_{mech} – which is a function of the ventilator inspiratory pressure, ventilator inspiratory cycle-off algorithm, and the time-constant of the respiratory system, increases the likelihood of patient-ventilator dyssynchrony.

Does the mismatching between the onset of TE_{neural} and mechanical expiratory time (TE_{mech}) contribute to patient-ventilator dyssynchrony? To quantify the mismatching between TE_{neural} and TE_{mech}, Parthasarathy and co-workers (1998) used a Starling resistor to induce airflow limitation in healthy subjects and measured the phase difference between the onset of TE_{neural} and TE_{mech} (Fig. 13.1), quantified as the phase angle (θ), expressed in degrees. A simultaneous onset of TE_{neural} and TE_{mech} has the phase angle of zero degrees. When the onset of TE_{neural} precedes TE_{mech}, it has a negative phase angle, and when it follows TE_{mech} it has a positive phase angle. The phase angle between the onset of TE_{neural} and TE_{mech} was greater in the breaths before the ineffective than before the effective triggering efforts when the PSV was set at 10 and 20 cmH$_2$O (Fig. 13.2). This suggests that the onset of expiratory muscle activation prior to termination of mechanical inflation interfered with the ability of the next inspiratory effort to trigger the ventilator. In the presence of high ventilatory demand, expiratory muscles may be recruited in late inspiration to optimize diaphragm muscle function. By reducing lung volume below the volume of equilibrium, the expiratory muscles share the work of the diaphragm during the next inspiration. However, the presence of airflow limitation may prevent the reduction in lung volume and hinder this sharing of work. In this regard, expiratory muscle activation may contribute to patient-ventilator dyssynchrony. On the other hand, with the continuation of mechanical inflation and prolonged TI_{mech}, the subject attempts to terminate the prolonged mechanical inspiration by recruiting the expiratory muscles, and this manifests as patient-ventilator dyssynchrony. It is unclear which of these two conditions predominates in patients with airflow limitation.

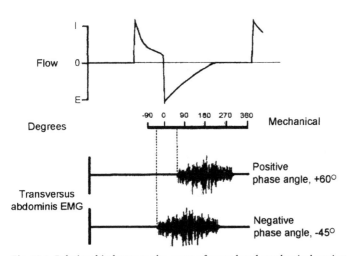

Fig. 13.1. Relationship between the onset of neural and mechanical expiratory time, measured as phase angle and expressed as degrees. If the onset of neural and mechanical expiratory time occurs simultaneously, the phase angle is zero degrees. If the onset of neural occurs prior to that of mechanical expiratory time, the phase angle is negative, but if the onset of neural follows that of mechanical expiratory time, the phase angle is positive. (Adapted from Parthasarathy et al. 1998, with permission)

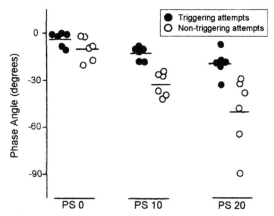

Fig. 13.2. Phase angles between onset of neural and mechanical expiratory time prior to effective triggering efforts (*closed circles*) and ineffective triggering efforts (*open circles*) at varying pressure support (*PS*) levels. At PS of 10 and 20 cmH$_2$O, the phase angle before the ineffective triggering efforts exceeded that before effective triggering efforts, indicating that neural expiratory time during mechanical inflation was longer before the ineffective triggering efforts than before the effective triggering efforts. This interfered with the ability of the next inspiratory effort to trigger the ventilator. (Adapted from Parthasarathy et al. 1998, with permission)

13.3.2 Respiratory System Mechanics

In the presence of airflow resistance, not only will P_{mus} increase (see equation 1), but it will also prolong TI_{mech} (Jubran et al. 1995). This is because in most of the ventilators, the algorithm for cycling-off inspiration with PSV is determined by a fixed flow rate (e.g., when flow rate is reduced to 5 l/min for Puritan Bennett 7200ae, or to 25% of peak flow for Siemens 900 C). Hence, with increased airflow resistance, substantial time is required for flow to decrease to its threshold value before the ventilator cycles off, lengthening TI_{mech}.

Dynamic hyperinflation is frequently associated with ineffective triggering effort in patients receiving mechanical ventilation (Appendini et al. 1996; Nava et al. 1995; Wilkes et al. 1999). It is commonly associated with high ventilatory demand, high airflow resistance, or short expiratory time. With dynamic hyperinflation the patient breathes at a high lung volume and elastic recoil pressure which is transmitted to the alveoli. The end-expiratory alveolar pressure is positive relative to the airway opening pressure. This positive pressure is termed intrinsic positive end-expiratory pressure (PEEPi). With PEEPi, the patient has to generate a substantial inspiratory effort, or P_{mus}, to overcome the high elastic recoil pressure before the ventilator delivers flow. If P_{mus} is inadequate, the patient generates ineffective triggering efforts. Studies (Nava et al. 1995; Wilkes et al. 1999) have shown that the application of external PEEP (PEEPe) titrated to static PEEPi reduced the frequency of ineffective triggering efforts and improved patient-ventilator interaction. Titration of PEEPe according to dynamic PEEPi (PEEPi$_{dyn}$) was less effective (Wilkes et al. 1999). This is because of the high breath-by-breath variability of PEEPi$_{dyn}$.

13.3.3 Ventilator-Related Factors

Previous studies have shown that, compared with pressure-triggering, flow triggering significantly reduces the pressure-time product of the inspiratory muscles (PTP) which reflects the oxygen consumption of the inspiratory muscles (Aslanian et al. 1998; Barrera et al. 1999). However, despite the reduced PTP, flow triggering has not been shown to reduce ineffective triggering efforts (Chao et al. 1997). In fact, the decreased PTP is associated with a decrease in respiratory drive, which could theoretically increase ineffective triggering efforts (Leung et al. 1997).

In some ventilators the PSV mode is equipped with adjustable pressure rise time to attain the target airway pressure (e.g., Siemens 300, Mallinckrodt Nellcor Puritan Bennett 840, Evita Drager). The more rapidly the set inspiratory pressure is reached, the higher is the initial flow rate and the less the patient's work of breathing (Bonmarchand et al. 1996, 1999). Varying the pressure rise time has no effect on tidal volume, respiratory frequency, or PEEPi. As mentioned above, the effects of high initial flow rate during PSV on ineffective triggering have not been studied. It is possible that as PTP decreases with high initial flow rate or rapid pressure rise time, respiratory drive decreases and wasted efforts increase. On the other hand, a slow rise time not only increases PTP but may also prolong TI_{mech}. When this is combined with increased airflow resistance, the likelihood of mismatching between TI_{neural} and TI_{mech} and of patient-ventilator dyssynchrony increases. Thus, both very rapid and very slow rise times are likely to increase ineffective triggering efforts, though this speculation remains to be proven.

Like inspiratory pressure rise time, the ability to vary flow thresholds for the ventilator to cycle off is also currently available in some ventilators (e.g., Mallinckrodt Nellcor Puritan Bennett 840). These flow thresholds are expressed as percentage of the peak flow. Because adjustment of flow thresholds influences TI_{mech}, one can predict that in patients with high airflow resistance the sooner the ventilator cycles off, the better matching of TI_{neural} and TI_{mech} will occur, with subsequent improvement of patient-ventilator interaction. Varying the cycle-off flow thresholds does not affect patient PTP or work of breathing. However, Santos and Mancebo (2000) showed that it altered the breathing pattern with reduced VT, higher frequency, and shorter TI when the flow threshold was 45% compared with 5% of peak flow.

The set inspiratory pressure of PSV has a definite influence on ineffective triggering efforts (Appendini et al. 1996; Chao et al. 1997; Leung et al. 1997; Giannouli et al. 1999). The higher the set pressure support (PS) level, the higher the peak flow and the longer it takes for the ventilator to cycle off with the resulting prolonged TI_{mech}. In addition, the higher the PS level, the greater is the unloading of inspiratory muscle work during the post-trigger phase (Leung et al. 1997). The latter, through feedback mechanisms, results in decreased respiratory center drive and probably contributes to the ineffective triggering efforts. As the PS level is decreased, ineffective triggering efforts are also reduced, but at the expense of increasing P_{mus} which may result in weaning failure if the patient is not yet ready for discontinuation of mechanical ventilation.

13.4 Approach to Improving Patient-Ventilator Dyssynchrony

The adverse effects of patient-ventilator dyssynchrony during weaning remain unclear. Nevertheless, the contraction of inspiratory muscles during exhalation and the contraction of expiratory muscles during inhalation are forms of eccentric contractions, which in limb muscles have resulted in muscle injury (Friden et al. 1991). Current advances in technology are underway to improve matching between TI_{neural} and TI_{mech}. These include: (a) Proportional assist ventilation (PAV), in which the applied ventilator pressure is proportional to patient effort. The use of PAV requires measurement and monitoring of respiratory system mechanics to determine the degree of machine unloading (Younes 1992; Younes et al. 1992). In addition, it requires an intact neural pathway from the respiratory center to the diaphragm. (b) Neural triggering with neurally adjusted ventilatory assist, in which diaphragm electrical activity is used to trigger the ventilator (Fig. 13.3) and provides a means

A. Airway pressure trigger B. Neural trigger

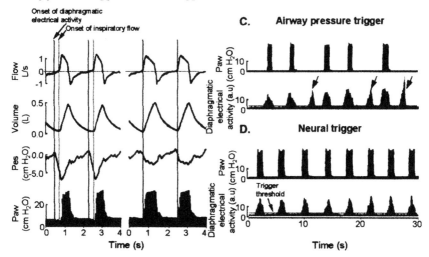

Fig. 13.3 A–D. Partial ventilatory support with conventional airway pressure and neural triggering in two patients with severe chronic obstructive pulmonary disease and acute respiratory failure. **A** Conventional airway pressure triggering: Mechanical ventilatory assistance starts when airway pressure decreases by a preset amount. The beginning of inspiratory effort (*solid line*) precedes inspiratory flow. This delay is due to intrinsic PEEP and occurs despite externally applied PEEP. A further delay from the onset of inspiratory flow (*vertical dashed line*) to the rise in positive airway pressure is present due to mechanical limitation of the ventilator trigger. **B** Neural triggering: The ventilator provides support as soon as diaphragmatic electrical activity exceeds a threshold level. The delay to onset of inspiratory flow and increase in airway pressure is almost eliminated. **C** Poor patient-ventilator interaction with conventional pressure triggering. Diaphragmatic electrical activity is poorly coordinated with the mechanical ventilatory support (indicated by increased airway pressure) and often results in completely wasted inspiratory efforts (*arrows*). **D** Implementation of neural triggering (same patient with identical ventilatory settings as in **C**, except for the trigger system) restores the interaction between the patient's neural drive and the ventilator support. *a.u.*, Arbitrary units. (From Sinderby et al. 1999, with permission)

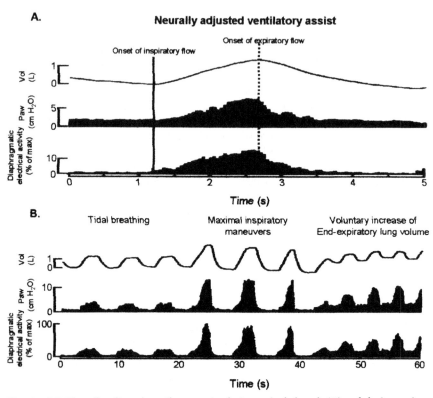

Fig. 13.4 A,B. Neurally adjusted ventilatory assist during a single breath (**A**) and during various breathing maneuvers (**B**). Continuous proportional adjustments of airway pressure (reflecting ventilatory assist) with changes in diaphragmatic electrical activity (reflecting neural drive) during changes in tidal and end-expiratory lung volumes. (From Sinderby et al. 1999, with permission)

of continuous ventilatory assist in proportion to the neural drive, both within a given breath and between breaths (Fig. 13.4; Sinderby et al. 1999). Neural triggering is not affected by PEEPi, and therefore does not require the application of PEEPe for triggering purposes. Like PAV, neurally adjusted ventilatory assist also requires an intact neural pathway to the diaphragm. Furthermore it requires measurement of diaphragm electrical activity using esophageal electrodes. It appears that with current filtering technology a clean diaphragm electromyogram signal can be obtained.

13.5 Summary

Patient-ventilatory dyssynchrony during weaning or acute respiratory failure occurs because of maladaptation of the ventilator to the patient's neural respiratory timing. An instantaneous, breath-by-breath adaptation of the ventilator to neural respiratory timing, such as that provided by PAV or neurally adjusted ventilatory assist (NAVA) (Figs. 13.3 and 13.4), eliminates the mismatch between neural respiratory and ventilator timing. Outcome studies which compare PAV and NAVA with conventional mechanical ventilation in terms of complications, the duration of mechanical ventilation, and length of ICU or hospital stay have yet to be conducted.

13.6 References

Appendini L, Purro A, Patessio A, Zanaboni S, Carone M, Spada E, Donner CF, Rossi A (1996) Partitioning of inspiratory muscle workload and pressure assistance in ventilator-dependent COPD patient. Am J Respir Crit Care Med 154:1301–1309

Aslanian P, El Atrous S, Isabey D, Valente E, Corsi D, Harf A, Lemaire F, Brochard L (1998) Effects of flow triggering on breathing effort during partial ventilatory support. Am J Respir Crit Care Med 157:135–1343

Barrera R, Melendez J, Ahdoot M, Huang Y, Leung D, Groeger JS (1999) Flow triggering added to pressure support ventilation improves comfort and reduces work of breathing in mechanically ventilated patients. J Crit Care 14:172–176

Bonmarchand G, Chevron V, Chopin C, Jusserand D, Girault C, Moritz F, Leroy J, Pasquis P (1996) Increased initial flow rate reduces inspiratory work of breathing during pressure support ventilation in patients with exacerbation of chronic obstructive pulmonary disease. Intensive Care Med 22:1147–1154

BonmarchandG, Chevron V, Menard JF, Girault C, Moritz-Berthelot F, Pasquis P, Leroy J (1999) Effects of pressure ramp slope values on the work of breathing during pressure support ventilation in restrictive patients. Crit Care Med 27:715–722

Brochard L, Rauss A, Benito S, Conti G, Mancebo J, Rekik N, Gasparetto A, Lemaire F (1994) Comparison of three methods of gradual withdrawal from ventilatory support during weaning from mechanical ventilation. Am J Respir Crit Care 150:896–903

Chao DC, Scheinhorn DJ, Stearn-Hassenpflug M (1997) Patient-ventilator trigger asynchrony in prolonged mechanical ventilation. Chest 112:1592–1599

Clark FJ, von Euler C (1972) On the regulation of depth and rate of breathing. J Physiol (Lond) 222:267–295

Davis S, Potgieter PD, Linton DM (1989) Mandatory minute volume weaning in patients with pulmonary pathology. Anaesth Intensive Care 17:170–174

Esteban A, Alia I, Ibanez J, Benito S, Tobin MJ (1994) Modes of mechanical ventilation and weaning. A national survey of Spanish hospitals. The Spanish Lung Failure Collaborative Group. Chest 106:1188–1193

Esteban A, Frutos F, Tobin MJ, Alia I, Solsona JF, Vallverdu I, Fernandez R, de la Cal MA, Benito S, Tomas R, Carried D, Mafias S, Blanco J (1995) A comparison of four methods of weaning patients from mechanical ventilation. Spanish Lung Failure Collaborative Group. N Engl J Med 332:345–350

Esteban A, Alia I, Gordon F, Fernandez R, Solsona JF, Vallverdu I, Mafias S, Allege JM, Blanco J, Carried D, Leon M, de la Cal MA, Taubate F, Gonzalez de Velasco J, Polyzoan E, Carrizosa F, Tomas R, Suarez J, Goldwasser RS (1997) Extubation outcome after spontaneous breathing trials with T-tube or pressure support ventilation. The Spanish Lung Failure Collaborative Group. Am J Respir Crit Care Med 156:459–465

Fernandez R, Mendez M, Younes M (1999) Effect of ventilator flow rate on respiratory timing in normal humans. Am J Respir Crit Care Med 159:710–719

Friden J, Lieber RL, Thornell LE (1991) Subtle indications of muscle damage following eccentric contractions. Acta Physiol Scand 142:523–524

Georgopoulos D (1998) Proportional assist ventilation: an alternative approach to wean the patient. Eur J Anaesthesiol 15:756–760

Giannouli E, Webster K, Roberts D, Younes M (1999) Response of ventilator-dependent patients to different levels of pressure support and proportional assist. Am J Respir Crit Care Med 159:1716–1725

Jubran A, Van de Graaff WB, Tobin MJ (1995) Variability of patient-ventilator interaction with pressure support ventilation in patients with chronic obstructive pulmonary disease. Am J Respir Crit Care Med 152:129–136

Leung P, Jubran A, Tobin MJ (1997) Comparison of assisted ventilator modes on triggering, patient effort, and dyspnea. Am J Respir Crit Care Med 155:1940–1948

Linton DM, Potgieter PD, Davis S, Fourie ATJ, Brunner JX, Laubscher TP (1994) Automatic weaning from mechanical ventilation using an adaptive lung ventilation controller. Chest 106:1843–1850

Nava S, Bruschi C, Rubini F, Palo A, Iotti G, Braschi A (1995) Respiratory response and inspiratory effort during pressure support ventilation in COPD patients. Intensive Care Med 21:871–879

Parthasarathy S, Jubran A, Tobin MJ (1998) Cycling of inspiratory and expiratory muscle groups with the ventilator in airflow limitation. Am J Respir Crit Care Med 158:1471–1478

Santos J, Mancebo J (2000) Effects of different cycling-off criteria (COC) during pressure support ventilation (PSV). (Abstract) Am J Respir Crit Care Med 161:A462

Sinderby C, Navalesi P, Beck J, Skrobik Y, Comtois N, Friberg S, Gottfried SB, Lindstrom L (1999) Neural control of mechanical ventilation in respiratory failure. Nat Med 5:1433–1436

Stocker R, Fabry B, Eberhard L, Haberthur C (1997) Support of spontaneous breathing in the intubated patient: automatic tube compensation (ATC) and proportional assist ventilation (PAV). Acta Anaesthesiol Scand [Suppl] 111:123–128

Vallverdu I, Calaf N, Subirana M, Net A, Benito S, Mancebo J (1998) Clinical characteristics, respiratory functional parameters, and outcome of a two-hour T-piece trial in patients weaning from mechanical ventilation Am J Respir Crit Care Med158:1855–1862

Wilkes WA, Jubran A, Tobin MJ (1999) Is ventilator non-triggering alleviated by the addition of external PEEP? (Abstract) Am J Respir Crit Care Med 159:A362

Younes M (1992) Proportional assist ventilation, a new approach to ventilatory support. Theory. Am Rev Respir Dis 145:114–120

Younes MK, Remmers JE (1981) Control of tidal volume and respiratory frequency. In: Horbein TF (ed) Regulation of breathing. Marcel Dekker, New York, NY, pp 621–671

Younes M, Puddy A, Roberts D, Light RB, Quesada A, Taylor K, Oppenheimer L, Cramp H (1992) Proportional assist ventilation. Results of an initial clinical trial. Am Rev Respir Dis 145:121–129

14 Weaning Criteria: Physiologic Indices in Different Groups of Patients

I. Vallverdú and J. Mancebo

14.1 Introduction

Intubation and mechanical ventilation are commonly employed to save the lives of critically ill patients with respiratory failure. However, selection of the most appropriate time for liberation (from the machine) and endotracheal extubation are among the most difficult decisions critical care physicians make. Roughly two thirds of patients can be successfully extubated after a brief period of breathing through a T-tube, once the problems which precipitated respiratory failure have been treated. However, about 30% of patients who require intubation and mechanical ventilation for longer than 24 h cannot tolerate initial attempts to breathe without the mechanical ventilator [1, 2].

Unnecessary prolongation of mechanical ventilation increases the risks of complications, including bronchopulmonary infections, barotrauma, cardiovascular compromise, tracheal injuries, and oxygen toxicity. At the same time, premature discontinuation of mechanical ventilation leading to reintubation may also increase morbidity [3], mortality [3, 4], duration of intensive care unit (ICU) stay, and the likelihood that patients will require transfer to a long-term ventilator unit [5]. Accordingly, clinicians should optimize weaning, that is, should seek to achieve successful liberation/extubation in the shortest possible time to maximize patient outcomes and to minimize costs associated with mechanical ventilation.

14.2 Common Disorders That Cause Respiratory Pump Insufficiency

Before weaning is considered, the underlying disease process responsible for the acute respiratory failure and mechanical ventilation should have improved. The patient must be hemodynamically stable (absence of myocardial ischemia, no need for vasopressors due to shock, no recent onset of arrhythmia) and adequately oxygenated (PaO_2 >60 mmHg with FiO_2 <0.4 and PEEP <5 cmH_2O), with no agitation, sepsis, or overt central nervous system depression. However, many patients satisfying these conditions fail to wean.

Unsuccessful weaning attempts usually indicate incomplete resolution of the illness that initially generated the need for mechanical ventilation. The most common mechanism of weaning failure is respiratory pump failure, caused by an imbalance between capabilities and demands [6, 7]. This is attributed to an imbalance between neuromuscular (pump) capacity and the loads on the respiratory muscles. Less commonly, weaning failure results from cardiovascular dysfunction, hypoxemia, or psychological dependence on the ventilator.

During spontaneous breathing, the inspiratory muscles must generate sufficient force to overcome the elastance of the lungs and chest wall (lung and chest wall elastic loads) as well as the airway and tissue resistances (resistive load). This requires generation of the signal in the respiratory centers of the brain stem, anatomic and functional integrity of nerves that conducted the signal, unimpaired neuromuscular transmission, and adequate muscle strength. The common disorders that alter the balance of capacity and load in critical illness are reduced neuromuscular capacity and/or increased muscle load.

14.3 Imbalance Between Capacity and Load in Critical Illness

14.3.1 Reduced Neuromuscular Capacity

Reduced output of the respiratory control centers may occur following administration of sedatives, the long-acting effects of some being enhanced in the presence of renal and/or hepatic failure [8]. An altered level of consciousness occurs in several nervous system disorders (including stroke, hemorrhage, infection, etc.), often associated with attenuated cough and upper airway protection reflexes, and depressed respiratory drive, all of which contribute to difficult weaning. Furthermore, severe metabolic alkalosis decreases the output of respiratory centers.

Phrenic nerve dysfunction can occur following diaphragmatic injuries or cardiac surgery [9]. Diaphragmatic dysfunction frequently follows upper abdominal surgery [10]. Critical illness polyneuropathy and myopathy, which are frequent complications of sepsis and multiple organ system failure [11], may also impede weaning. Neuromuscular blocking agents (with or without concomitant corticosteroids) and aminoglycosides, may also contribute to weaning failure [12–17]. Hepatic and/or renal dysfunction, which frequently complicates critical illness, leads to reduced clearance of such medications, further magnifying their deleterious effect.

The strength and/or endurance of respiratory muscles decreases in many clinical conditions. Dynamic hyperinflation generates an elastic threshold load and places the diaphragm in a mechanically disadvantageous position [18]. Malnutrition, deconditioning due to prolonged bed rest, and increased muscle catabolism can induce severe muscle dysfunction. Moreover, patients with poor muscle mass, chronic heart failure [19], chronic renal failure, and severe emphysema may present with pre-existing muscle dysfunction. Finally, abnormalities in respiratory muscle dysfunction are exacerbated by decreased oxygen supply [20], metabolic acidosis, electrolyte deficiencies, and endocrinological disorders (e.g., hypothyroidism). Besides, in some cases of flail chest, muscle contraction can be completely inefficient because diaphragmatic contraction leads to paradoxical inward movement of the chest wall.

14.3.2 Increased Muscle Loads

Increased work of breathing results from increased mechanical loads (elastic and/or resistive) or from processes that require higher minute volumes. Increased ventilatory (minute volume) requirements are quite common in critically ill patients, particularly during periods of hyperthermia, sepsis, metabolic acidosis, or hyperventilation (that can be related to anxiety and/or pain). Overfeeding also increases carbon dioxide production, increasing the minute volume required to maintain a constant $PaCO_2$. Finally, an increase in the dead space/tidal volume ratio (e.g., when using heat and moisture exchangers) is another source of increased ventilatory needs.

Increased elastic workloads occur when lung (e.g., pulmonary edema, extreme hyperinflation during an acute asthmatic attack, pulmonary fibrosis) and/or chest wall (abdominal distension, obesity, trauma, thoracic deformities) compliance is reduced. Pulmonary dynamic hyperinflation, causing intrinsic PEEP (PEEPi), is another example of increased elastic workload and is a relatively common phenomenon, especially in patients with chronic obstructive pulmonary disease (COPD).

Increased resistive work of breathing is caused by bronchospasm, excessive secretions, endotracheal tube resistance (which increases with kinking and deposition of secretions), ventilatory valve/circuits and humidifiers, especially when conditioning of inspired gases is provided with heat and moisture exchangers.

14.3.3 Cardiovascular Dysfunction

The presence of cardiovascular dysfunction may contribute to weaning failure by augmenting loads and by reducing neuromuscular capacity. A study by Epstein [21] showed that as many as one third of weaning failures resulted solely or in part from congestive heart failure, whereas fewer (14%) failures were due to cardiovascular reasons in other studies [22]. Cardiovascular dysfunction results from physiological changes that occur during the resumption of spontaneous unassisted breathing [23]. Several factors contribute to this phenomenon. In the process of weaning, intrathoracic pressure during inspiration changes from positive to negative, which increases left ventricular preload and afterload. Cardiac loading is thus expected to be most marked in patients with large mechanical respiratory muscle loads (e.g., patients with severe obstructive or restrictive respiratory disease) who require relatively large negative pleural pressures to inspire. A significant decrease in left ventricular ejection fraction [24] has been described during spontaneous breathing trials in COPD patients without coronary artery disease (CAD).

An increase in catecholamine release during weaning further augmented preload, afterload and myocardial inotropy. Increased myocardial loading may be sufficient, especially when coupled with left ventricular noncompliance, to precipitate congestive heart failure (which stiffens the lungs and further increases loads). Moreover, increased heart loads augment myocardial oxygen demand and may precipitate myocardial ischemia in patients with CAD [24]. Chatila et al. [25]

found electrocardiographic evidence of myocardial ischemia during weaning in 6% of patients. Ischemia was detected more frequently (in 10% of patients with a history of CAD) and was associated with weaning failure in 22% of these patients. Myocardial ischemia causes left ventricular dysfunction that may potentiate acute pulmonary edema and arterial hypoxemia [26]. This can lead to a vicious circle of myocardial ischemia increasing work of breathing leading to increased catecholamines and increased myocardial loads.

Clinically, many critically ill patients with respiratory failure have both COPD and CAD, which predispose to this combined cardiopulmonary pathogenesis of weaning failure. Since electrocardiography is relatively insensitive with regard to detecting myocardial ischemia, this reason for weaning failure should be suspected in susceptible patients. To assess the relationship of hemodynamic performance, global tissue oxygen delivery, and weaning outcomes, Jubran et al. [27] recently examined hemodynamics and mixed venous saturations in patients during weaning trials. Successful patients demonstrated increases in cardiac oxygen and oxygen transport compared with values during mechanical ventilation. An increase in cardiac index is the anticipated response to discontinuation of mechanical ventilation in patients with intact cardiovascular function/reserve. Patients who failed weaning also failed to increase O_2 delivery, due partly to elevated right and left-ventricular afterloads. Patients who failed also increased peripheral oxygen extraction which, combined with relative decreases in O_2 delivery, resulted in reduced mixed oxygen saturations.

14.4 Weaning Parameters

Because the etiology of weaning failure is multifactorial, it is highly desirable to have objective measurements – indices that can help in making the decision to wean a patient from the ventilator. The main purpose of weaning indices is to differentiate between those patients who can maintain spontaneous breathing indefinitely and those who are unable to do so, in order to avoid both premature discontinuation of ventilatory support and unnecessarily long periods of mechanical ventilation. From a physiological point of view, these indices can be the following: (a) those that assess simple ventilatory parameters, such as vital capacity (VC) and minute ventilation (MV) [28, 29]; (b) those that assess oxygenation, such as the ratio of arterial oxygen tension to the fraction of oxygen in the inspired air (PaO_2/FiO_2); (c) those that attempt to assess respiratory muscle strength, such as maximal inspiratory pressure (MIP) and maximal expiratory pressure (MEP) [2, 28]; (d) those that try to asses the central respiratory drive, such as $P_{0.1}$ (the airway pressure developed 100 ms after the beginning of inspiration against an occluded airway) [30]; (e) those that measure respiratory muscle reserve, such as maximal voluntary ventilation/minute ventilation (MVV/MV) [29] or mean transdiaphragmatic pressure per breath over maximal transdiaphragmatic pressure (Pdi/Pdimax) [31]; (f) those that record and analyze the pattern of spontaneous breathing in terms of tidal volume (V_T), respiratory rate (f), or f/V_T [32] – a measure of rapid shallow breathing; (g) those that assess the work of breathing; and finally (h) composite indices, such as $P_{0.1} \times f/V_T$, that integrate different variables of respiratory function [33].

The multifactorial nature of the pathophysiology of weaning failure has been demonstrated in a prospective study of patients who had initially failed to wean from mechanical ventilation but were successfully liberated later [34]. In this study, it was observed that during episodes of weaning failure, patients had markedly elevated inspiratory loads (as evidenced by a greater PEEPi), inspiratory resistance, and ratio of mean to maximum inspiratory pressure (Pi/Pimax). At the same time, their ability to generate inspiratory pressure (Pimax) was reduced. The energy demand, or tension-time index (TTI), was elevated and the breathing pattern was more rapid and shallow. Multiple logistic regression analyses revealed that the TTI and ratio of respiratory frequency:tidal volume (f/V_T) were independently associated with weaning failure. A high TTI is believed to signal an imbalance between respiratory muscle energy supply and demand. Rapid, shallow breathing during weaning failure may represent the response of the central respiratory controller to loaded breathing [35], and/or it may signal impending inspiratory muscle fatigue [32].

Recent randomized controlled trials have shown that the duration of mechanical ventilation [36, 37], as well as the time spent on weaning, can be reduced by the adoption of specific strategies. These include the systematic daily screening of respiratory function, followed (when appropriate) by trials of spontaneous breathing to identify as early as possible when a patient is able to wean, and the implementation of ventilatory protocols for difficult-to-wean patients instead of relying on physicians' personal preferences. However, the existence of so many different indices simply implies that no index has yet proven to be ideal, that is, to be highly predictive of weanability. Classical respiratory parameters such as VC, MIP, and VE are useful in patients who have been receiving respiratory support for a short period of time [38], but their value as weaning predictors in prolonged mechanical ventilation, in COPD, and in the elderly has not been demonstrated [32]. These weaning parameters have been reported to delay extubation in some patients [39], whereas in others, reintubation will be necessary within the first few hours [40, 41]. De Haven and co-workers [42] found that 105 of 589 extubated patients had a pre-extubation respiratory rate >30 breaths/min, which was considered a reason for failure. Of these 105 patients, 97 were successfully extubated, thus indicating that tachypnea per se is sensitive but not sufficiently specific.

New indices integrating different physiologic variables have been proposed in an attempt to achieve greater outcome. The frequency-to-tidal volume ratio (f/V_T) has shown greater predictive power than MIP or VE [32]. The study by Sassoon and Mahutte [33] has shown a high sensitivity and specificity for both $P_{0.1}$ and f/V_T and for their combination ($P_{0.1} \times f/V_T$). Yang and Tobin studied the predictive power of weaning indices [32] and showed that the rapid and shallow ratio (f/V_T) was the best. In their study, 95% of patients with a ratio f/V_T greater than 105 failed during a test of spontaneous breathing. However, a more recent study has not confirmed these results. On the one hand, the rapid and shallow breathing index does not predict extubation outcome. Epstein et al. [21, 43] found that between 27% and 40% of patients with an f/V_T ratio above 100 could be successfully extubated, while some patients with an f/V_T below 100 were reintubated due to processes unrelated with the original respiratory process. Many of the causes of extubation failure noted by these investigators would not be expected to increase the f/V_T. These data indicate that some patients with an $f/V_T \geq 100$ can be successfully extubated. Moreover, a rapid and shallow breathing index during a weaning trial with the patients receiving partial ventilatory support [21, 44] does not preclude successful extubation. Gandia and Blanco [45] found that the breathing pattern in successfully extubated patients was not stable after discontinuation of ventilatory support. An increase in VE and frequency was observed 15 min after the beginning of a weaning trial. Therefore, predictors of the outcome of a weaning trial could theoretically be less accurate if the criteria used were determined too early. Accordingly, serial measurements of the rapid shallow breathing index in elderly medical patients during a spontaneous breathing trial can accurately predict successful weaning from mechanical ventilation. Using an $f/V_T \leq 130$ as the threshold value for prospectively predicting successful weaning, Krieger et al. [46] showed that diagnostic accuracy increased significantly when measurements were made at the beginning of the weaning trial as compared with 3 h later. It has been demonstrated that women, especially when breathing through small endotracheal tubes, have higher f/V_T than men, independent of extubation outcome [43].

The value of $P_{0.1}$ as an index to predict the weaning outcome is not widely accepted, probably because its measurement requires additional equipment. There is also high interindividual and intraindividual variability, and the $P_{0.1}$ value also depends on end-expiratory lung volume [47], which makes comparisons difficult. In the study by Sassoon and co-workers performed in 12 patients with COPD, a $P_{0.1}$ higher than 6 cmH_2O showed a sensitivity and specificity of 100%. Herrera et al. [48] found that a $P_{0.1}$ above 4.2 cmH_2O has a sensitivity of 78% and a specificity of 100%. Sassoon and Mahutte [33] recently showed that the predictive power of $P_{0.1}$ in patients with respiratory failure of various etiologies who failed a weaning trial is nearly as high as both the f/V_T index and the product $f/V_T \times P_{0.1}$. When analyzing the overall population and the COPD and ARF patient subgroups, Vallverdú et al. [2], found significantly lower values of $P_{0.1}$ in successfully extubated patients in comparison to patients who failed weaning, but no differences in $P_{0.1}$ values were observed in neurological patients.

The variable performance of the same index in different studies has several explanations. The duration of ventilatory support varies widely, and indices usually work better as the duration of mechanical ventilation becomes shorter. The moment at which the patients are studied is also important. An index that correctly predicts the outcome of weaning cannot correctly predict the extubation outcome, thus indicating that pathophysiologic bases for weaning failure are probably different from those responsible for extubation failure. Outcome of weaning is also influenced by different unit-to-unit clinician practice, i.e., regarding sedation, analgesia, and muscle paralysis. The ventilatory techniques (T-piece trial, pressure support, intermittent mandatory ventilation) and the protocols for these techniques are not the same and can influence the weaning and extubation outcome. The highly variable definition of weaning outcome justifies, at least in part, the discrepancy in the studies. Weaning success is usually defined as successful spontaneous ventilation for at least 24 h; nevertheless, many investigators require either shorter or much longer (i.e., 72 h) observation periods. Different authors also use different end points to define weaning failure; some set strict objective criteria (i.e., measurement of arterial blood gases), while others use subjective clinical criteria (i.e., anxiety, agitation, or diaphoresis). The absence of standardized criteria of weaning outcome makes it difficult to compare the performance of weaning indices in different studies, because patients judged to have failed a weaning trial in one study might have been classified as successfully weaned in another, and vice versa. Finally, the differences in patient populations regarding number, age, and disease process can also strongly influence the weaning outcome. Weaning studies have usually included patients with different clinical conditions (chronic obstructive pulmonary disease, heart failure, neurological disease, etc.), and it has recently been reported that the weaning outcome and the respiratory parameters studied as weaning predictors vary considerably depending on the underlying disease [2].

Vallverdú et al. [2] studied 217 patients on mechanical ventilation who met standard weaning criteria ($V_T \geq 5$ ml/kg, f ≤ 35 breaths/min, and MIP lower than -20 cmH$_2$O) and who underwent a 2-h T-piece weaning trial. Before the T-piece trial was begun, functional respiratory parameters were measured. If the spontaneous breathing trial was well-tolerated clinically, patients were extubated. If clinical tolerance to the T-piece trial was poor, patients were reconnected to ventilatory support. Weaning was considered a failure when patients needed reintubation within 48 h or did not tolerate spontaneous breathing and required reconnection to mechanical ventilation. Weaning was considered successful if spontaneous breathing was sustained for more than 48 h after extubation. Figure 14.1 shows the evolution of these 217 patients according to the etiology of respiratory failure i.e., COPD, neurological conditions, and acute respiratory failure (ARF) of varying etiology. Reintubation was required in 35.7% (15 of 42) of the neurological patients and in 8.6% (eight of 93) of the patients with ARF, but it was unnecessary in all patients with COPD ($p<0.001$). On the other hand, the ventilatory support was resumed because of intolerance to the T-piece trial in 60.6% of

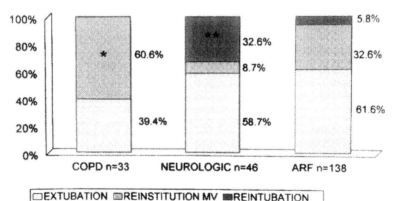

Fig. 14.1. Distribution of the 217 patients according to their evolution and etiology: of 33 with COPD, 13 (39.4%) were successfully extubated and 20 (60.6%) required progressive withdrawal of mechanical ventilation; 46 had a neurological disease, of whom 27 (58.7%) were successfully extubated, four (8.7%) required progressive withdrawal from mechanical ventilation, and 15 (32.6%) were reintubated; and 138 had ARF of various etiologies, with 85 (61.6%) being successfully extubated, 45 (32.6%) requiring progressive withdrawal of mechanical ventilation, and eight (5.8%) being reintubated. (From Vallverdú et al. 1988, with permission)

COPD patients, in whom progressive withdrawal of mechanical ventilation was needed. In these patients, the best predictive indices were f/V_T and $P_{0.1}$. Tables 14.1 and 14.2 show the respiratory functional parameters and the clinical characteristics of patients studied. The authors also found that the number of days they had received mechanical ventilation (DMV) before the weaning trial was started was significantly higher in the weaning-failure group (12±12) than in the weaning-success group (7±7), $p<0.001$. The length of time on mechanical ventilation before the weaning trial could indirectly indicate the severity of the initial injury that led to intubation and mechanical ventilation, and also the different clinical approach regarding practices such as sedation, analgesia, and muscle paralysis.

Another interesting finding in this study [2] was that the weaning trial failed in a high percentage of neurological patients because of extubation failure (35.7%). The need for reintubation in these patients was neither clinically suspected nor suggested by abnormal physiologic indices. Hence, for patients with mental status changes or neurological impairment, other tools need to be developed and prospectively evaluated in order for the clinician to decide on the appropriate time to withdraw mechanical ventilation. The data obtained by Vallverdú et al. suggest that, from a clinical point of view, it is important to evaluate the ability to cough and clear secretions, especially in neurological patients. In the study mentioned, only MIP and MEP values were significantly lower in those patients for whom weaning failed. Additionally, the discriminant analysis selected MEP, MIP, and $f/V_T \times P_{0.1}$ as predictors of weaning outcome with a diagnostic accuracy of 74%. It has been suggested that MEP is related to the ability to cough

Table 14.1. Clinical characteristics and functional respiratory parameters obtained in the total group of patients according to the clinical evolution

| | All patients ($n=217$) | |
	SW ($n=125$)	FW ($n=92$)
Age (years)	55±17	59±15
DMV	7±7	12±12*
f (breaths/min)	24±6	29±8*
V_T (ml)	432±143	378±134**
V_E (l)	11±10	10±3
MIP (cmH$_2$O)	65±21	53±17*
MEP (cmH$_2$O)	53±25	37±17*
$P_{0.1}$ (cmH$_2$O)	3.6±1.5	5±2.4*
f/V_T (breaths/min/l)	65±30	88±44*
VC (ml)	1634±642	1297±512*
$f/V_T \times P_{0.1}$ (cmH$_2$O breaths/min/l)	241±177	452±363*
$P_{0.1}$/MIP (%)	6.3±3.2	10.3±5.6*

*$p<0.001$, **$p<0.01$, successfully weaned versus failed to wean.
Abbreviations: *SW*, successful weaning; *FW*, failure of weaning; *DMV*, days of mechanical ventilation before weaning trial; *f*, frequency; V_T, tidal volume; V_E, expired minute volume; *MIP*, maximal inspiratory pressure; *MEP*, maximal expiratory pressure; $P_{0.1}$, occlusion pressure; *VC*, vital capacity. (From Vallverdú et al. 1988, with permission).

Table 14.2. Clinical characteristics and functional respiratory parameters obtained in COPD patients, neurological patients, and patients with ARF, according to clinical evolution

| | ARF (n=138) | | COPD (n=33) | | Neurological (n=46) | |
	SW (n=85)	FW (n=53)	SW (n=13)	FW (n=20)	SW (n=27)	FW (n=19)
Age (years)	58±16	58±15	61±11	68±8	47±20	55±18
DMV	6±7	13±13*	5±3	9±10	10±8	13±10
f (breaths/min)	25±7	29±7**	19±5	30±8*	25±6	29±8
V_T (ml)	428±125	404±145	422±209	291±90**	452±164	401±105
V_E (l)	10±3	11±3	7.6±2	8.4±3	15±20	11±3
MIP (cmH_2O)	64±21	52±18**	60±19	59±16	70±19	58±13**
MEP (cmH_2O)	55±27	36±16*	48±21	48±17	50±23	31±8*
$P_{0.1}$ (cmH_2O)	3.7±1.6	4.9±2.3*	3.2±1.2	5.6±3.1**	3.7±1.5	4.3±2.1
f/V_T (breaths/min/l)	64±32	84±37**	59±32	110±50**	59±22	82±52
VC (ml)	1598±632	1206±507*	1491±851	1289±431	1808±525	1542±526
$f/V_T \times P_{0.1}$ (cmH_2O breaths/min/l)	252±189	425±314*	217±193	595±431**	223±119	413±457
$P_{0.1}$/MIP (%)	6.1±3.2	10.2±6.1*	6.3±3.8	12.6±8.7**	5.7±2.8	7.8±4.3

*$p<0.001$, **$p<0.05$ successfully weaned versus failed to wean.
Abbreviations: *ARF*, acute respiratory failure; *COPD*, chronic obstructive pulmonary disease; *SW*, successful weaning; *FW*, failure of weaning; *DMV*, days of mechanical ventilation before weaning trial; *f*, frequency; V_T, tidal volume; V_E, expired minute volume; *MIP*, maximal inspiratory pressure; *MEP*, maximal expiratory pressure; $P_{0.1}$, occlusion pressure; *VC*, vital capacity. (From Vallverdú et al. 1988, with permission)

[49]. This can be assessed objectively by measuring MEP. Alteration of expiratory muscles and coordination between inspiratory and expiratory muscles can make coughing and clearing of respiratory secretions difficult, possibly leading to progressive hypoxemia and hypercapnia, and ultimately warranting reintubation. Furthermore, MEP values in neurological patients and patients with ARF who failed the weaning trial were significantly lower than those in the successful weaning trial group, but this was not so for patients with COPD. One possible explanation could be that most patients with COPD present a constant expiratory muscular activity [50], which aids the adequate clearance of secretions.

Regarding the patients with neurological disease as a cause of ARF, Koh et al. [51] performed a retrospective study of 49 neurosurgical patients who were mechanically ventilated for more than 48 h. In this study, 32 patients were successfully extubated (group I), nine patients underwent tracheotomy after one or more failed extubations (group II), and eight patients underwent elective tracheotomy (group III). The incidence of reintubation was found to be 22% (nine of 41) despite the fact that the patients met the conventional criteria. Glasgow Coma Scale scores at extubation were 11.3±2.8 for group I, vs 7.8±2.7 for group II ($p=NS$) and 5.4±2.3 at elective tracheotomy (group III). The incidence of ventilator-associated pneumonia was 35% in group I vs 100% in groups II and III ($p<0.05$). Active pneumonia with tracheal secretions and poor Glasgow Coma Score were found to be important predictors of the likelihood of failed extubation. Their results also showed that elective tracheotomy, when performed on selected neurosurgical patients, was beneficial in terms of shorter ICU stay and more rapid weaning from mechanical ventilation, thus contributing to reduced hospital costs.

In a more recent study, Coplin and co-workers studied the variation in extubation of brain-injured patients [52]. Their data provide no justification for delaying extubation of patients whose only indications for prolonged intubation are a depressed level of consciousness. They found that timely extubation of these patients who meet standard weaning criteria appears to be safe (no increased risk of reintubation or subsequent tracheotomy), potentially beneficial (associated with a lower incidence of pneumonia), and less expensive (shorter ICU stay and lower hospital costs). In this study reintubation was done in 17 of 99 patients (17.2%) without extubation delay and seven of 37 (18.9%) with extubation delay ($p=0.8$). Reintubation for airway or pulmonary dysfunction was not related to extubation delay or to coma at the time of extubation. Only two components of the semi-quantitative assessment of need for airway care were associated with successful extubation: spontaneous cough ($p=0.01$) and suctioning frequency ($p=0.001$). In summary, in neurological patients, the need for reintubation is not usually detected by standard weaning criteria, but extubation should not be delayed when the only reason to maintain mechanical ventilation is a depressed level of consciousness. In these patients, who usually present a high reintubation rate, suffer severe neurological impairment, and have longer periods of intubation and greater difficulties with control of airway secretions, the measurement of MEP could be very useful for determining the timing of extubation and/or the timing of tracheotomy if the neurological damage is so severe that extubation cannot be considered.

Finally, liberation of patients with COPD from mechanical ventilation can be particularly difficult. Elevated resistive and elastic (due to hyperinflation) loads are coupled frequently with respiratory muscle weakness (which is aggravated by treatment with corticosteroids). Moreover, malnutrition and other comorbidity, such as renal failure or CAD, are quite common in COPD patients with ARF. In some studies, COPD has been a principal cause of prolonged weaning duration [53, 54], and in others, COPD patients needed progressive withdrawal from respiratory support more frequently than other patients with different underlying disease [2].

Purro et al. [53] investigated the pathophysiologic mechanism of ventilator dependence in 28 COPD patients and 11 post-cardiac surgery (PCS) patients receiving long-term mechanical ventilation during a spontaneous breathing trial, and in 20 stable spontaneously breathing patients matched for age and disease. COPD patients with ventilator dependence demonstrated a lower minute ventilation, tidal volume, maximal inspiratory pressure, and Pdimax and higher PEEPi, $P_{0.1}$, lung resistance, and tension-time index of the diaphragm (TTIdi). PCS patients with ventilator dependence demonstrate reduced tidal volume, MIP, and Pdimax and higher respiratory frequency and $P_{0.1}$. The authors concluded that in the presence of a high drive to breathe, the imbalance between increased work load and reduced inspiratory muscle strength causes respiratory distress and CO_2 retention. Another major contribution of this study is the observation that respiratory frequency may be significantly underestimated when untriggered breaths are not appreciated. This may result in an underestimation of the degree of rapid and shallow breathing and provide another explanation for why some patients fail weaning trials despite a "favorable breathing pattern". Noninvasive measurements (breathing pattern, $P_{0.1}$, $P_{0.1}/V_T/T_i$) may provide a better insight into weaning failure and could be useful in clinical decision-making, particularly for those patients with COPD who do not show rapid shallow breathing (56% in their study).

Based on the available evidence, it appears that a negative weaning parameter may not be sufficient justification for either delaying weaning trials or delaying extubation after a patient has successfully completed a spontaneous breathing trial. However, because in some circumstances clinical judgment alone is not sufficiently accurate to predict weaning outcome, it seems reasonable, from a practical standpoint, to combine weaning predictors and clinical judgment. Indeed, the accuracy of some weaning predictors can be improved by clinical evaluation (for example, in patients with COPD), and, conversely, the use of some weaning predictors can improve the accuracy of clinical judgment (for example, in neurological patients).

14.5 References

1. Esteban A, Alía I, Gordo F, et al (1997) Extubation outcome after spontaneous breathing trials with T-tube or pressure support ventilation. Am J Respir Crit Care Med 156:459–465
2. Vallverdú I, Calaf N, Subirana M, et al (1998) Clinical characteristics, respiratory parameters, and outcome of a two-hour T-piece trial in patients weaning from mechanical ventilation. Am J Respir Crit Care Med 158:1855–1862
3. Torres A, Gatell JM, Aznar E (1995) Re-intubation increases the risk of nosocomial pneumonia in patients needing mechanical ventilation. Am J Respir Crit Care Med 152:137–141
4. Epstein SK, Ciubotaru R (1997) Effect of failed extubation on the outcome of mechanical ventilation: Chest 112:186–192
5. Epstein SK, Ciubotaru R (1998) Independent effects of etiology of failure and time to reintubation on outcome for patients failing extubation. Am J Respir Crit Care Med 158: 489–493
6. Marini JJ (1991) Weaning from mechanical ventilation. N Engl J Med 324:1496–1498
7. Vassilakopoulos T, Roussos CH, Zakynthinos S (1999) Weaning from mechanical ventilation. J Crit Care 14:39–62
8. Wheeler AP (1993) Sedation, analgesia, and paralysis in the intensive care unit. Chest 104:566–577
9. Diehl JL, Lofaso F, Deleuze P, et al (1994) Clinically relevant diaphragmatic dysfunction after cardiac operations. J Thoracic Cardiovasc Surg 107:487–498
10. Dureuil B, Viires N, Cantineua JP, et al (1986) Diaphragmatic contractility after upper abdominal surgery. J Appl Physiol 61:1775–1780
11. Maher J, Rutledge F, Remtulla H, et al (1995) Neuromuscular disorders associated with failure to wean from the ventilator. Intensive Care Med 21:737–743
12. Decramer M, Lacquet LM, Fagard R, et al (1994) Corticosteroids contribute to muscle weakness in chronic airflow obstruction. Am J Respr Crit Care Med 150:11–16
13. Gallagher CG (1994) Respiratory steroid myopathy. Am J Respr Crit Care Med 150:4–6
14. Hansen-Flaschen, Cowen J, Raps EC, et al (1993) Neuromuscular blockade in the intensive care unit: more than we bargained for. Am Rev Respir Dis 147:234–236
15. Hunter JM (1995) New neuromuscular blocking drugs. N Engl J Med 332:1691–1699
16. Laghi F, D'Alfonso N, Tobin MJ (1995) Pattern of recovery from diaphragmatic fatigue over 24 hours. J Appl Physiol 79:539–546
17. Lee C (1995) Intensive care unit neuromuscular syndrome? Anesthesiology 83:237–240

18. Rossi A, Polese G, Brandi G (1991) Dynamic hyperinflation. In: Marini JJ, Roussos C (eds) Update in intensive care and emergency medicine: Ventilatory failure. Springer-Verlag, Berlin Heidelberg New York, pp 199–218
19. McParland C, Krishnan B, Wang Y, et al (1992) Inspiratory muscle weakness and dyspnea in chronic heart failure. Am Rev Respir Dis 146:467–472
20. Aubier M (1993) Respiratory muscles. Working or wasting? Intensive Care Med 19:564–568
21. Epstein SK (1995) Etiology of extubation failure and the predictive value of the rapid shallow breathing index. Am J Respir Crit Care Med 152:545–548
22. Stroetz RW, Hubmayr RD (1995) Tidal volume maintenance during weaning with pressure support. Am J Respir Crit Care Med 152:1034–1040
23. Lemaire F, Teboul JL, Cinotti L, et al (1988) Acute left ventricular dysfunction during unsuccessful weaning from mechanical ventilation. Anesthesiology 69:171–179
24. Richard C, Teboul JL, Archambaud F, et al (1994) Left ventricular function during weaning of patients with chronic obstructive pulmonary disease. Intensive Care Med 20:181–186
25. Chatila W, Ani S, Guaglianone D, et al (1996) Cardiac ischemia during weaning from mechanical ventilation. Chest 109:1577–1583
26. Teboul JL, Lenique L (1994) Comment ventiler un patient atteint d'oedeme pulmonaire cardiogenique ? In: Brochard L, Mancebo J (eds) Ventilation artificielle. Principes et applications. Amette, Paris, pp 313–330
27. Jubran A, Mathru M, Dries D, et al (1998) Continuous recordings of mixed venous oxygen saturation during weaning from mechanical ventilation and the ramifications thereof. Am J Respir Crit Care Med 158:1763–1769
28. Hilberman M, Kamm B, Lamy M, et al (1976) An analysis of potential predictors of respiratory adequacy following cardiac surgey. J Thorac Cardiovasc Surg 71:711–719
29. Tahvanainen J, Salmenpera M, Nikki P (1983) Extubation criteria after weaning from intermittent mandatory ventilation and continuous positive airway pressure. Crit Care Med 11:702–707
30. Le Bourdelles G, Viires N, Boezkowski J, et al (1994) Effects of mechanical ventilation on diaphragmatic contractile properties in rats. Am J Respr Crit Care Med 149:1539–1544
31. Pourriat JL, Lamberto C, Hoang P, et al (1986) Diaphragmatic fatigue and breathing pattern during weaning from mechanical ventilation in COPD patients. Chest 90: 703–707
32. Yang KL, Tobin MJ (1991) A prospective study of indexes predicting the outcome of trials of weaning from mechanical ventilation. N Engl J Med 324:1445–1450
33. Sassoon, CSH., Mahutte CK (1993) Airway occlusion pressure and breathing pattern as predictors of weaning outcome. Am Rev Respir Dis 148:860–866
34. Vassilakopoulos T, Zakynthinos S, Roussos CH (1998) The tension-time index and the frequency/tidal volume ratio are the major pathophysiologic determinants of weaning failure and success. Am J Respir Crit Care Med 158:378–385
35. Tobin MJ, Pérez W, Guenther SM, et al (1986) The pattern of weaning during successful and unsuccessful trials of weaning from mechanical ventilation. Am Rev Respir Dis 134:1111–1118
36. Ely, E. W, Baker AM, Dunagan DP, Burke HL, Smith AC, Kelly PT, Johnson MM, Browder RW, Bowton DL, Haponik EF (1996) Effect on the duration of mechanical ventilation of identifying patients capable of breathing spontaneously. N Engl J Med 335:1864–1869
37. Saura P, Blanch L, Mestre J, et al (1996) Clinical consequences of the implementation of a weaning protocol. Intensive Care Med 157:1052–1056
38. Tomilson, JR., Miller KS, Lorch DG, Smith L, Reines HD, Sahn SA (1989) A prospective comparison of IMV and T-piece weaning from mechanical ventilation. Chest 96:348–352
39. DeHaven, CB, Hurst JM, Branson RD (1986) Evaluation of two different extubation criteria: attributes contributing to success. Crit Care Med 14:92–94
40. Brochard L, Rauss A, Benito S, et al (1994) Comparison of three methods of gradual withdrawal from ventilatory support during weaning from mechanical ventilation. Am J Respir Crit Care Med 150:896–903
41. Esteban A, Frutos F, Tobin MJ, et al (1995) A comparison of four methods of weaning patients from mechanical ventilation. N Engl J Med 332:345–350

42. De Haven CB, Kirton OC, Morgan JP, Hart AML, Shatz DV, Civetta JM (1996) Breathing measurement reduces false-negative classification of tachypneic preextubation trial failures. Crit Care Med 24:976–980
43. Epstein SK, Ciubotaru R (1995) Influences of gender and endotracheal tube size on preextubation breathing pattern. Am J Respir Crit Care Med 152:545–549
44. Lee K.H, Hui KP, Chan TB, Tan WC, Lim TK (1994) Rapid shallow breathing (frequency-tidal volume ratio) did not predict extubation outcome. Chest 105:540–543
45. Gandía, F, Blanco J (1992) Evaluation of indexes predicting the outcome of ventilator weaning and value of adding supplemental inspiratory load. Intensive Care Med 18: 327–333
46. Krieger BP, Isber J, Breitenbucher A, Throop G, Ershowsky P (1997) Serial measurements of the rapid-shallow-breathing index as a predictor of weaning outcome in elderly medical patients. Chest 112:10029–1034
47. Fernández R, Blanch LL, Artigas A (1991) Respiratory center activity during mechanical ventilation. J Crit Care 6:102–111
48. Herrera M, Blasco J, Venegas J, Barba R, Doblas A, Márquez E (1985) Mouth occlusion pressure ($P_{0.1}$) in acute respiratory failure. Intensive Care Med 11:134–139
49. Truwit JD, Marini JJ (1988) Evaluation of thoracic mechanics in the ventilated patient. Part I: primary measurements. J Crit Care 3:133–150
50. Ninane V, Yernault JC De Troyer A (1993) Intrinsic PEEP in patients with chronic obstructive pulmonary disease. Role of expiratory muscles. Am Rev Respir Dis 148:1037–1042
51. Koh WY, Lew TWK, Chin NM, Wong MFM (1997) Tracheostomy in a neuro-intensive care setting: indications and timing. Anaesth Intensive Care 25:365–368
52. Coplin WM, Pierson J, Cooley KD, Newell DW, Rubenfeld GD (2000) Implications of extubation delay in brain-injured patients meeting standard weaning criteria. Am J Respir Crit Care Med 161:1530–1536
53. Purro A, Appendini L, De Gaetano A, Gudjonsdottir M, Donner CF, Rossi A (2000) Physiologic determinants of ventilator dependence in long-term mechanically ventilated patients. Am J Respir Crit Care Med 161:1115–1123
54. Capdevila X, Perrigault PF, Ramonatxo M, Roustan P, Peray P, d'Athis F, Prefaut C (1998) Changes in breathing pattern and respiratory muscle performance parameters during difficult weaning. Crit Care Med 26:79–87

15 How Should We Interpret Weaning-Predictive Indices?

S.K. Epstein

15.1 Introduction

For the past three decades investigators have employed numerous physiologic and clinical parameters in an attempt to predict weaning and extubation outcome:

1. Measures of oxygenation and gas exchange (P_aO_2/F_IO_2, P_aO_2/P_AO_2, oxygenation index, alveolar-arterial O_2 gradient, dead-space fraction, pH)
2. Simple measures of capacity and load (vital capacity, tidal volume; respiratory rate; minute ventilation; maximal voluntary ventilation; negative inspiratory force (NIF) or maximal inspiratory pressure (MIP); static or dynamic compliance; maximal expiratory pressure)
3. Integrative indices (frequency–tidal volume ratio or f/V_T; CROP index; weaning index; inspiratory effort quotient)
4. Complex measurements of capacity and load requiring special equipment (airway occlusion pressure or $P_{0.1}$; $P_{0.1}/P_Imax$; gastric intramucosal pH; work of breathing; Pdi/Pdimax; P_I/P_Imax)

To date, several hundred papers have been published and more than 50 individual parameters have been studied. Only recently have investigators turned their attention to the study of how weaning predictors should be used to improve clinical decision-making. In evaluating the utility of these parameters it is crucial to consider the outcome being examined (e.g., weaning versus extubation), the patient population (e.g., medical, surgical), and the disease process (e.g., acute lung injury, cardiac disease, COPD, neurologic disease) under investigation. The methodology, timing, and reproducibility of the measurements must be carefully analyzed. In addition, numerous major limitations have been identified. For example, nearly all studies are observational, with parameters measured and then correlated with outcome. In the majority of studies physicians performing weaning and extubation were not completely blinded to the results of the predictor. Under these circumstances, the parameter itself may have influenced the decision to wean or extubate (or not) and therefore contaminated the results. Perhaps the most compelling question is whether or not parameters provide additional predictive data that lead to improvements in outcome, such as a decrease in weaning and extubation failures or avoidance of prolonged mechanical ventilation. In uncontrolled fashion, many investigators have used one or more weaning parameters to decide whether or not to initiate weaning trials (Brochard et al. 1994; Esteban et al. 1997; Esteban et al. 1999; Esteban et al. 1995). Similarly, randomized controlled trials of protocol-directed weaning have included standard parameters as part of a multi-component screen but have not investigated the precise role of these tests (Ely et al. 1999). This has raised the important question: Can spontaneous breathing trials be initiated when standard clinical criteria are satisfactory (e.g., hemodynamic stability, adequate oxygenation), or must further measurements (e.g., weaning parameters) be used before proceeding? The potential "dark side" of weaning parameters is best illustrated by a study demonstrating that nearly one third of patients who never passed a daily screen, often because of the weaning parameter alone, were still successfully extubated (Ely et al. 1999). The implication of these observations is that overly strict application of a parameter could result in needless prolongation of mechanical ventilation for a sizable fraction of patients. Undeniably, physiologic measurements provide insight into the mechanisms of weaning failure and ventilator dependence. In this chapter I will focus on how to interpret the literature on parameters and how to apply them in clinical practice. Although these tests are used to predict the outcome of trials of spontaneous breathing (e.g., liberation or weaning) or extubation, for simplicity I will refer to them collectively as weaning predictors, parameters, or tests.

15.2 What Outcome Should Be Predicted?

There are several sentinel points where clinicians may seek to predict outcome, including identifying the earliest time that a trial of minimal ventilatory support can be undertaken, the result of such a spontaneous breathing trial (SBT), and the likelihood of tolerating extubation. In general, spontaneous breathing trials are considered when the process leading to respiratory failure has substantially improved or resolved, other clinical criteria are deemed acceptable, and, typically, when one or more physiologic variables (e.g., weaning parameters) are satisfactory (Table 15.1). These latter variables have often included the negative inspiratory force, tidal volume, vital capacity, and respiratory frequency. Yet few of these criteria have been critically assessed. More commonly, patients not fulfilling criteria are kept on ventilatory support while those satisfying criteria are given an opportunity to breathe on their own. Large prospective trials demonstrate that approximately 70% of patients satisfying these criteria will tolerate a spontaneous breathing trial (Brochard et al. 1994; Esteban et al. 1997; Esteban et al. 1999; Esteban et al. 1995; Vallverdu et al. 1998). In contrast, the percentage of patients satisfying only a portion of the criteria but still capable of passing a spontaneous breathing trial has not been investigated.

The greatest emphasis has been placed on predicting whether patients deemed capable of initiating spontaneous breathing will actually tolerate the trial. These trials of minimal (PSV, CPAP) or no (T-piece) ventilatory support typically vary in duration from 30 min to 24 h. The criteria used to determine the tolerance for such trials are both subjective and objective (Table 15.1). In either case, the criteria applied are often nonspecific and may reflect factors unrelated to the under-

Table 15.1. Weaning trial criteria

Criteria to be met before weaning trials are initiated
1. Resolution of (or significant improvement in) the cause for requiring mechanical ventilation
2. Hemodynamic stability
3. Adequate oxygenation
4. Adequate neurologic status
5. Ability to protect airway and manage respiratory secretions
6. Acceptable hemoglobin level*
7. Absence of fever*

Criteria for tolerating weaning trials
1. Oxygenation (PaO_2 $\geq$60 mmHg or SaO_2 $\geq$90% on FiO_2 $\leq$0.40–0.50)
2. Ventilation ($PaCO_2$ increase $\leq$10 mmHg or pH decrease $\leq$ 0.10)
3. Blood pressure (systolic blood pressure $\geq$90 or $\leq$180 mmHg; increase or decrease $\leq$20%)
4. Heart rate ($\geq$50 or $\leq$140 beats/min; increase or decrease $\leq$20%)
5. Respiratory rate (f $\leq$35 breaths/min)
6. No sign of excessive respiratory work (absence of thoracoabdominal paradox, respiratory alternans, or accessory respiratory muscle action)
7. No diaphoresis, agitation, depressed mental status, or distress

*Some authors include these factors.

lying pathophysiology of weaning failure. Tolerance for the SBT results in extubation if the patient has adequate respiratory drive and the capacity to protect the airway. As many as 20% of extubated patients fail and require reintubation within 24–72 h (Epstein 2000a), for reasons that are often distinct from those leading to weaning intolerance (Epstein 1995). Most investigators analyzing the predictive accuracy of weaning parameters have combined weaning and extubation failure into a single outcome. A number of recent investigations have appropriately categorized weaning and extubation outcome as separate and distinct outcomes. The rationale for this is bolstered by the realization that many patients "failing" spontaneous breathing trials are in fact ready for liberation (DeHaven et al. 1996; Epstein et al. 2000).

15.3 The Rationale for Predicting Outcome

Before deciding how to predict outcome it is important to investigate the rationale for prediction. Although mechanical ventilation can be a life-saving intervention it is also associated with many complications including ventilator-associated pneumonia (VAP), sinusitis, gastrointestinal bleeding, thromboembolism, barotrauma, airway injury, and respiratory muscle atrophy. The risk for complications, especially VAP, increases with duration of mechanical ventilation (Fagon et al. 1989). Using a Cox proportional hazards model, one study also raised the possibility that increasing duration of mechanical ventilation was associated with increased mortality, though survival subsequently improved for patients ventilated for more than 21 days (Ely et al. 1999). Therefore, an important goal in the clinical application of weaning predictors is to identify the earliest time that patients can be liberated from the ventilator in order to minimize the exposure to these complications.

Another reason cited for using predictive indices is to avoid premature trials of minimal ventilatory support. Several investigators have found that many patients failing T-piece trials demonstrate an elevated tension-time index (Capdevila et al. 1998; Jubran and Tobin 1997; Vassilakopoulos et al. 1998) or an electromyographic pattern suggestive of respiratory muscle fatigue (Brochard et al. 1989; Cohen et al. 1982; Murciano et al. 1988). In a study of healthy volunteers, fatigue was induced by inspiratory threshold loading and the subjects subsequently took more than 24 h to recover (Laghi et al. 1995). Furthermore, animal models indicate that structural injury to the respiratory muscles can result from prolonged breathing against a high inspiratory workload (Reid et al. 1994). A major ramification of these observations is that a failed trial of spontaneous breathing will adversely affect future weaning efforts, especially if insufficient rest is provided before embarking on the next trial. The end result could be further deterioration in the balance between respiratory load and capacity and an unnecessary prolongation of the duration of mechanical ventilation. Several studies raise important questions about the validity of this hypothesis. First, a recent investigation found that respiratory muscle fatigue may recover more rapidly (<<24 h) than previously suggested and therefore would not be anticipated to delay subsequent weaning attempts (Travaline et al. 1997). Second, a preliminary study using phrenic nerve stimulation found evidence of contractile fatigue to be fairly uncommon in patients failing T-piece trials (Laghi et al. 2000). Most persuasively, a well-done study of weaning modes found no difference in outcome between once-daily and multiple daily T-piece trials (Esteban et al. 1995). If failed weaning trials adversely affected future attempts, one would have predicted that the multiple daily group would experience a lower success rate and ultimately a longer duration of mechanical ventilation.

Another concern is that a weaning trial, especially a premature one, could precipitate cardiac failure or ischemia in patients with underlying cardiac disease (Lemaire et al. 1988). Conversely, the development of ischemia during weaning may result in weaning failure and consequently prolonged ventilator dependence. In fact, the incidence of ischemia was low (6.4%) in a large prospective study conducted in an MICU/CCU (Chatila et al. 1996a), and a clinically relevant adverse impact on outcome was not demonstrated. Therefore, at the present time there is no definitive evidence that a failed trial of spontaneous breathing negatively impacts outcome. Further study of this issue is of paramount importance, because much of the rationale for prediction is based on the desire to avoid the adverse impact of a failed weaning trial. The rationale for trying to accurately predict extubation outcome is even more compelling, because many studies have now demonstrated that patients failing extubation have a significantly increased mortality (Epstein 2000a; Esteban et al. 1997; Esteban et al. 1999).

15.4 Testing of Parameters

15.4.1 General Principles of Test Interpretation

Unfortunately, many investigations of weaning predictors have compared only mean values for success and failure patients, which precludes application to bedside clinical decision-making. A more useful approach relates the presence or absence of a predictor (using a threshold value) to the outcome under investigation (e.g., weaning success or failure) (Epstein and Picken 1997). This process is best achieved by constructing a two-by-two table, permitting direct comparison of the test results to the "gold standard". For example, in Fig. 15.1, the test result (e.g., f/V_T) is displayed on the left, with positive and negative results determined using a preselected threshold value, while the gold standard (e.g., the actual outcome) is displayed across the top. A true positive (TP) is present when the test is positive (e.g., $f/V_T \leq 105$ breaths/l/min) and the patient is successfully weaned. A false positive (FP) is present when the test is positive but the patient fails. A negative test (e.g., $f/V_T > 105$ breaths/l/min) is considered a true negative (TN) when the patient fails weaning and a false negative (FN) when the patient succeeds.

The ratio of true positives to the sum of true positives plus false negatives is the sensitivity (TP/TP+FN). The sensitivity refers to the proportion of successfully weaned patients who will have a positive test. The ratio of true negative to the sum of true negative and false positives is the specificity (TN/TN+FP). The specificity refers to the proportion of patients failing weaning who have a negative test. The two-by-two table also yields the expressions positive predictive value (PPV) and negative predictive value (NPV). The PPV (TP/TP+FP) refers to the proportion of patients with a positive test (e.g., predicted to succeed) who are successfully weaned. In contrast, the NPV (TN/TN+FN) refers to the proportion of patients with a negative test (e.g., predicted to fail) who fail weaning. While sensitivity and specificity are properties of the test itself, independent of the particular patient sample in whom the test is used, the PPV and NPV depend on the prevalence of weaning success.

	Successful Weaning	Failed Weaning
Positive Test ($f/V_T < 105$)	True Positive (TP)	False Positive (FP)
Negative Test ($f/V_T > 105$)	False Negative (FN)	True Negative (TN)

Fig. 15.1. Two-by-two table comparing results of a weaning parameter (f/V_T) with the actual results of the weaning trial. (From Epstein and Picken 1997, with permission)

15.4.2 Pre-Test and Post-Test Probability, Bayes Theorem, and Likelihood Ratios

A quintessential concept in diagnostic test interpretation is full consideration of the prevalence (e.g., the prior or pre-test probability) of the condition under examination. This approach is familiar to pulmonary physicians who use this strategy when interpreting ventilation-perfusion scans, PPD skin testing, and solitary pulmonary nodules. Only recently have investigators demonstrated the importance of the pre-test probability of weaning or extubation success in interpreting and using predictors (Epstein and Picken 1997; Jaeschke et al. 1997; Sassoon and Mahutte 1993). By combining the pre-test probability of success (P[D+]) with the true-positive rate (TPR or sensitivity) and the false-positive rate (FPR, 1-specificity) of the weaning predictor, a post-test probability can be generated using Bayes' theorem. The probability of weaning success with a positive test (P[D+T+]) can be determined by applying the equation,

$$P[D+T+]= \frac{(P[D+])\times(TPR)}{[(P[D+])\times(TPR)] +[(1-P[D+])\times(FPR)]}$$

The probability of weaning success with a negative test (P[D+T-]) can be calculated from the equation,

$$P[D+T-]= \frac{(P[D+])\times(1-TPR)}{[(P[D+])\times(1-TPR)] +[(1-P[D+])\times(1-FPR)]}$$

With a very high pre-test probability of weaning success, a positive test results in only a minimal increase in the post-test probability of success. A positive test will significantly increase the probability of success when the pre-test probability is very low, but failure may remain the most likely outcome (e.g., post-test probability of success is <0.50). Similar effects will occur when patients with negative tests are examined. With a very high pre-test probability of success, the probability of success may remain significant even with a negative test. In contrast, a negative test minimally effects the post-test probability when the pre-test probability of success is very low. Therefore, at the extremes of probability the post-test probability may differ little from the pre-test value, even for a reasonably accurate weaning test. Another axiom is that identical test results (e.g., two patients with a positive test, $f/V_T \leq 105$ breaths/l/min) can result in very different post-test probabilities, 23% and 96%, when the pre-test probabilities are divergent, 10% and 90%, respectively. Conversely, patients with different f/V_T values may demonstrate identical post-test probabilities of weaning success (e.g., 47%) when the pre-test probabilities are very different, 25% (in a patient with a positive test) and 95% (in a patient with a negative test, $f/V_T >105$ breaths/l/min) (Epstein and Picken 1997).

The likelihood ratio (LR) is a statement of the odds that a specific test result will be present in a patient with a specific condition (e.g., weaning success) when compared with a patient without the condition (e.g., weaning failure). The LR+ is the odds that a patient with weaning success will have a positive test ($f/V_T \leq 105$ breaths/l/min) compared with the odds that a patient with weaning failure will

Table 15.2. Application of likelihood ratios[a]

LR+=sensitivity/(1–specificity)
(example: LR+[f/$V_T \leq 105$]=2.69)
LR–=(1–sensitivity)/specificity
(example: LR–[f/V_T>105]=0.05)

[a]Using data from the study of Yang and Tobin (sensitivity 0.97; specificity 0.64), (Yang and Tobin 1991).

demonstrate a positive test. The LR– is the odds that a patient with weaning success will have a negative test (f/V_T>105 breaths/l/min) compared with the odds that a patient with failure will have a negative test. Compared with PPVs and NPVs, the likelihood ratio provides a number of advantages for test interpretation. First, the ratios are derived exclusively from the sensitivity and specificity of the test, and are therefore independent of prevalence (Table 15.2). Second, the ratios can be calculated for different ranges of a test result. For example, using the original data from Yang and Tobin, LRs of 7.53 (f/V_T<80 breaths/l/min), 0.77 (f/V_T = 80–100 breaths/l/min) and 0.004 (f/V_T >100 breaths/l/min) can be calculated (Jaeschke et al. 1997). Third, the post-test probability of success can be easily calculated after the pre-test probability has been converted to the pre-test odds using the equation: pre-test probability / 1– (pre-test probability) = pre-test odds. The pre-test odds are then multiplied by the LR to generate the post-test odds. The post-test odds can be converted to post-test probability using the equation: post-test odds/ (post-test odds +1) = post-test probability. By using the pre-test probability, the LR, and a simple nomogram the post-test probability can be rapidly determined without mathematical calculation (Jaeschke et al. 1997). Fourth, the LR provides meaningful insight into the clinical relevance of a test because it conveys information on the magnitude of change in probability of success or failure with a given test result. For example, an LR of 1 indicates that the test is of no value because post-test probability will be identical to pre-test probability. Although the probability of success increases when LR>1 and decreases when LR<1, the magnitude of change may vary. For example, although an LR of 1.5 indicates an increased probability of success, the change from the pre-test probability is small and unlikely to be clinically relevant. More moderate changes in probability, which may or may not be clinically important, are associated with LRs of 2–5 or 0.2–0.5. Larger, usually clinically relevant changes in probability occur when the LR of a test is either >5 or <0.2. Unfortunately, the latter LRs are not commonly seen for tests used as weaning parameters.

Weaning predictor tests are most often measured by a continuous function. For this information to be applied at the bedside to weaning and extubation decision-making, a threshold value should be selected to determine when a test will be considered positive or negative (Fig. 15.2). This selection process entails an interesting trade-off: A high threshold increases the false-positive rate because more patients who fail have a positive test. In contrast, although selection of a low threshold value decreases the number of false positives, this comes at the cost of a lower true-positive rate (or higher false-negative rate). The trade-off between false positives and true positives can be depicted by plotting

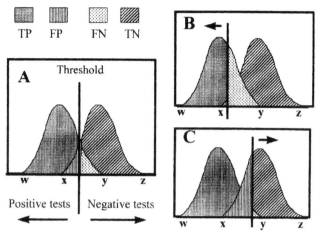

Fig. 15.2. Selection of a threshold value for a test. The distribution from *w* to *y* indicates patients with weaning success. The distribution from *x* to *z* indicates patients with weaning failure. In *panel A*, the threshold selected results in equal numbers of false positives (*FP*) and false negatives (*FN*). In *panel B*, the threshold has been shifted to the left, resulting in a decrease in FPs and an increase in FNs. In *panel C*, the threshold has been shifted to the right, resulting in an increase in FPs and a decrease in FNs. *TP*, True positives, *TN*, true negatives. (From Epstein 2000b, with permission)

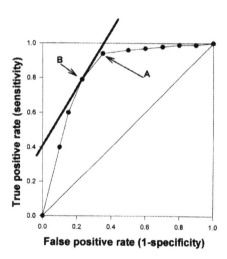

Fig. 15.3. Receiver operating characteristic curve. A threshold value is usually selected by identifying the point that maximizes the true-positive rate without further increasing the false-positive rate (*arrow A*). More appropriately, a threshold should be selected that also takes into account the cost of a false positive [C], the benefit of a true positive [B], and the pre-test probability of weaning success p[D]. By using the equation C/B x (1-p[D])/p[D], the slope of a line is derived that identifies the optimal threshold value (*arrow B*). (From Epstein 2000b, with permission)

the TPR and FPR for all test results (e.g., varying the threshold value) and creating a receiver operating characteristic (ROC) curve (Fig. 15.3). The ROC curve serves several functions: When different weaning tests are compared, the predictor with the greatest area under the ROC curve is considered the preferred parameter, independent of the threshold value selected. A test that results in no change in the post-test probability is characterized by an area under the ROC curve of 0.50. In contrast, a "perfect" test, with both sensitivity and specificity of 1, will have an area of 1.0.

ROC curves can also be used to optimize selection of the threshold value. Traditionally, threshold values have been chosen based on the point on the ROC curve that minimizes both false positives and false negatives (e.g., the point yielding the highest TPR without further increasing FPR). This approach gives equal weight to false positives and false negatives and disregards the pre-test probability of weaning success. In truth, the adverse impact of a failed weaning trial or failed extubation, i.e., the cost (C) of a false positive and the benefit (B) of avoiding unnecessary prolongation of mechanical ventilation, are often not equivalent. The best threshold value, weighing the trade-off between false positives and false negatives, can be determined using the equation $C/B \times (1-p[D])/p[D]$, where p[D] is the pre-test probability of success (Sox et al. 1988). The equation yields the slope of a line which, when placed tangent to the ROC curve, yields the best threshold (Fig. 15.3). Under circumstances where the cost of weaning or extubation failure markedly exceeds the benefit of avoiding additional time on mechanical ventilation (e.g., $C/B \gg 1$), an f/V_T cutoff of 60 breaths/l/min would be optimal (e.g., a value that decreases the chance of a false positive, though false negatives may increase). Conversely, when the benefit of avoiding excess time on mechanical ventilation outweighs the cost of failed weaning or extubation (e.g., $C/B < 1$), the resulting point on the ROC curve corresponds to a higher f/V_T value. In either case, the pre-test probability of success remains a crucial influence, with a rising p[D] leading to selection of higher cutoff values.

15.5 Weaning Parameters

If clinical assessment by ICU practitioners were adequate, objective weaning parameters would be unnecessary. Although some epidemiologic information, including increased duration of mechanical ventilation prior to weaning onset (Capdevila et al. 1995; Del Rosario et al. 1997; Lee et al. 1994; Vallverdu et al. 1998) and disease category (e.g., COPD) (Nava et al. 1994; Vallverdu et al. 1998), indicate increased risk for weaning failure, the impact on decision-making is unstudied. An older study of post-cardiac surgery patients, observed a PPV 0.83 and an NPV 0.67 for the nurses' assessment of whether patients would pass their initial weaning trial (Hilberman et al. 1976). Subsequently, Stroetz and Hubmayr noted that even experienced intensivists were frequently incorrect about a patient's readiness to tolerate unassisted breathing (sensitivity 0.35, specificity 0.70, PPV 0.67, NPV 0.50) (Stroetz and Hubmayr 1995). Even when qualitative clinical measures appear to have some degree of accuracy, the vague nature of the criteria makes it difficult to apply them outside the center conducting the study. Therefore, clinical gestalt appears insufficiently exact, and objective measurements may have the potential to improve predictive accuracy.

If an objective weaning parameter is to be used it is desirable that the measurement technique be safe, be easy to perform at the bedside, and not require special equipment. Measurements that are independent of patient cooperation are favored because variability in patient effort can influence the result of some tests. A high degree of test reproducibility is essential with a low coefficient of variation, but this goal has been more difficult to achieve when multiple operators (Multz et al. 1990), rather than a single or small group of operators, are involved (Baumeister et al. 1997; Yang 1992). Ideally the parameter would have a sound "physiologic" basis for predicting outcome and provide insight into the mechanisms of failure.

Numerous possible parameters are available and have been extensively studied, including indices of oxygenation and gas exchange and simple measures of capacity and load (see Table 15.1). The principal focus here will be on the two most comprehensively studied predictors, the maximal inspiratory pressure and the frequency–tidal volume ratio.

15.5.1 Maximal Inspiratory Pressure (Negative Inspiratory Force)

A determination of respiratory muscle strength may identify patients at increased risk for weaning failure (Table 15.3). The maximal inspiratory pressure (MIP) or negative inspiratory force (NIF) can be measured by attaching an aneroid manometer to the endotracheal tube and instructing the patient to maximally inspire against an occluded airway. What accounts for the very wide range of reported positive predictive (0.55–1.0) and negative predictive values (0–1.0) seen with this parameter? Why are some patients with apparently severe respiratory muscle weakness (e.g., unable to generate -20 cmH_2O) able to be successfully liberated? The MIP depends upon numerous factors including muscle strength, coordination, chest wall compliance, lung volume, respiratory drive, patient effort/cooperation, and investigator technique. Some factors are difficult to control in patients on mechanical ventilation and poor values may result, not from true respiratory muscle weakness but from one of these other considerations. By using a 20-s occlusion and a one-way valve that allows expiration but not inspiration, a reproducible and reliable maximal effort is generated (Truwit and Marini 1992; Yang 1992). Although reproducibility is good when a single investigator takes measurements on a single day, a much higher coefficient of variation (32%) has been noted when different investigators study the same patient on the same day (Multz et al. 1990). Why does an adequate MIP (e.g., more negative than -20 to -30 cmH_2O) fail to ensure weaning success? First, a single maneuver may not adequately reflect respiratory muscle strength and does not ensure satisfactory endurance capacity. Second, even if muscle strength is satisfactory it does not take into account the load against which the muscles must contract. Third, many investigators have restricted weaning efforts to patients able to generate a minimum of -20 cmH_2O of pressure during the MIP maneuver. Under these circumstances, when the prevalence of weaning failure is high, the number of false positives will

Table 15.3. Studies examining the predictive value of negative inspiratory force or maximal inspiratory pressure

Reference	Threshold value (cmH$_2$O)	Sensitivity	Specificity	PPV	NPV
Sahn and Lakshminarayan (1973)	−25	1.0	1.0	1.0	1.0
Tahvanainen et al. (1983)	−30	0.67	0	0.74	0
Krieger et al. (1989)	−20	NR	NR	0.91	0.22
	−30	NR	NR	0.92	0.21
Yang and Tobin (1991)	−15	1.0	0.11	0.59	1.00
	−20	1.0	0.14	0.60	1.00
	−30	0.86	0.21	0.58	0.55
Gandia and Blanco (1992)	−23	0.82	0.75	0.88	0.64
Yang (1993)	−15	1.00	0.13	0.55	1.00
Sassoon and Mahutte (1993)	−20	0.91	0.3	0.82	0.50
Mohsenifar et al. (1993)	−20	1.00	0.09	0.64	1.00
Capdevila et al. (1995)	−50	0.80	0.41	0.86	0.31
Chatila et al. (1996b)	−20	0.90	0.26	0.67	0.60
	−30	0.67	0.69	0.78	0.55
Leitch et al. (1996)	−20	0.97	0	0.99	0
Jacob et al. (1997)	−20	0.96	0.07	0.92	0.14

PPV, positive predictive value; *NPV*, negative predictive value; *NR*, not reported.

increase. In summary, although maximal inspiratory pressure is better than most of the other simple parameters, it illustrates how differences in technique and considerations of underlying pathophysiology may confound interpretation and yield a wide range of predictive values.

15.5.2 Frequency–Tidal Volume Ratio, f/V$_T$

Although numerous weaning predictors have been studied, the f/V$_T$ is the most thoroughly examined and provides the best paradigm for investigating the utility of these parameters. The theoretical, physiologic, and clinical foundations for using breathing pattern as a predictor of weaning outcome initially appeared to be reasonably robust. For example, it was demonstrated that patients failing weaning manifested a breathing pattern similar to that of patients studied shortly after the onset of acute respiratory failure (Del Rosario et al. 1997). Furthermore, the relationship between respiratory load and respiratory muscle capacity was found to be a prime determinant of weaning outcome (Jubran and Tobin 1997; Vassilakopoulos et al. 1998). When imbalance or respiratory muscle fatigue existed in non-mechanically ventilated patients, a pattern of rapid and shallow breathing was often observed (Roussos 1984). Yet Tobin and colleagues found that patients ultimately failing weaning trials breathed rapidly and shallowly immediately upon discontinuation of mechanical ventilation, suggesting the existence of mechanisms other than fatigue (Tobin et al. 1986). Similarly, in a study of healthy subjects, respiratory muscle fatigue led to rapid shallow breathing only when simultaneously combined with an increased respiratory load (Mador and Acevedo 1991). More recently, even this relationship between f/V_T and respiratory load has been questioned because no correlation between f/V_T and the tension-time index was found among patients failing weaning trials (Jubran and Tobin 1997; Vassilakopoulos et al. 1998). In addition, a large number of other factors have been associated with a pattern of rapid shallow breathing, including anxiety, female gender, narrow endotracheal tube size, sepsis or pneumonia, older age, supine positioning, increased body temperature, and preceding lung disease (Epstein 2000b).

In a landmark paper, Yang and Tobin demonstrated that the area under the ROC curve for the f/V_T was greater than that measured for other weaning parameters (minute ventilation, respiratory frequency, tidal volume, maximal inspiratory pressure, compliance, oxygenation), indicating that it was the most accurate test available (Yang and Tobin 1991). Since that original report, numerous published investigations have examined the predictive capacity of the f/V_T (Table 15.4). Although the PPV of an $f/V_T \leq 105$ breaths/l/min has been consistently reported in the range of 0.75 and above, the very high NPV (0.95) originally noted has been more difficult to reproduce. Numerous explanations have been offered to explain differing results, including differences in the lack of blinding, the prevalence of weaning success, variable presence of confounding factors that influence breathing pattern, and the use of respiratory frequency as a criterion for weaning failure (Epstein and Picken 1997; Jaeschke et al. 1997). Many investigators require a respiratory rate <35 breaths/min or a tidal volume >4–5 ml/kg before allowing a patient to proceed with a weaning trial. This confounds study of predictor accuracy because patients not satisfying these criteria cannot be evaluated. Similarly, few if any studies have truly blinded the clinicians to the test results, thus raising the possibility that these parameters influenced decisions on weaning and extubation. Changes in prevalence of weaning success will also influence the positive and negative predictive values for a given parameter (Epstein and Picken 1997). When the prevalence of success is very high, the positive predictive value increases (e.g., there are few false positives) and the negative predictive value decreases (e.g., there a few true negatives, which magnifies the effect of false negatives) (Chatila et al. 1996b; Jacob et al. 1997; Krieger et al. 1989; Leitch et al. 1996; Levy et al. 1995; Vallverdu et al. 1998). Some studies have focused exclusively on weaning outcome, or extubation outcome, or on a combination of the two (Epstein and Picken 1997; Jaeschke et al. 1997). The high prevalence of extubation success among patients tolerating spontaneous breathing trials helps to explain, in part, why weaning parameters perform poorly in predicting extubation outcome.

Although the majority of recent studies have employed objective criteria for determining tolerance for a spontaneous breathing trial, these have been poorly standardized. The subjective nature of the criteria for weaning failure may offer

Table 15.4. Studies examining the predictive value of the frequency-tidal volume (f/V$_T$) ratio

Reference	Number of patients studied	Outcome evaluated (%EF)	Threshold value (breaths/l/min)	Sensitivity	Specificity	PPV	NPV	LR+ LR−	Comments
Yang and Tobin (1991)	100	W, E (NR)	105	0.97	0.64	0.78	0.95	2.69 0.05	
Gandia and Blanco (1992)	40	W	96	0.82	0.83	0.92	0.66	4.82 0.22	Measured 15 min after disconnection
Yang (1993)	31	W	100	0.94	0.73	0.79	0.92	3.48 0.08	
Sassoon and Mahutte (1993)	45	W, E	100	0.97	0.40	0.85	0.78	1.62 0.08	
Mohsenifar et al. (1993)	29	W, E (27)	105	1.00	0.27	0.69	1.00	1.37 0	Measured on PSV
Lee et al. (1994)	52	E	105	0.72	0.11	0.79	0.08	0.81 2.55	Measurements made on CPAP or PSV
Shikora et al. (1994)	28	W	100	0.40	0.52	0.15	0.80	0.83 1.15	Failure defined as not extubated within 2 weeks
Stroetz and Hubmayr (1995)	31	W	60	0.79	0.71	NR	NR	2.72 0.30	Measurements on PSV
Epstein (1995)	94	E	100	0.92	0.22	0.83	0.40	1.18 0.36	
Capdevila et al. (1995)	67	E	60 100	0.73	0.75	0.92	0.36	2.92 0.36	Measured after 20 min of T-piece
Chatila (1996b)	100	W, E (16)	100	0.89	0.41	0.72	0.68	1.51 0.27	
Dojat et al. (1996)	38	W, E (24)	100	0.94	0.81	0.80	0.94	4.95 0.07	

Table 15.4. *Continued.*

Reference	Number of patients studied	Outcome evaluated (%EF)	Threshold value (breaths/l/min)	Sensitivity	Specificity	PPV	NPV	LR+ LR−	Comments
Epstein and Ciubotaru (1996)	218	E	100	0.86	0.23	0.86	0.28	1.12 / 0.61	
Leitch et al. (1996)	163	E	100	0.96	0	0.98	0	0.96 / NA	Measurements made on PSV; >20% used non-invasive ventilation immediately post-extubation
Bouachour et al. (1996)	26	W	105	1.00	0.4	0.77	1.00	1.67 / 0	
Baumeister et al. (1997)	47	E	11 (per kg)	0.79	0.78	0.94	0.45	3.59 / 0.27	Measurements made on IMV + PSV
Rivera and Weissman (1997)	40	W, E (17)	65	0.90	0.80	0.90	0.70	4.5 / 0.13	Measurements made on CPAP+PSV
Krieger et al. (1997)	49	W, E (NR)	105	0.74	0.73	0.90	0.44	2.74 / 0.36	
Jacob et al. (1997)	183	W, E (53)	100	0.97	0.33	0.94	0.50	1.45 / 0.09	
Vallverdu et al. (1998)	217	W, E (25)	100	0.90	0.36	0.66	0.73	1.41 / 0.28	
Farias et al. (1998)	84	W, E (57)	11 (per kg)	0.86	0.48	0.83	0.53	1.65 / 0.29	
Maldonado et al. (2000)	27	W	105	0.93	0.75	0.89	0.89	3.72 / 0.09	

W, weaning; *E*, extubation; *%EF*, percentage of failures that were extubation failures; *PPV*, positive predictive value; *NPV*, negative predictive value; *LR+*, likelihood ratio for positive test; *LR−*, likelihood ratio for negative test; *NR*, not reported.

some explanation for differences in reported accuracy. For example, two large studies reported that one third of patients failed because of diaphoresis, agitation, or subjective distress (Chatila et al. 1996b; Vallverdu et al. 1998). Jubran and Tobin were unable to detect a pathophysiologic cause for weaning failure in 3/17 patients with COPD, despite exhaustive investigation. Leitch et al. considered patients successfully extubated even though 21% needed mask CPAP after extubation (Leitch et al. 1996). Other authors have explicitly considered such patients failures (Lee et al. 1994).

Another reason for discrepancy between studies is that different techniques have been employed to measure breathing pattern. As originally described, the quantification of breathing pattern is relatively simple and very reproducible, with a low coefficient of variation, at least when a single investigator performs the maneuver (Yang and Tobin 1991). One advantage over the MIP is that the measurement is independent of patient effort or cooperation. To perform the test, the patient is disconnected from the mechanical ventilator and a spirometer is then attached to the endotracheal or tracheostomy tube. The minute ventilation (V_E) is measured by the apparatus as the patient breathes spontaneously for 1 min. The respiratory frequency (f) is determined by physical examination and the tidal volume (V_T) is calculated using the simple equation $V_T = V_E/f$. To calculate the f/V_T, the respiratory rate is divided by the tidal volume (in liters). For example, if the respiratory rate is 40 and tidal volume is 0.20 l, the f/V_T is 200 breaths/l/min. When compared with measurements made without ventilatory support, those made on positive pressure are characterized by lower respiratory rate, higher tidal volume, and therefore a lower f/V_T ratio. Lee and co-workers noted a trend toward higher f/V_T measured on CPAP compared with those on pressure support ventilation (PSV) (86 vs 69, $p=0.16$), suggesting that the type of positive pressure is also important (Lee et al. 1994). Nevertheless, weaning-success patients have been noted to have lower tidal volumes and higher respiratory rates over a range of PSV levels compared with patients with weaning failure. Stroetz and Hubmayr noted ROC areas of 0.66, 0.79, 0.80, 0.78 and 0.82 for f/V_T measurements made on PSV 20, 15, 10, 5 and CPAP 5, respectively (Stroetz and Hubmayr 1995). Recently, Rivera and Weissman determined the f/V_T during IMV (4/min) and PSV (5 cmH_2O) using the spontaneous rate and tidal volume (Rivera and Weissman 1997). Although a lower threshold was identified, predictive accuracy was comparable to that of studies using the technique of disconnection from the ventilator. One advantage of this approach is that it does not require removing the patient from mechanical ventilation to make the measurements. Caution must be exercised, because using the digital display data may significantly underestimate the respiratory rate in patients with untriggered breaths.

A further consideration is the time at which the breathing pattern measurements are made. The majority of studies report values determined within the first few minutes of spontaneous breathing. The pattern of breathing may be unstable in the first minute of disconnection from the ventilator and may require approximately 3 min to achieve a steady state. More recently, others investigators have examined this parameter during the weaning trial (Capdevila et al. 1995; Chatila et al. 1996b; Gandia and Blanco 1992; Krieger et al. 1997; Vassilakopoulos et al.

1998). Chatila and colleagues noted higher PPVs (0.83 vs. 0.72) and NPVs (0.94 vs. 0.68) for the f/V_T measured 30–60 min into a SBT compared with a determination made in the first minute (Chatila et al. 1996b). These authors noted that the f/V_T tended to decrease in successfully extubated patients and increased in those who failed. In contrast, Gandia and Blanco found that measurements of f/V_T made at 60 and 120 min did not improve accuracy over measurements made after 15 min of disconnection (Gandia and Blanco 1992). In a study of patients >70 years old, predictive accuracy increased when f/V_T measurements (threshold value of 130) were made 3 h into the weaning trial (Krieger et al. 1997). In contrast, a study of surgical patients found no difference in accuracy for measurements made at 1 min and those made at 30 min (Jacob et al. 1997). There are several problems inherent in considering measurements made during the weaning trial. The logic behind using a weaning parameter is to avoid failed trials of minimal ventilatory support. A determination made 30–180 min into the trial will not protect the patient against the negative consequences of a failed trial. Analysis for measurements such as the f/V_T may be particularly problematic, because an elevated respiratory frequency is typically used as a criterion of weaning failure (Chatila et al. 1996b; Vallverdu et al. 1998).

Using a single threshold value for a weaning parameter is not ideal and encompasses a number of trade-offs. Single cutoff values for a parameter are unlikely to accurately discriminate between low- and high-risk patients. Ideally, different threshold values or ranges of values are applied (Khan et al. 1996). Chatila et al. noted that six of 11 patients with f/V_T between 101 and 125 were successfully extubated, compared with only 1/11 patients with f/V_T >125 (Chatila et al. 1996b). Similarly, Krieger et al. noted that accuracy increased using an f/V_T threshold of 130 rather than 105 for patients greater than 70 years of age (Krieger et al. 1997). In a post-hoc analysis, Epstein and Ciubotaru found that a threshold of 140 increased predictive accuracy for extubation outcome (Epstein and Ciubotaru 1996). Recently, Alvisi et al. found that predictive accuracy was significantly better for COPD when a lower f/V_T threshold (84 breaths/l/min) was used (Alvisi et al. 2000).

In summary, based on the available evidence, the f/V_T appears to be the most accurate of the easily measured weaning predictors. In assessing the vast literature on this (and all) weaning parameters, it becomes evident that a broad range of test characteristics have been reported. Explanations for this variability between studies include differences in patient populations, the outcome being examined, prevalence of weaning success, duration of mechanical ventilation prior to weaning, criteria for success or failure, timing and technique of measurement, and the applied thresholds. The often striking differences in methodology emphasize the difficulty in combining data from the various studies to generate meta-analyses and more meaningful guidelines. For example, pooling data from the studies in Table 15.4 would be highly problematic, given differences in outcomes assessed (e.g., weaning alone, extubation alone, or the combination of both), the populations studied (e.g., medical, surgical, or mixed), and the techniques used to make the f/V_T measurement (e.g., unassisted off the ventilator through a spirometer, on the ventilator and assisted with either PSV, CPAP, or IMV).

15.5.3 Other Integrative Parameters

Because predictive parameters dissociated from the pathophysiologic cause for failure may perform poorly, investigators have examined the utility of other, more complex integrative parameters. These multi-component tests often combine measurements of oxygenation, minute ventilation (or its elements), compliance, and inspiratory muscle strength. The various resulting combinations have been termed the inspiratory effort quotient (Milic-Emili 1986), the weaning index (Jabour et al. 1991), and the CROP index (Yang and Tobin 1991). At the present time the absence of sufficient confirmatory prospective studies and the highly complex nature of the measurements indicate that it is unlikely that these parameters will find widespread application.

15.6 Complex Measurements Requiring Special Equipment

With advances in technology, it is now possible to directly or indirectly assess numerous complex physiologic parameters including neuromuscular drive, respiratory muscle blood flow, respiratory muscle function and fatigue, and various aspects of the work of breathing.

15.6.1 Airway Occlusion Pressure

Airway occlusion pressure measured at 100 ms (P_{100} or $P_{0.1}$) has been used to assess respiratory drive and demand (mechanical load) on the respiratory system. Although independent of respiratory system resistance and compliance, the measurement is influenced by lung volume, chest wall configuration, and respiratory muscle strength. While the determination of $P_{0.1}$ previously required a manually operated apparatus, some modern ventilators have automated the process by taking advantage of the time delay between initial pressure generation by the respiratory muscles and the opening of a demand valve (Conti et al. 1992). During weaning failure the $P_{0.1}$ is elevated, indicating increased neuromuscular drive in response to imbalance between respiratory load and respiratory muscle capacity (Sassoon and Mahutte 1993). After correction for respiratory muscle strength (e.g., $P_{0.1}$/MIP) predictive accuracy, especially NPV, increases substantially (Capdevila et al. 1995; Gandia and Blanco 1992). In general, although the $P_{0.1}$ is a reasonably good predictor of weaning outcome, overall accuracy appears similar to that seen with the more simply determined f/V_T.

15.6.2 Gastric Intramucosal pH

It has been postulated that diversion of splanchnic blood to the respiratory muscles during unsuccessful weaning may lead to gastric mucosal ischemia and may therefore be detectable by measuring gastric intramucosal pH (pHi) (Mohsenifar et al. 1993). Several techniques have been used, including saline tonometry (Bouachour et al. 1996), gastric juice pHi, and gas tonometry (Maldonado et al. 2000). In general, weaning failure has been associated with lower gastric pHi and increased $PgCO_2$ measured 20 min into the trial, though one study in COPD found significant differences in gastric pHi, $PgCO_2$, and PCO_2 gap ($PgCO_2$-$PaCO_2$) during mechanical ventilation before the onset of a SBT. A more recent study found $PgCO_2$ to be a good predictor, though it was less accurate than the f/V_T in predicting liberation outcome (Maldonado et al. 2000).

15.6.3 Measurements of Respiratory Muscle Function

While some studies noted electromyographic changes suggestive of diaphragmatic fatigue among patients failing weaning trials (Brochard et al. 1989; Cohen et al. 1982; Murciano et al. 1988), true reductions in contractile function were more difficult to demonstrate (Sassoon et al. 1987; Swartz and Marino 1985). More recently, several investigators demonstrated that, in contrast to successfully weaned patients, those who fail frequently develop a tension-time index (TTI) exceeding the 0.15 threshold associated with a fatiguing load (Jubran and Tobin 1997; Vassilakopoulos et al. 1998). Because these measurements require esophageal and gastric balloons to determine Pdi and Pdimax, a simpler technique for determining P_I/P_Imax has been proposed (Yang 1993.) Unfortunately, this parameter was less accurate than the f/V_T and when combined with the latter did not significantly improve predictive accuracy.

15.6.4 Work of Breathing

Work of breathing (WOB), as assessed by oxygen cost of breathing (O_2COB) or determining pressure volume changes (the energy required to breath spontaneously), appears to be significantly greater in patients who fail weaning. That said, the degree of overlap between weaning success and failure patients can be considerable, thereby limiting clinical application. Another limitation in using WOB is that either an esophageal manometry system or a metabolic cart to determine VO_2 is necessary. It is difficult to foresee regular application of a complicated technique to determine readiness for weaning when the majority of patients will pass a spontaneous breathing trial as long as simple clinical criteria are satisfied. One potential use is to identify patients ready for liberation despite failing weaning trials based exclusively on subjective or nonspecifically objective assessment. For example, DeHaven et al. measured mechanical WOB in surgical trauma patients who manifested a respiratory rate >30 breaths/min during a room-air CPAP trial. Approximately 90% of these patients were successfully extubated when either total WOB (WOB_{TOT}) was ≤1.1 J/l or WOB_{TOT} minus imposed WOB was ≤0.8 J/l (DeHaven et al. 1996).

15.6.5 Summary

Although complex measurements of neuromuscular drive, respiratory muscle function, and WOB provide valuable insight into the pathophysiologic basis for weaning failure, the need for specialized equipment makes it unlikely that these techniques will find widespread application.

15.7 How Should Weaning Parameters Be Used? Implications for Future Research

Though they have been extensively studied, the direct impact of weaning parameters on outcome remains ill-defined. The goal of using a weaning parameter is to reduce the duration of mechanical ventilation (e.g., liberate as soon as possible) while avoiding the adverse consequences of failed weaning or extubation trials. Among the simply determined parameters, the respiratory rate–tidal volume ratio (f/V_T) is most accurate, but even for this predictor the range of reported predictive values is very wide. In deciding whether to use a test (and which test to use) we must ask how accurate the weaning parameter should be. Among the numerous investigations of the f/V_T, relatively few yield likelihood ratios that translate into large changes in the probability of failure or success (e.g., LR >5.0 or <0.10). Does application of a test that leads to only small or moderate changes in the probability of success or failure improve clinical care? To answer this question, one must also factor in the risk of each unnecessary day of mechanical ventilation and the adverse impact of a failed weaning trial. Unfortunately, only limited quantitative information is available, especially for the latter. In fact, these risks are likely to vary from patient to patient.

To address these issues randomized controlled trials specifically examining the role of weaning parameters are needed. Does use of a weaning parameter shorten the duration of mechanical ventilation, reduce the length of stay, reduce ventilator-associated complications, or improve mortality? In a preliminary study, Nevins et al. screened patients daily for measures of oxygenation, cough and secretions, adequacy of mental status, hemodynamic stability, and the f/V_T ratio (Nevins et al. 2000). One hundred patients were randomized to two groups: in one the f/V_T was used to determine eligibility for a daily spontaneous breathing trial and in the other it was measured but not used. No other weaning parameters were measured and the clinicians were blinded as to group assignment and f/V_T results. The investigators noted no differences in reintubation rate, mortality, or need for tracheostomy. Although it did not achieve statistical significance, the investigators found a trend toward an increase in duration of mechanical ventilation in patients in whom the weaning parameter was used for weaning decision-making. Lastly, complex decision-analytic models can be used to address the following question: For a given set of risks (e.g., of prolonged mechanical ventilation, of a failed weaning trial, of failed extubation), how accurate does the weaning parameter have to be and what threshold should be used (Cardinal et al. 2000)?

15.8 Conclusions

Numerous weaning parameters have been investigated, ranging from easily performed tests such as measuring breathing pattern to complex maneuvers requiring special equipment such as the mechanical work of breathing. Based on the available evidence, it appears that a negative weaning parameter may not be sufficient justification for either delaying weaning trials or delaying extubation after a patient has successfully completed a spontaneous breathing trial. It is imperative that clinicians wishing to use parameters must be aware of the limitations of these tests. They should consider adjusting the thresholds used based on individual patient characteristics, including the estimated risks of each additional day of mechanical ventilation and perceived risk of a failed trial of weaning or extubation. They must also be aware of the testing methodology and the patient population on which it is applied. In the case of a patient repeatedly failing weaning trials, parameters may help elucidate the mechanism for failure, thereby providing a target for therapeutic intervention leading to successful liberation.

15.9 References

Alvisi R, Volta C, Righini E, et al (2000) Predictors of weaning outcome in chronic obstructive pulmonary disease patients. Eur Respir J 15:656–662

Baumeister BL, el-Khatib M, Smith PG, et al (1997) Evaluation of predictors of weaning from mechanical ventilation in pediatric patients. Pediatr Pulmonol 24:344–352

Bouachour G, Guiraud MP, Gouello JP, et al (1996) Gastric intramucosal pH: an indicator of weaning outcome from mechanical ventilation in COPD patients. Eur Respir J 9:1868–1873

Brochard L, Harf A, Lorino H, et al (1989) Inspiratory pressure support prevents diaphragmatic fatigue during weaning from mechanical ventilation. Am Rev Respir Dis 139:513–521

Brochard L, Rauss A, Benito S, et al (1994) Comparison of three methods of gradual withdrawal from ventilatory support during weaning from mechanical ventilation. Am J Respir Crit Care Med 150:896–903

Capdevila XJ, Perrigault PF, Perey PJ, et al. (1995) Occlusion pressure and its ratio to maximum inspiratory pressure are useful predictors for successful extubation following T-piece weaning trial. Chest 108:482–489

Capdevila X, Perrigault PF, Ramonatxo M, et al (1998) Changes in breathing pattern and respiratory muscle performance parameters during difficult weaning. Crit Care Med 26:79–87

Cardinal P, Hutchinson T, Tousignant P, et al. (2000) Should we use the RR/Vt ratio when deciding to extubate? Am J Respir Crit Care Med 161:A792

Chatila W, Ani S, Guaglianone D, et al (1996a) Cardiac ischemia during weaning from mechanical ventilation. Chest 109:1577–1583

Chatila W, Jacob B, Guaglionone D, et al (1996b) The unassisted respiratory rate-tidal volume ratio accurately predicts weaning outcome. Am J Med 101:61–67

Cohen CA, Zagelbaum G, Gross D, et al (1982) Clinical manifestations of inspiratory muscle fatigue. Am J Med 73:308–316

Conti G, De Blasi R, Pelaia P, et al (1992) Early prediction of successful weaning during pressure support ventilation in chronic obstructive pulmonary disease. Crit Care Med 20:366–371

DeHaven CB, Kirton OC, Morgan JP, et al (1996) Breathing measurement reduces false negative classification of tachypneic preextubation trial failures. Crit Care Med 24:976–980

Del Rosario N, Sassoon CS, Chetty KG, et al (1997) Breathing pattern during acute respiratory failure and recovery. Eur Respir J 10:2560–2565

Dojat M, Harf A, Touchard D, et al (1996) Evaluation of a knowledge-based system providing ventilatory management and decision for extubation. Am J Respir Crit Care Med 153: 997–1004

Ely EW, Baker AM, Evans GW, et al. (1999) The prognostic significance of passing a daily screen of weaning parameters. Intensive Care Med 25:581–587

Epstein SK (1995) Etiology of extubation failure and the predictive value of the rapid shallow breathing index. Am J Respir Crit Care Med 152:545–549

Epstein SK (2000a) Endotracheal extubation. Respir Care Clin N Am 6:321–360

Epstein SK (2000b) Weaning parameters. Respir Care Clin N Am 6:253–301

Epstein SK, Ciubotaru RL (1996) Influence of gender and endotracheal tube size on preextubation breathing pattern. Am J Respir Crit Care Med 154:1647–1652

Epstein SK, Picken H (1997) Application of decision analysis principles to predicting weaning and extubation outcome. Clin Pulm Med 4:283–291

Epstein SK, Nevins ML, Chung J (2000) Effect of unplanned extubation on outcome of mechanical ventilation. Am J Respir Crit Care Med 161:1912–1916

Esteban A, Frutos F, Tobin MJ, et al (1995) A comparison of four methods of weaning patients from mechanical ventilation. N Engl J Med 332:345–350

Esteban A, Alia I, Gordo F, et al (1997) Extubation outcome after spontaneous breathing trials with T-tube or pressure support ventilation. Am J Respir Crit Care Med 156:459–465

Esteban A, Alia I, Tobin M, et al (1999) Effect of spontaneous breathing trial duration on outcome of attempts to discontinue mechanical ventilation. Am J Respir Crit Care Med 159:512–518

Fagon JY, Chastre J, Domart Y, et al (1989) Nosocomial pneumonia in patients receiving continuous mechanical ventilation. Prospective analysis of 52 episodes with use of a protected specimen brush and quantitative culture techniques. Am Rev Respir Dis 139:877–884

Farias JA, Alia I, Esteban A, et al (1998) Weaning from mechanical ventilation in pediatric intensive care patients. Intensive Care Med 24:1070–1075

Gandia F, Blanco J (1992) Evaluation of indexes predicting the outcome of ventilator weaning and value of adding supplemental inspiratory load. Intensive Care Med 18:327–333

Hilberman M, Kamm B, Lamy M, et al (1976) An analysis of potential physiological predictors of respiratory adequacy following cardiac surgery. J Thorac Cardiovasc Surg 71:711–720

Jabour ER, Rabil DM, Truwit JD, et al (1991) Evaluation of a new weaning index based on ventilatory endurance and the efficiency of gas exchange. Am Rev Respir Dis 144:531–537

Jacob B, Chatila W, Manthous C (1997) The unassisted respiratory rate/tidal volume ratio accurately predicts weaning outcome in postoperative patients. Crit Care Med 25:253–257

Jaeschke R, Meade M, Guyatt G, et al (1997) How to use diagnostic test articles in the intensive care unit: diagnosing weanability using the f/Vt. Crit Care Med 25:1514–1521

Jubran A, Tobin MJ (1997) Pathophysiologic basis of acute respiratory distress in patients who fail a trial of weaning from mechanical ventilation. Am J Respir Crit Care Med 155:906–915

Khan N, Brown A, Venkataraman ST (1996) Predictors of extubation success and failure in mechanically ventilated infants and children. Crit Care Med 24:1568–1579

Krieger BP, Ershowsky PF, Becker DA, et al (1989) Evaluation of conventional criteria for predicting successful weaning from mechanical ventilatory support in elderly patients. Crit Care Med 17:858–861

Krieger BP, Isber J, Breitenbucher A, et al (1997) Serial measurements of the rapid-shallow-breathing index as a predictor of weaning outcome in elderly medical patients. Chest 112:1029–1034

Laghi F, D'Alfonso N, Tobin MJ (1995) Pattern of recovery from diaphragmatic fatigue over 24 hours. J Appl Physiol 79:539–546

Laghi F, Jubran A, Parthasarathy S, et al (2000) Can patients who fail a weaning trial develop diaphragmatic fatigue? Am J Respir Crit Care Med 161:A790

Lee KH, Hui KP, Chan TB, et al (1994) Rapid shallow breathing (frequency-tidal volume ratio) did not predict extubation outcome. Chest 105:540–543

Leitch EA, Moran JL, Grealy B (1996) Weaning and extubation in the intensive care unit. Clinical or index-driven approach? Intensive Care Med 22:752–759

Lemaire F, Teboul J-L, Cinotti L, et al (1988) Acute left ventricular dysfunction during unsuccessful weaning from mechanical ventilation. Anesthesiology 69:171–179

Levy MM, Miyasaki A, Langston D (1995) Work of breathing as a weaning parameter in mechanically ventilated patients. Chest 108:1018–1020

Mador MJ, Acevedo FA (1991) Effect of respiratory muscle fatigue on breathing pattern during incremental exercise. Am Rev Respir Dis 143:462–468

Maldonado A, Bauer T, Ferrer M, et al (2000) Capnometric recirculation gas tonometry and weaning from mechanical ventilation. Am J Respir Crit Care Med 161:171–176

Milic-Emili J (1986) Is weaning an art or a science? Am Rev Respir Dis 134:1107–1108

Mohsenifar Z, Hay A, Hay J, et al (1993) Gastric intramural pH as a predictor of success or failure in weaning patients from mechanical ventilation. Ann Intern Med 119:794–798

Multz AS, Aldrich TK, Prezant DJ, et al (1990) Maximal inspiratory pressure is not a reliable test of inspiratory muscle strength in mechanically ventilated patients. Am Rev Respir Dis 142:529–532

Murciano D, Boczkowski J, Lecocguic Y, et al (1988) Tracheal occlusion pressure: a simple index to monitor respiratory muscle fatigue during acute respiratory failure in patients with chronic obstructive pulmonary disease. Ann Intern Med 108:800–805

Nava S, Rubini F, Zanotti E, et al (1994) Survival and prediction of successful ventilator weaning in COPD patients receiving mechanical ventilation for more than 21 days. Eur Respir J 7:1645–1652

Nevins M, Hendra K, Epstein S (2000) Randomized controlled trial of the use of the f/V$_T$ ratio in a weaning protocol. Am J Respir Crit Care Med 161:A792

Reid WD, Huang J, Bryson S, et al. (1994) Diaphragm injury and myofibrillar structure induced by resistive loading. J Appl Physiol 76:176–184

Rivera L, Weissman C (1997) Dynamic ventilatory characteristics during weaning in postoperative critically ill patients. Anesth Analg 84:1250–1255

Roussos C (1984) Ventilatory muscle fatigue governs breathing frequency. Bull Eur Physiopathol Resp 20:445–451

Sahn SA, Lakshminarayan S (1973) Bedside criteria for discontinuation of mechanical ventilation. Chest 63:1002–1005

Sassoon CS, Mahutte CK (1993) Airway occlusion pressure and breathing pattern as predictors of weaning outcome. Am Rev Respir Dis 148:860–866

Sassoon CSH, Te TT, Mahutte CK, et al. (1987) Airway occlusion pressure: an important indicator for successful weaning in patients with chronic obstructive pulmonary disease. Am Rev Respir Dis 135:107–113

Shikora SA, Benotti PN, Johannigman JA (1994) The oxygen cost of breathing may predict weaning from mechanical ventilation better than the respiratory rate to tidal volume ratio. Arch Surg 129:269–274

Sox HC, Blatt MA, Higgins MC, et al (1988). Medical decision-making. Butterworths, Boston

Stroetz RW, Hubmayr RD (1995) Tidal volume maintenance during weaning with pressure support. Am J Respir Crit Care Med 152:1034–1040

Swartz MA, Marino PL (1985) Diaphragmatic strength during weaning from mechanical ventilation. Chest 88:736–739

Tahvanainen J, Salmenpera M, Nikki P (1983) Extubation criteria after weaning from intermittent mandatory ventilation and continuous positive airway pressure. Crit Care Med 11:702–707

Tobin MJ, Perez W, Guenther SM, et al (1986) The pattern of breathing during successful and unsuccessful trials of weaning from mechanical ventilation. Am Rev Respir Dis 134:1111–1118

Travaline JM, Sudarshan S, Criner GJ (1997) Recovery of PdiTwitch following the induction of diaphragm fatigue in normal subjects. Am J Respir Crit Care Med 156:1562–1566

Truwit JD, Marini JJ (1992) Validation of a technique to assess maximal inspiratory pressure in poorly cooperative patients. Chest 102:1216–1219

Vallverdu I, Calaf N, Subirana M, et al (1998) Clinical characteristics, respiratory functional parameters, and outcome of two-hour T-piece trial in patients weaning from mechanical ventilation. Am J Respir Crit Care Med 158:1855–1862

Vassilakopoulos T, Zakynthinos S, Roussos C (1998) The tension-time index and the frequency/tidal volume ratio are the major pathophysiologic determinants of weaning failure and success. Am J Respir Crit Care Med 158:378–385

Yang KL (1992) Reproducibility of weaning parameters; a need for standardization. Chest 102:1829–1832

Yang KL (1993) Inspiratory pressure/maximal inspiratory pressure ratio: a predictive index of weaning outcome. Intensive Care Med 19:204–208

Yang KL, Tobin MJ (1991) A prospective study of indexes predicting the outcome of trials of weaning from mechanical ventilation. N Engl J Med 324:1445–1450

16 Timing and Criteria for Beginning Weaning

R. Fernandez

Mechanical ventilation (MV) is a supportive tool for critically ill patients which saves lives worldwide each day. Nevertheless, this advantage is obtained at the cost of additional morbidity and mortality. The classical side effects of MV are widely recognized in the form of tracheal damage, need for sedatives, and hemodynamic disturbances. In the 1980s, the impact of pulmonary infections, so-called ventilator-associated pneumonia, was the target of substantial research in the field of adverse consequences of MV. In the 1990s, the focus was directed to the direct damage caused by MV on the lungs, and such terms as "barotrauma", "volotrauma", and recently "biotrauma" were tailored to define different problems directly related to the use of life-saving MV.

The recognition of such iatrogenic problems fueled the research in methods to reduce their intensity (e.g. reducing airway pressure, reducing tidal volumes), but also to reduce the time of exposure to these agents by reducing the length of MV. In a frequently cited study, Esteban et al. [1] showed that a large proportion of the time spent under MV was dedicated to weaning. At that time, in 1992, as much as 40% of the time under MV was related to weaning. In a more recent report [2], the same investigator chaired a 1-day prevalence study of 412 ICUs from North America, South America, Spain, and Portugal. The study involved 1638 ventilated patients, 520 (32%) of whom were being weaned at that moment. This means that a high proportion of the workload dedicated to MV patients is devoted to weaning, and that the most common approach to weaning is still a progressive reduction of ventilatory support. Nevertheless, in the past decade we have learned that the majority of patients do not need such a progressive withdrawal of MV [3]. In these patients, prolonging MV will be of no benefit, while the deleterious effects of MV appeared as unacceptable from a risk/benefit ratio.

At this point, we can summarize the field of decisions about weaning in terms of "when to start weaning" and "how to proceed with weaning". In both issues, we can suggest two opposite approaches, i.e. the more "conservative" method and the more "aggressive" method. In the "conservative" approach to starting weaning a physician waits for physiological parameters to return to "normal" values before attempting to evaluate whether the patient is able to resume spontaneous ventilation, in other words, for the patient to "fully" recover from the initial condition requiring MV. In this scenario, wide variability exists regarding the minimal values that a patient "must" exhibit before weaning can be started. In contrast, the "aggressive" approach to starting weaning will consider a patient able to be weaned as early as possible, i.e. when he or she does not show signs of life-threat-ening worsening after MV is stopped. Again, what can be described as "clinically significant" worsening remains to be clarified.

There are also two different approaches to reducing ventilatory support.. First, the "conservative" method (from now on, the "less stressful" approach) argues for a progressive reduction within hours or days, trying to avoid abrupt changes in the clinical condition of the patients. Conversely, the "aggressive" method (from now on, the "less iatrogenic" approach) supports fast withdrawal of MV to avoid the iatrogenic effects of prolonged MV.

Overview: Different approaches to starting and performing weaning

When to start?

- The "full recovery" approach: Only when a patient has returned to almost normal physiological function may the physician approach weaning.
- The "less iatrogenic" approach: MV must be withdrawn as early as possible; any data suggesting successful restoration of spontaneous breathing may be enough to start weaning.

How to proceed?

- The "less stressful" approach: Spontaneous ventilation has to be resumed progressively to avoid stress to the patient.
- The "less iatrogenic" approach: If spontaneous ventilation can be resumed quickly, any delay in withdrawn MV may induce further complications.

In the realization that medical practice shows wide variability in approaches to weaning, this chapter will explore the available data supporting each type of approach.

16.1 The "Full Recovery" vs. the "Less Iatrogenic" Approaches to Starting Weaning

Common textbooks of critical care medicine state that a minimum of physiolog-ic variables should return to "normal" values before weaning is attempted. Wide consensus exists about the inconvenience of starting weaning in patients with high fever, low level of consciousness, severe hypotension, or uncontrolled arrhythmia. This common sense has been translated into research studies, which ordinarily have excluded patients with these conditions. Actually, most of the recently published papers on weaning do not mention exclusion criteria such as agitation, fever, arrhythmia, and myocardial ischemia. Although we are unable to ascertain whether these kinds of patients were studied or not, we can assume that most physicians refuse to think about weaning when patients are unstable. The fact that these physicians probably would not intubate patients because of agitation, fever, arrhythmia, or myocardial ischemia seems to contradict the "full recovery" approach. In other words, if these conditions (fever, agitation, etc.) per se are not indications for MV, why are such conditions to be used as criteria for not attempting MV withdrawal?

Other required physiological parameters frequently suggested in reviews about weaning are: adequate hemoglobin (Hb) levels, appropriate neurological and muscular status, correction of metabolic and/or electrolyte disorders, and adequacy of sleep [4]. Again, the terms adequate and appropriate are vague enough to allow wide variability when approaching weaning capabilities. But all these suggestions are based on clear common sense. When a patient is going to experience a stressful situation, as weaning can sometimes be, the physician prefers to reduce the amount of other loads for the patient. Anemia is known to force the heart to work hard in order to maintain oxygen delivery to the tissues and, importantly, to the respiratory muscles during weaning. Accordingly, the physician commonly orders packed red cells to avoid significant anemia. Nevertheless, the suggested 10 g Hb/dl concentration needs to be reviewed in light of the results of recent studies on transfusion strategies. In a Canadian study [5], patients treated without transfusion until Hb went down to 7–8 g/dl were more likely to survive than those who managed to maintain the 10 g Hb/dl level during their complete stay in the ICU. Whether the transfusion strategy may behave differently during weaning has not been evaluated, but no reasons can be anticipated to reduce the side effects of transfusion, mainly its immunosuppressant effect.

It would appear to be more difficult to ensure that patients have experienced adequate sleep during their stay in the ICU, but it may be expected that most patients will suffer some level of sleep deprivation after being mechanically ventilated. One must take into account that the lethargy or agitation that frequently prevent weaning can be due to sleep deprivation. Nevertheless, even if we can diagnose sleep deprivation, it is unrealistic to delay weaning until patients achieve a "normal" sleep pattern.

When neurological deficit arises from brain injury, the issue of timing for extubation is controversial. In a very recent study, Coplin et al. [6] hypothesized that clinicians would vary considerably in the timing for extubating brain-injured patients once these patients were capable of spontaneous breathing. Further, they hypothesized that many patients could be extubated promptly and safely despite such ostensibly poor predictive factors as coma, absence of a gag reflex, and the presence of respiratory tract secretions, and that patients in whom extubation was delayed would have worse outcomes in terms of pneumonia, length of stay, or costs. Of 136 patients, 99 (73%) were extubated within 48 h of meeting defined readiness criteria. The other 37 (27%) remained intubated for a median of 3 days The important results were that patients with delayed extubation developed more pneumonia (38 vs. 21%) and had longer ICU (8.6 vs. 3.8 days) and hospital (19.9 vs. 13.2 days) stays. They conclude that "the study does not support delaying extubating patients when impaired neurologic status is the only concern prolonging intubation in brain-injured patients".

The issue of electrolyte disturbances during weaning has been extensively studied. The fact that low blood levels of calcium, phosphorus, potassium, and magnesium reduce the contractility of the respiratory muscles is undoubtedly proved. In 1985, Aubier et al. [7] studied the effect of hypophosphatemia in eight patients with acute respiratory failure who were artificially ventilated. In all the patients, increasing serum phosphorus was accompanied by a marked increase in transdiaphragmatic pressure during phrenic stimulation, the increase for eight patients averaging 70%. Given the frequent association of respiratory muscle weakness or fatigue with weaning failure, it seems logical to correct any condition associated with low performance of the respiratory muscles. As a routine, it is suggested that the blood level of these electrolytes be monitored in order to supplement any observed deficit [8].

Acidosis is another common clinical condition in ventilated critically ill patients. Acidosis increases the amount of minute ventilation needed to normalize arterial pH, with associated increases in the work of breathing requirements. Moreover, in an animal model, respiratory acidosis worsened diaphragmatic performance, whereas lactic acidosis did not [9]. The depressant effect of severe respiratory acidosis (pH 7.10, $PaCO_2$ 80 mmHg) was observed in both maximal pressure (Pdi) and relaxation rate of the diaphragm. Nevertheless, even in this extreme condition, diaphragmatic force development was reduced only to 30% of baseline. Again, before starting weaning, it appears advisable to treat conditions that induce acidosis.

Respiratory muscle function is declared to be one of the fundamental physiological parameters that must be restored before weaning is attempted. Enough evidence has demonstrated the association between indexes of respiratory muscle weakness or fatigue and unsuccessful weaning. One of the most elegant studies in this field was published by Murciano et al. [10]. They studied the EMG pattern of the diaphragm in COPD patients during the course of MV, showing that all patients exhibit EMG diagnosis of diaphragmatic fatigue in the first day of MV. Those patients showing recovery of the fatigue pattern were successfully extubated, while those patients who remained in fatigue needed reintubation. These results suggest that weaning is very unlikely to succeed in patients with respiratory muscle fatigue. Interestingly, the EMG pattern of fatigue was closely correlated with elevated occlusion pressure ($P_{0.1}$), allowing diagnosis of fatigue at the bedside. Nevertheless, we do not know how long the resting period should be to recover from diaphragmatic fatigue or how much diaphragmatic strength is required to sustain spontaneous ventilation. Regarding the time needed for recovery, Laghi et al. [11] showed that normal subjects recover almost normal function in 1 day, but the Murciano study demonstrate that some patients may remain in fatigue even under mechanical ventilatory support. Whether different clinical conditions such as COPD may behave differently with regard to the incidence and recovery time of respiratory muscle fatigue is still unknown. The issue of the minimum fatigue recovery needed to resume spontaneous ventilation is intriguing. The Laghi study suggests restoration of 50% of the diaphragmatic function in 8–12 h, and one clinical trial demonstrated that patients who fail a trial of spontaneous ventilation may succeed the trial after 24 h of rest under MV [12]. It is possible that in case of suspicion of respiratory muscle fatigue and intolerance to a trial of spontaneous ventilation, 1 day of rest under full ventilatory support may be enough to restore diaphragmatic function.

Another physiological parameter frequently recommended to be normalized before attempting weaning is respiratory mechanics. Nevertheless, some recent studies found very little differences in respiratory mechanics between patients able and those unable to sustain spontaneous ventilation. Jubran and Tobin [13] reported the passive mechanics of the respiratory system in 12 patients who went on to fail a weaning trial and in 12 patients who were successfully weaned. The unweanable patients had a tendency to worse airway resistance, lung elastance, and PEEPi, but the differences achieved statistical significance only when they were integrated as dynamic elastance (35 vs. 27 cmH_2O/l). The authors conclude that "mechanics of the respiratory system did not satisfactorily discriminate between patients who failed a weaning trial and those successfully weaned, and, thus, are unlikely to be useful in signaling a patient's ability to tolerate the discontinuation of MV".

In spontaneous ventilation, respiratory muscles have to cope with the loads imposed by the respiratory system. Moreover, high elastic and resistive loads during the weaning trial have been correlated with poor weaning outcomes. In a recent study [14], COPD patients who fail a weaning trial exhibited higher work of breathing (WOB) than successfully extubated patients. This increase in the WOB was due to both elastic and resistive components of the load, but, interestingly, the majority was attributable to the increase in autoPEEP. Additionally, not only mechanics, but also gas-exchange derangements were responsible for the adverse outcome. When the authors combined respiratory effort against mechanics with inefficient CO_2 clearance, as the product of PTP and $PaCO_2$, this index was more than twice as high in the failure group than in the success group at the end of the trial. Nevertheless, no clear-cut level of any of these physiological parameters anticipates the failure of weaning in a more convincing way than the spontaneous respiration trial.

Proposals for speeding up the process of weaning have been the topic of many recent papers in intensive care literature. A hallmark of this issue was the study of Ely et al. [15] in 1996. They reported that daily screening of the respiratory function of patients receiving mechanical ventilation, followed by trials of spontaneous breathing prior to extubation, could reduce the duration of mechanical ventilation and the cost of intensive care. They conducted a randomized, controlled trial of 300 adult patients receiving MV in medical and coronary ICUs. All the patients underwent daily screening of their respiratory function to determine whether they could breathe without assistance. Five simple weaning criteria were screened: a PaO_2/FiO_2 ratio greater than 200; PEEP less than 5 cmH_2O; adequate airway reflexes; an f/V_T ratio less than 105 bpm/l; and no infusion of vasopressor agents or sedative drugs. In the patients of the intervention group who met these criteria, a 2-h trial of spontaneous ventilation was performed and physicians were notified when their patients successfully completed such a trial. Patients in the control group were also screened daily, but they did not undergo trials of spontaneous breathing. In both groups, the decision to discontinue MV was made by the attending physician. The percentage of patients who had successful screening did not differ between groups (76% in the intervention group and 68% in the control group, $p=0.14$). The time that elapsed from the initiation of MV until successful screening tests was 3 days vs. 2 days, respectively. Forty-eight hours after patients had successful screening tests, 57% of patients in the intervention group were successfully extubated, as compared with 23% in the control group. The median duration of MV was 4.5 days in the intervention group and 6 days in the control group. The main suggestion of this study was that an objective and protocolized approach to weaning might speed up the process in the average ICUs.

Because of the wide variability in terms of availability of intensivists, expertise, and resources in different ICUs, one can argue that the impact of such an approach may be less in dedicated ICUs. This contention was also rejected in our experience, as reported by Saura et al. [16]. In our ICU with a team experienced in weaning issues, we compared our results in the period of recruitment of patients to one of the studies of the Spanish Lung Failure Collaborative Group with those of the previous year. The fact that participation in that study forced us to follow a very strict protocol for screening patients' ability to breathe spontaneously allows for comparison with a similar population of patients managed by the same team, very close in time. The groups were comparable in terms of age, APACHE II score, and main cause of acute respiratory failure. Number of days on MV up to the weaning trial was similar in the two groups (8.4 in the protocol group vs. 7.5 in the control group). The most interesting result was that most of the patients (80%) in the protocol group were directly extubated without a weaning technique, unlike the control group (10%). Total duration of MV was shorter in the protocol group (10.4±11.6 days) than in the control group (14.4±10.3 days). As a result, the ICU stay was reduced by using the weaning protocol (16.7±16.5 days vs. 20.3±13.2 days in the control group). The incidence of complications showed a nonsignificant tendency to be lower in the protocol group. These results support the suggestion that even experienced physicians tend to be very conservative and needlessly prolong MV while waiting for "maximal improvement" in patients' clinical condition.

Again, a close look at these results shows that, when a weaning technique was used, the weaning time was similar in the two groups (3.5 days vs. 3.6 days), irrespective of the fact that most patients in the control group probably could be directly extubated. It suggests that the time needed for extubation, when a method of progressive withdrawal of MV is used, depends more on the pacing of the attending team than on the clinical condition of the patient. This aspect is indirectly confirmed by one study on the influence of the quality of nursing on the duration of weaning [17]. In this report, the mean duration of MV in COPD patients was less than 10 days when the number of qualified nurses was sufficient, but it increased to 15–20 days when the nursing workforce was downsized. Dramatic results appeared during the year of the strongest financial cutbacks, reaching a 40-day average duration of MV. While patients exhibited a similar degree of severity on admission, the lengthened duration of ICU stay was followed by an increase in tracheotomy rate (50% vs. 6%). An encouraging finding was that duration of MV for such sick patients returned to "normal" values following recruitment of more qualified nursing personnel.

Advantages and disadvantages of prolonging mechanical ventilation in an attempt to obtain better "full recovery" before weaning may be investigated in different ways. In a very recent paper, Kress et al. [18] conducted a randomized, controlled trial involving 128 adult patients who were receiving mechanical ventilation and continuous infusions of sedative drugs in a medical intensive care unit. In the intervention group, the sedative infusions were interrupted until the patients were awake, on a daily basis; in the control group, the infusions were interrupted only at the discretion of the clinicians in the ICU. The main results were a reduction in the median duration of mechanical ventilation from 7.3 to 4.9 days and in the median length of stay in the ICU from 9.9 to 6.4 days. Complications attributable to mild sedation were similar in both groups. Based on this study, we can speculate that heavy sedation and long periods of MV did not improve recovery of respiratory function, at least in terms of outcome. Another look at this investigation suggests that sedation tailored according to patients' needs is probably better than deep continuous sedation for the average population of ICU patients.

Difficulty with integrating all the physiological parameters involved in respiratory failure, and the cumbersome task of diagnosing it, have fueled research in the field of "weaning parameters". The idea behind all these weaning parameters is that, regardless of the precipitating factor, the respiratory system would adopt a common response to weaning failure. Since many factors can be responsible for the failure of an attempt to wean a patient from mechanical ventilation, Yang and Tobin [19] reasoned that accurate prediction is more likely with an index that integrates a number of physiological functions. They developed two new indexes. The first was the ratio of respiratory frequency to tidal volume, which quantifies the extent of rapid shallow breathing, a common finding in patients who fail a weaning trial. The second index (CROP index) incorporates a measure of pulmonary gas exchange and an assessment of the relation between the demands placed on the respiratory system and the capacity of the respiratory muscles to handle them. They compared these new indexes with traditional ones with regard to accuracy. The predictive power of each of the two new indexes of weaning outcome, the f/V_T ratio and the CROP index, was considerably greater than that of traditional indexes, such as minute ventilation and PImax. The precise pathophysiologic basis of an elevated f/V_T ratio in patients who fail a weaning trial is unknown, but it is suggested that it is a stress response reflecting an imbalance between respiratory neuromuscular reserve and respiratory demands. As a predictor, the f/V_T ratio has several attractive features: it is easy to measure, it is independent of the patient's effort and cooperation, it has high predictive power, and, fortunately, it has a "rounded-off" threshold value (100) that is easy to remember. Of the primary indexes, V_T was the most accurate in predicting weaning outcome. Since V_T is determined by the interaction between the amount of inspiratory pressure generated for each breath and the load placed on the respiratory system (i.e. $V_T = P_I \times C_{dyn}$), it is not too surprising that it proved to be a relatively accurate predictor.

Subsequent studies tried to validate the results of Yang and Tobin, with varying results. In a prospective, observational, noninterventional study, Epstein [20] followed 249 adult patients during weaning. He found that, in agreement with Yang and Tobin, an f/V_T <100 has a high positive predictive value (0.83) for extubation success. His results also demonstrate that a rapid shallow breathing pattern identifies patients in whom an underlying respiratory process increases the work of breathing beyond the capacity of the respiratory muscle pump. In 13 of 14 patients with an f/V_T <100 (false-positive rate 0.17) in whom extubation failed, it did so because of a process distinct from or in addition to an underlying respiratory process. This suggests that this predictive index may be less accurate when it fails to reflect the pathophysiological cause for extubation failure or when that cause is not detectable at the time the index (f/V_T) is measured.

Thus, we can view f/V_T <100 as a necessary but insufficient parameter to measure before attempting weaning; i.e. patients with f/V_T >100 are very unlikely to succeed, but patients with f/V_T <100 still have a 10%–20% chance to fail the weaning process. Most of the recent trials of weaning have confirmed this rate of reintubation. In 1997, Esteban et al. [21] studied 484 patients during a spontaneous breathing trial with two different approaches, T-tube and pressure-support ventilation. They found a 17%–19% rate of reintubation irrespective of the method used for testing. The fact that the median f/V_T ratio was 51 (25th–75th percentiles 35–73) indicates the low specificity of this index to detect weaning failure. Another important conclusion of this investigation works against the "full recovery" approach. In their study, the intended alleviation of the work imposed by the endotracheal tube by using pressure-support ventilation did not improve the ability to tolerate the spontaneous breathing trial, or the likelihood of remaining extubated after 48 h. Again, after screening for very simple respiratory data, only a trial of spontaneous breathing can tell us which patients will be able to resume spontaneous ventilation [22].

The fact that the reintubation rate is also similar in the group of patients submitted to progressive reduction in ventilatory support [12, 21] emphasizes the low accuracy of any weaning parameter to detect extubation failure [20].

16.2 Conclusion

We have explored the rationale behind the different approaches to starting and performing weaning. While no strong data preclude the use of any method, those available data suggest that accelerating the withdrawal of MV is as safe as more conservative approaches. Its advantage is to reduce the likelihood of deleterious side effects, with reduction in the length of stay in the ICU, and associated hospital costs.

Recent randomized, controlled trials have demonstrated that the ability to resume spontaneous ventilation can be more successfully explored by daily testing of simple clinical parameters. Moreover, most patients can be successfully disconnected from MV in a single step, the tolerance test. The duration of this test can be as short as 30 min, and it may be performed with either a T-tube or low-level pressure-support ventilation.

16.3 References

1. Esteban A, Alía I, Ibáñez J, Benito S, Tobin MJ, Spanish Lung Failure Collaborative Group (1994) Modes of mechanical ventilation and weaning: a national survey of Spanish hospitals. Chest 106:1188–1193
2. Esteban A, Anzueto A, Alia I, Gordo F, Azpeteguia C, Palizas F, et al (2000) How is mechanical ventilation employed in the intensive care unit? An international utilization review. Am J Respir Crit Care161:1450–1458

3. Alia I, Esteban A, Gordo F (1998) What have we learned about weaning over the last five years? In: Vincent JL (ed) Yearbook of intensive care and emergency medicine. Springer, Berlin Heidelberg New York, pp 505–516
4. Mancebo J (1996) Weaning from mechanical ventilation. Eur Respir J 9:1923–1931
5. Hebert PC, Wells G, Blajchman MA, Marshall J, Martin C, Pagliarello G, et al (1999) A multicenter, randomized, controlled clinical trial of transfusion requirements in critical care. N Engl J Med 340:409–417
6. Coplin WM, Pierson DJ, Cooley KD, Newell DW, Rubenfeld GD (2000) Implications of extubation delay in brain-injured patients meeting standard weaning criteria. Am J Respir Crit Care Med 161:1530–1536
7. Aubier M, Murciano D, Lecocguic Y, et al (1985) Effect of hypophosphatemia on diaphragmatic contractility in patients with acute respiratory failure. N Engl J Med 313:420–424
8. Aubier M, Viires N, Piquet J, et al (1985) Effects of hypocalcemia on diaphragmatic strength generation. J Appl Physiol 58:2054–2061
9. Yanos J, Wood LDH, Davis K, Keamy M (1993) The effect of respiratory and lactic acidosis on diaphragm function. Am Rev Respir Dis 147:616–619
10. Murciano D, Boczkowski J, Lecocguic Y, Milic-Emili J, Pariente R, Aubier M (1988) Tracheal occlusion pressure: a simple index to monitor respiratory muscle fatigue during acute respiratory failure in patients with chronic obstructive pulmonary disease. Ann Intern Med 108:800–805
11. Laghi F, D'Alfonso N, Tobin MJ (1995) Pattern of recovery from diaphragmatic fatigue over 24 h. J Appl Physiol 79: 539–546
12. Esteban A, Frutos F, Tobin MJ, Alía I, Solsona JF, Valverdú I, et al (1995) A comparison of four methods of weaning patients from mechanical ventilation. N Engl J Med 332:345–50
13. Jubran A, Tobin MJ (1997) Passive mechanics of lung and chest wall in patients who failed or succeeded in trials of weaning. Am J Respir Crit Care Med 155:916–921
14. Jubran A, Tobin MJ (1997) Pathophysiologic basis of acute respiratory distress in patients who fail a trial of weaning from mechanical ventilation. Am J Respir Crit Care Med 155:906–915
15. Ely EW, Baker AM, Dunagan DP, et al (1996) Effect on the duration of mechanical ventilation of identifying patients capable of breathing spontaneously. N Engl J Med 335:1864–1869
16. Saura P, Blanch Ll, Mestre J, Vallés J, Artigas A, Fernandez R (1996) Clinical consequences of the implementation of a weaning protocol. Intensive Care Med 22:1052–1056
17. Thorens JB, Kaelin RM, Jolliet P, Chevrolet JC (1995) Influence of quality of nursing on the duration of weaning from mechanical ventilation in patients with chronic obstructive pulmonary disease. Crit Care Med 23:1807–1815
18. Kress JP, Pohlman AS, O'Connor MF, Hall JB (2000) Daily interruption of sedative infusions in critically ill patients undergoing mechanical ventilation. N Engl J Med 342:1471–1477
19. Yang KL, Tobin MJ (1991) A prospective study of indexes predicting the outcome of trials of weaning from mechanical ventilation. N Engl J Med 324:1445–1450
20. Epstein SK (1995) Etiology of extubation failure and the predictive value of the rapid shallow breathing index. Am J Respir Crit Care Med 152:545–549
21. Esteban A, Alia A, Gordo F, Fernandez R, Solsona JF, Vallverdu I, et al (1997) Extubation outcome after spontaneous breathing trials with T-tube or pressure support ventilation. Am J Respir Crit Care Med 156:459–465
22. Tobin MJ (2000) Weaning from mechanical ventilation: what have we learned? Respir Care 45:417–431

17 The Importance of Clinical Algorithms to Facilitate Weaning and Extubation

E.W. Ely

17.1 Introduction

The strength of evidence now available to direct clinical decisions regarding weaning from mechanical ventilation has improved dramatically over recent years. Decisions can now be made using strong recommendations based on evidence gained from well-conducted, randomized trials. For the Agency for Healthcare Policy and Research (AHCPR) and the McMaster Evidence-Based Medicine working group, Cook et al. [1] recently performed an exhaustive review of the literature on weaning. After initially reviewing 5653 investigations carried out over the past 30 years, they decided, based on study design and quality of the investigation, to use only 154 articles. This AHCPR report and its conclusions represent a fresh look at the state of the art in this field, and will be used to direct my comments in this chapter.

Specifically, the AHCPR directed the McMaster Evidence-Based Weaning working group to answer the following five questions, which I will address succinctly at the conclusion of the chapter based upon the data presented:
1. When should weaning be initiated?
2. What criteria should be used to initiate the weaning process?
3. What are the most effective methods of weaning?
4. What are the optimal roles of non-physician health-care professionals (HCPs) in facilitating safe and expeditious weaning?
5. What is the value of clinical practice algorithms and computers in expediting weaning?

Despite the popularity of the term "weaning", one of the most important concepts to arise from recent prospective, randomized, controlled trials (RCTs) is that a gradual reduction in ventilator support may unnecessarily delay extubation of patients who have recovered from respiratory failure [2]. With increasing recognition of the complications of MV, and growing attention being paid to resources consumed in the care of patients with respiratory failure, a change in the clinical paradigm is warranted. Evidence supports the liberation of patients from MV [3–6]. That is, the rapid identification of patients who have recovered from respiratory failure is more important than manipulation of MV in an attempt to accelerate recovery.

Several investigators have set out to investigate the utility of protocols in liberating patients from MV. Medical centers have felt increasing pressures to encourage physicians to be even more effective and efficient in the management of patients. We have spent the past 5 years studying the development, implementation, and efficacy of ventilator management protocols for patients with respiratory failure. We have shown that using a simple two-step protocol incorporating daily screening (DS) followed by spontaneous breathing trials (SBTs), one can improve upon the best practices of board-certified intensivists and cardiologists safely and in a way which actually reduces complication rates.

17.1.1 Prospective Randomized Controlled Trials

A survey of MV in Spain determined that "weaning time" accounted for over 40% of total ventilator time [7], demonstrating a considerable opportunity for improvement. Despite numerous efforts to determine the best method of weaning patients from MV, it was not until 1994 that any RCT showed one method (pressure-support ventilation, or PSV) to be superior to others [8]. The following year, however, another well-performed RCT showed seemingly conflicting results, with SBTs leading to earlier extubation among mechanically ventilated patients [5] (Fig. 17.1). Although these investigations reached contradictory conclusions, they showed that (a) weaning strategies influence the duration of MV; (b) the specific criteria used to initiate changes in ventilatory support influence outcome; and (c) the most ineffective approach was intermittent mandatory ventilation, previously a widely used strategy.

In general, physicians do not discontinue MV efficiently. In the above-cited studies [5, 8], 69%–76% of patients evaluated for enrollment were judged ready for immediate extubation. In addition, as many as half of the patients who extu-

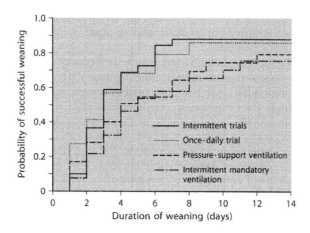

Fig. 17.1. Kaplan-Meier curves of the probability of successful weaning with four different techniques. After adjustment for baseline characteristics in a Cox proportional-hazards model, the rate of successful weaning with a once-daily trial of spontaneous breathing was 2.83 times higher than that with intermittent mandatory ventilation ($p<0.006$) and 2.05 times higher than that with pressure-support ventilation ($p<0.04$). (From [5] with permission)

bate themselves prematurely do not require reintubation within 24 h [9, 10]. Physicians' predictions of whether patients can have MV successfully discontinued are inaccurate, with positive and negative predictive values of only 50% and 67%, respectively [11].

The above-mentioned studies did not include a non-protocol "control" group, which left clinicians without assurance that protocols were superior to their individual decision-making at the bedside. In order to address this issue, we enrolled 300 mechanically ventilated medical and nonsurgical cardiac patients into an RCT in which the treatment group was "weaned" to extubation using a two-step process of screening by respiratory care practitioners (RCPs), followed by SBTs when recovery was sufficient to "pass" the DS [6]. Of course, this screening process can be performed by nursing staff as well. In this and the chapter that follows, RCPs and nursing staff are used as synonymous because in Europe, in general, there are no RCPs. The DS and SBT are defined below. We also incorporated a written and verbal physician prompt into the treatment arm, which notified them when a patient had successfully passed an SBT.

Importantly, the physicians involved in our investigations were all board-certified intensivists or cardiologists operating in "closed" intensive care units. A survey taken prior to initiating the investigation indicated that the majority (68%) doubted that their practice style could be improved by routine objective measurements along with increased input from RCPs. That is, they had confidence in their level of efficiency in removing patients from MV and felt that the protocol would not lead to improved outcomes. However, the outcomes of the investigation included: removal from MV 2 days earlier in the protocol-directed group despite a higher severity of illness, 50% fewer complications, and a reduction in the cost of intensive care unit stay by US $5000 per patient (Table 17.1) [6]. Kaplan-Meier survival analysis (Fig. 17.2) and the Cox proportional-hazards model demonstrated that subjects assigned to the intervention group had MV successfully discontinued earlier (relative rate of successful extubation = 2.13, 95% confidence interval, 1.58–2.86; $p<0.0001$).

The protocol encouraged extubation as soon as recovery was documented, and we expected a higher rate of complications (particularly reintubation) in the intervention group. In fact, the risk of nonlethal complications was lower in the intervention group. The reintubation rate in our institution prior to initiation of this investigation was 8%, comparable to that seen in our controls. The intervention group experienced a lower rate of reintubation (4%), perhaps because of careful objective screening prior to extubation. Because reintubation is associated with an increased risk of nosocomial pneumonia [12], this finding may prove especially important if confirmed. The reintubation rates in this trial compare favorably to those rates in two recent large weaning trials, 7.3% [8] and 17.7% [5]. Subsequent implementation of this protocol in 530 patients at another large medical center was associated with a similar reintubation rate (i.e., 6%) and no increased risk of mortality [13].

This protocol has been found to be broadly applicable not only in university hospitals, but also in community hospital settings (A.M. Baker, personal communication). The techniques and measurements require no special monitoring or equipment, no additional expenditures beyond staffing, and no laboratory stud-

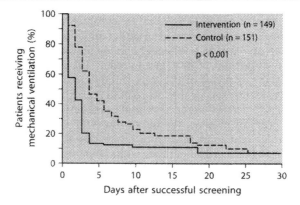

Fig. 17.2. Kaplan-Meier curves of the risk of remaining mechanically ventilated in protocol vs. control groups. After adjusting for baseline characteristics using covariates that described severity of illness (APACHE II), age, gender, race, ICU location, and duration of intubation prior to enrollment, a Cox proportional-hazards analysis demonstrated that subjects in the protocol group were removed from mechanical ventilation more rapidly than controls (relative rate of successful extubation = 2.13, 95% confidence interval, 1.55–2.92, $p<0.001$). (From [6] with permission)

Table 17.1. Improved ventilator days, complication rates, and cost of care in protocol-directed weaning. (From [6])

	Intervention group (n=149)	Control group (n=151)	p-value
APACHE II	19.8	17.9	0.01
Weaning days	1	3	0.0001
Ventilator days	4.5	6	0.003
Reintubation (%)	6 (4)	15 (10)	0.04
Mech. ventilation >21 days (%)	9 (6)	20 (13)	0.04
Any complication (%)	30 (20)	62 (41)	0.001
Total ICU costs	$15,740	$20,890	0.03

ies (arterial blood gases are optional). It has been recommended that ICUs either adopt or adapt the methods of this validated protocol or establish their own protocols with similar goals [14]. Use of the protocol to manage just four patients would result in one individual being off MV after 48 h who otherwise would not have been. In addition, if the protocol were used in six patients, one less complication would be expected.

Kollef and colleagues [15] conducted another RCT (n=357) of protocol-directed versus physician-directed weaning in four ICUs (two medical and two surgical). This investigation incorporated three separate "weaning" protocols due to difficulty in achieving consensus among different units, thereby underscoring the practical challenges facing implementation of protocols. The protocol-directed group incorporated an amalgam of SBTs, PSV, and synchronized intermittent mandatory ventilation protocols and demonstrated an earlier initiation of weaning efforts and a median duration of MV of 35 h versus 44 h in the physician-directed group.

Prospective investigations of strategies to reduce the cost of intensive care are few. In our study, the total cost of ICU care throughout the study period for the control group was $4,297,024, for the intervention group $3,855,001, representing a savings of $442,023. The 25% reduction in the cost of ICU care associated with the use of this protocol presents the opportunity for sizable financial savings when applied throughout an institution or health-care system. If applied only to medical and nonsurgical cardiac patients within our institution, the annualized cost savings for ICU care were estimated at greater than $700,000. Kollef et al. [15] reported a savings of $42,960 in their protocol-directed weaning group.

During implementation of our protocol, physician time commitment appeared to be minimal, since respiratory therapists and nurses who were already caring for the patients did most of the monitoring. Personnel expenses are thought to account for more than 50% of the cost of MV [16]. While we did not formally assess time spent by the respiratory therapists and nurses instituting the protocol, the DS generally required only a few minutes per patient per day and was incorporated readily into respiratory therapists' routines. Some investigators have advocated the use of a weaning team [17], though RCTs of this strategy are lacking. Future RCTs demonstrating the superiority of protocolized care being delivered via a weaning team vs. physicians, nurses, and therapists will help elucidate the optimal approach.

17.2 The Two-Step Process of Liberation

17.2.1 Daily Screening Techniques

It has been suspected (but not proven) that a DS tool could, if applied from the day of initiation of MV, greatly accelerate progress toward extubation. Physicians often fail to identify patients who can be successfully extubated, and they tend to underestimate the probability of successful discontinuation of MV [18]. In one investigation, physicians' clinical judgment had a specificity of 35% and a likelihood ratio of 1.5 [11], values that indicate little clinical utility without the use of objective monitoring parameters. We hypothesized that the busy clinician was unable to systematically accomplish the appropriate screening of patients while burdened with so many other individual patient concerns and professional duties.

Many weaning parameters have been proposed to identify patients ready for extubation [18–30]; they range from simple maneuvers such as counting and measuring breaths [19] to more complicated techniques requiring the insertion of esophageal or gastric balloons [20, 21] or the use of computerized decision-support models [18]. Eloquently performed investigations of difficult-to-wean patients have determined that in addition to the frequency/tidal volume ratio (f/V_T) [19], physiologic measurements including an airway occlusion pressure at 0.1 s ($P_{0.1}$) above 4.5 cm H_2O [9, 23, 31] and a tension-time index above 0.15 [30, 32] are helpful determinants of diaphragmatic fatigue and weaning failure. In general, these tests confirm that the load imposed on the inspiratory muscles is in excess of the neuromuscular capacity. Historic reliance on such measures is appealing because of their scientific basis and the potential theoretically to limit risks to the patient. However, these technically demanding tests are neither necessary nor practical for widespread use in the majority of patients within the confines of a protocol. Until recently, no RCT had documented that application of any tools produced better outcomes than physician judgment alone [6].

Manthous et al. [3] arrived at the following summary statements regarding three commonly used weaning parameters: (a) Maximal inspiratory pressure or NIF – the area under a receiver-operating-characteristic (ROC) curve (i.e., sensitivity vs 1-specificity) was 0.61–0.68. (b) Spontaneous minute ventilation shows an even poorer predictive combination, with ROC curve area of 0.40 to 0.54, and (c) f/V_T or rapid shallow breathing index yielded an ROC curve area of 0.75–0.89. Jaeschke et al. [33] eloquently discussed a process to determine whether these parameters are clinically useful to diagnose weanability. The f/V_T threshold level of 105 breaths/min/l chosen by Yang and Tobin [19] has a relatively high ROC curve area and appeared useful in our screening, at least in part because it is followed by a second step – SBTs. In fact, many patients with a ratio between 80 and 105 may fail SBTs [31, 33]. While alterations in the diagnostic thresholds for different components of the DS (e.g., the best "cutoff" for the f/V_T) may be appropriate, this will be discussed below and in the following chapter.

After reviewing the literature, we chose a set of five simple parameters to use as a DS to be performed on all patients. In the original investigation, a daily screening test was obtained on all 300 enrolled patients each morning between 06:00 a.m. and 07:00 a.m. by the unit's respiratory therapist. The results of the DS were not available to physicians caring for study patients. In this investigation, the DS required only about 2 min to perform.

In order to "pass" the DS, all of the following criteria had to be met:

1. $PaO_2/F_IO_2 \geq 200$ (P/F ratio) – e.g., PaO_2 of $100/F_IO_2$ of 0.5=200
2. Positive end-expiratory pressure (PEEP) ≤ 5 cmH$_2$O
3. Adequate cough during suctioning (i.e., intact airway reflexes)
4. Patient could not be receiving any vasopressor drips or sedatives by continuous infusion. Dopamine was allowed if dosed <5 μg/kg/min, and intermittent dosing of sedatives was allowed.
5. Frequency/tidal volume ratio (f/V_T) ≤ 105. This is also known as the rapid shallow breathing index (RSBI), measured after 1 min of spontaneous breathing with ventilator rate set to 0 and pressure support set to 0. Average V_T calculated by dividing f into V_E ($V_T = V_E / f$), alternatively: $f/V_T = f^2 / V_E$; e.g., rate (f) of 20,V_E of 10 l/min: (20×20) divided by 10 = f/V_T of 40. To measure the f/V_T, the patient was placed on continuous positive airway pressure with no mandatory ventilator breaths and with pressure support removed for 1 min [19]. Minute ventilation and respiratory rate were recorded as measured by the Puritan-Bennett 7200 or Siemens 900 mechanical ventilator, and tidal volume (V_T) was obtained by dividing the minute ventilation by respiratory frequency (f).

In our original investigation, it took these MICU and CCU patients an average of 2–3 days to pass the DS [6]. While 75% of our patients eventually passed the screen, another recent report found 290 of 537 (54%) of patients passed the same screening tool [13]. During DS assessments in over 1500 patients, there were no complications detected (e.g., during f/V_T) such as temporally associated self-extubation, prolonged desaturation, or hemodynamic instability. During our hospital-wide implementation of the protocol, of those patients who had once passed the DS ($n=722$), 41% ($n=298$) consistently passed the DS while 59% ($n=424$) fluctuated between passing and not passing [34]. When the DS was passed and an SBT was obtained, patients would pass the SBT 75.4% of the time, a rate that did not vary over the 12-month period of implementation or among services and units ($p=0.297$). Overly rigid interpretation of the "rules" of the protocol seemed counterproductive. For example, determining on consecutive days that a patient failed the DS because the PaO_2/F_IO_2 ratio was 198 (rather than being >200) or their f/V_T was 107 (rather than being <105) was felt to be inappropriate because some patients do not fit within the confines of specified "cutoffs" or thresholds [26, 33, 35, 36]. Continuing to advance patients through the protocol at this point and assessing their ability to breathe with an SBT may prove successful in many such circumstances.

17.2.2 Spontaneous Breathing Trials

Because of the heterogeneity of patients with respiratory failure and the dynamic interplay of multiple factors determining their need for ventilatory support, we believe there are inherent limitations to any current measures used to determine whether the patient can be liberated. Rather, allowing the patient to breathe spontaneously for a predetermined time trial during close monitoring (i.e., an SBT) is the optimum confirmation of the patient's readiness for extubation.

What Is an SBT and Who Receives One?
An SBT is a trial of spontaneous breathing for a predetermined amount of time (e.g., 30–120 min) using "flow-by" mode or T-piece, with ventilator rate set to 0 and pressure support set to 0. A patient who passes the DS is a candidate for an SBT.

Who Performs the SBT?
- RCPs (or nurses) perform DS and either initiate or prompt a physician to order an SBT.
- RCPs (or nurses) initiate the SBT, monitor the patient during the trial (in conjunction with the nurse), and re-initiate MV if criteria for trial termination are met.
- An ICU nurse monitors the patient with regard to criteria for trial termination and notifies the RCP (or the physician in charge) if they are met.

When is an SBT Terminated?
- If the patient successfully tolerates the SBT for up to 2 h, or...
- When one of the following conditions is met:
  - Respiratory rate >35 for more than 5 min
  - SaO_2 <90% during more than 30 s of good quality measurement

- 20% increase or decrease in heart rate for >5 min
- Systolic blood pressure (SBP) >180 or SBP <90 during at least 1 min of continuous recording or repeated measurements
- Agitation, anxiety, or diaphoresis confirmed as a change from baseline and present for more than 5 min

Some investigators have repeated the f/V_T after 30 min to 3 h of spontaneous breathing (for example) and found that this approach raised the accuracy by about 10% [36, 37].

What Does It Mean if a Patient Passes an SBT?

Successful completion of a 2-h SBT indicates a 90% chance of successfully staying off of MV for 48 h [6]. The median length of time a patient remained on the ventilator after passing an SBT was 1 day, a rate that did not vary among different patient populations or ICUs [34].

The SBT described above was used in the aforementioned investigations [5, 6] and further validated by other investigators [31]. In a preliminary report, Wood and colleagues [13] found that of 275 patients passing the DS who were selected for an SBT, 264 (96%) passed, with 232 of 264 (88%) extubated, and 217 of these patients (94%) remaining extubated for 3 days. This experience confirms the low reintubation rates described previously. Esteban and the Spanish Lung Failure Collaborative Group have defined practical aspects of the SBT. These investigators showed in an RCT of 526 patients that successful extubation was achieved equally effectively with SBTs lasting 30 min or 120 min [38]. In a previous study, they had documented that the SBT could be conducted with either a low level of PSV or a T-piece [39]. In our studies, SBTs were performed with either standard T-tube circuits or flow-triggered openings of the demand valve without additional support. Incorporating flow triggering during the SBT was a convenience that minimized respiratory therapist involvement, and it had not been investigated by others. Taken together, these investigations support institutional variations in the specific method of conducting an SBT. In fact, individual physicians may wish to tailor the technique and duration of SBTs for individual patients.

Not only is passing an SBT clinically important; failing an SBT also has major prognostic implications. First of all, most patients who failed a breathing trial did so fairly early, with a median duration of the SBT until failure of around 20 min [38]. Vallverdu et al. [31] have studied outcomes of a 2-hour T-piece trial and found that the mean time to failure (among those who were unable to sustain 120 min of spontaneous breathing) was 39 min (Fig. 17.3). However, 36% of patients failed after the first 30 min of successfully breathing on their own. None of seven weaning parameters consistently predicted time to failure. Because of the morbidity and mortality associated with reintubation, indices need to be developed to identify patients who can sustain spontaneous breathing without distress, but who nonetheless will require reintubation after extubation [38].

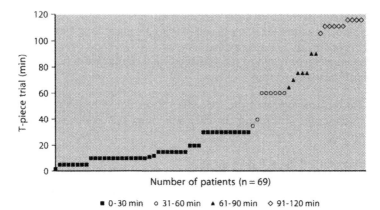

Fig. 17.3. Time to failure of spontaneous breathing trial among 69 patients with failed attempt. Distribution of patients according to the time of spontaneous breathing in the weaning trial before reconnection to mechanical ventilation. (From [31] with permission)

17.3 Controlling the Delivery of Sedatives Reduces Time on the Ventilator

The goals of sedation for mechanically ventilated patients usually include the following: (a) alleviation of agitation to a safe, tolerable level of movement by the patient and (b) alleviation of distress (pain, anxiety, dyspnea, and delirium). One randomized, controlled investigation, using a nursing-implemented protocol to manage the delivery of sedation, showed a reduction in the duration of mechanical ventilation by 2 days (p=0.008) and in the length of stay in the ICU by 2 days (p<0.0001), and controlled sedation was also associated with a significantly lower tracheostomy rate among the treatment group (6% vs 13%, p=0.04) [40]. This investigation presents important evidence that the management of sedation in the ICU can be improved by protocolized care, yet it did not seek to measure the impact on cognitive impairment rates or cost of care and reported only short-term follow-up. A more recently published investigation of 150 mechanically ventilated patients [41] implemented a protocol in which a treatment group had sedatives discontinued daily until they were awake and following commands, while the control group was managed according to the managing physicians preferences. In the treatment group, the duration of mechanical ventilation was reduced by 2 days (p=0.004), and ICU length of stay was reduced by 3.5 days (p=0.02). Overall complications and length of hospital stay were similar in both groups, and the approach to daily cessation of sedatives appeared safe in this medical ICU population.

These two investigations alert us to the fact that the administration of psychoactive medications to mechanically ventilated patients should attain higher focus in future investigations. An important component of the care of these patients, that often goes unrecognized, has to do with ongoing cognitive impairment or delirium. Delirium is associated with prolonged hospital stay, institutionalization, and death but has been poorly studied in the ICU setting. Key elements of delirium, such as inattention and altered consciousness, are difficult to assess in ICU settings due to the impaired ability of the patient to communicate. Unfortunately, there are no validated instruments available for ICU nurses or physicians to monitor delirium. We recently designed and prospectively tested a 5-min, multi-component, bedside delirium assessment that incorporated the Confusion Assessment Method (CAM) [42]. We consecutively enrolled 48 patients (24 of whom were mechanically ventilated), excluding those with underlying dementia or psychosis [43]. Two study nurses and two ICU physicians, using CAM, and two geriatric psychiatrists, using the Diagnostic and Statistical Manual of Mental Disorders (DSM-IV) for delirium as the reference standard, performed evaluations over 201 patient days. Coma was present in 27% of patient evaluations, stupor in 15%, and delirium in 27%. The sensitivity and specificity of CAM for delirium were 94% and 90% with high inter-rater reliability ($\kappa=0.83–0.93$, 179 paired evaluations). The likelihood ratio for a positive test (CAM+) was >30. Delirium was associated with an average of 3 ± 4 additional days of hospitalization ($p= 0.03$), and the duration of CAM+ days correlated highly with the duration of stay ($r=0.84$, $p<0.0001$). Despite the exclusion of dementia on enrollment, 52% of patients had severely impaired cognitive function according to the Folstein mental status examination at hospital discharge. In conclusion, delirium was associated with adverse outcomes, including prolonged stay and persistent neurological impairment. This system of delirium assessment [43], which appears valid and reliable in the hands of nurses and physicians, deserves further study and may prove useful for clinical and research applications in efforts to optimize the delivery of mechanical ventilation.

17.4 The Prognostic Significance of Weaning Parameters

The McMaster Evidence Based report on weaning scrutinized the available literature regarding weaning parameters [1]. Pooled results regarding the utility of traditional parameters in predicting successful extubation are presented in Table 17.2, along with data from the DS described above from our trial. While the conclusion of the McMaster report was that most weaning parameters have poor

Table 17.2. Pooled results regarding clinical utility of weaning parameters for predicting successful extubation. (From [1, 49])

Predictor	Likelihood ratio	Sensitivity (%)	Specificity (%)
Minute ventilation (10–12 l)	1.2	50	40
Respiratory rate (30–35 bpm)	1.6	97	31
Tidal volume (325 ml)	1.5	76	36
f/V_T (100 b/min/l)	2.8	84	42
NIF (–25 to –30 cmH$_2$O)	1.5	60	47
Daily screen (Ely et al.)	2.7	88	67
$P_{0.1}$/MIP or CROP	3–16	70	80–92

overall predictive power, we believe that incorporating these as a screen each morning of mechanical ventilation has merit and perhaps even potential prognostic significance. The following discussion will explore varying aspects of using a daily screen of weaning parameters within the context of a weaning protocol.

17.4.1 Identification of Patients

It is difficult to identify those patients in whom prolonged MV will or will not be necessary. Patients who require prolonged MV are best managed in a long-term, acute-care (LTAC) facility. Scheinhorn and colleagues reported successful weaning in 56% of 1123 LTAC patients requiring prolonged MV, with 1-year survival rates of 38% among discharged patients [44]. The management of chronically ventilated patients beyond their acute stay in the ICU has been addressed recently in other reports [45], including a consensus statement by the ACCP [46]. The following discussion will focus on the prognostic significance of our DS of weaning parameters during the initial ventilator course.

During the development of the APACHE III system, an analysis was performed of data collected on 5915 mechanically ventilated patients in an attempt to predict the duration of MV. Using logistic regression, it was determined that duration is primarily a function of the admitting diagnosis and the degree of physiologic derangement as measured by the acute physiology score [47]. While the predictive equation may help as a research tool, it was not meant for clinical use at the bedside. Others have concluded that a lung injury score <1 is predictive of MV less than 15 days [48], but that if the LIS is ≥1, "nothing further about the expected duration of MV can be said."

17.4.2 Prognosis Over Time Post-Intubation

We recently published data examining the relationship of patients' ability to pass a DS of weaning variables with hospital survival [49]. The percentage of patients who survived until discharge was higher for those who had passed the DS than for those who had not yet passed (78% vs. 50%, $p=0.001$), and for those who had been successfully extubated than for those who still required MV (84% vs. 60%, $p=0.001$). While the difference in survival between patients who had passed the DS and those who had not passed it was significant ($p=0.001$) at 3 days post-intubation, this difference decreased over time and was no longer statistically significant by 12 days post-intubation ($p=0.18$). Proportional-hazards analysis of time until in-hospital death confirmed the beneficial effect of passing the DS during the first 10 days ($p=0.01$), after adjustment for differences in severity of illness, age, race, gender, diagnosis, and treatment assignment.

The relationship between duration of MV and survival was significant (Fig. 17.4, $p=0.02$), with mortality increasing steadily throughout the first 3 weeks: the mortality was 33% (95% confidence interval of 26%–40%) for those on MV for 1–7 days, 48% for those on MV for 8–14 days (35%–59%), and 62% for those on MV 15–21 days (39%–78%). Patients on MV for more than 21 days had a low-

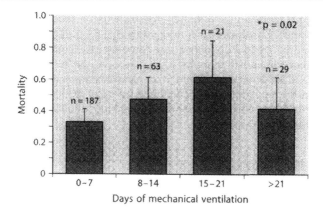

Days of mechanical ventilation

Fig. 17.4. Duration of mechanical ventilation and survival. There was a significant relationship between the number of days of mechanical ventilation and survival (p=0.02). The mortality increased steadily from 1 to 3 weeks of ventilator usage and then dropped for those requiring more than 21 days of mechanical ventilation. Proportional-hazards analysis of time until in-hospital death confirmed the relationship between survival and duration of mechanical ventilation even after adjustment for differences in severity of illness, age, race, gender, diagnosis, and treatment assignment (p=0.001). (From [50] with permission)

er mortality of 41% (24%–57%) [50]. Proportional-hazards analysis of time until in-hospital death confirmed this relationship between survival and duration of MV even after adjustment for differences in severity of illness, age, race, gender, diagnosis, and treatment assignment (p=0.001). This observation supports both long-standing anecdotal impressions and findings of a previous report of a multicenter registry of acute respiratory distress syndrome patients, in which 85% of the nonsurvivors had died by the fourth week and the subsequent mortality was much lower than that of the population as a whole [50]. While at least one other investigation has found an association between mortality and the duration of MV [51], we believe that the independent relationship between MV and survival requires further prospective study.

Although reducing the length of time that patients spend on MV is essential, neither the predictors of liberation from the ventilator (i.e., use of weaning parameters) nor the number of days on MV have previously been associated independently with survival. Our data provided additional new information regarding the prognostic value of the daily screening of ventilated patients by RCPs and/or physicians. The DS predicted the likelihood of successful extubation with an accuracy of 82%, and its sensitivity and positive predictive values both approached 90%. While liberation from MV was predictive of survival at any time during the hospital stay (p=0.001), the prognostic significance of the DS for hospital survival was related to how early after intubation it was passed. The difference in survival between patients who had passed and those who had not passed the DS was significant for 10 days post-intubation, but progressively decreased over time.

These data provide several other important insights. Because passing the DS was associated with a reduced incidence of prolonged MV (3% vs. 30%, p=0.0001), this monitoring technique may have useful triage implications for patients being considered for referral to regional weaning centers or for timing of tracheostomy in anticipation of a need for chronic airway support [52]. For example, if the DS becomes positive, a physician may delay tracheostomy and/or triage to a chronic ventilator facility. Although a negative screen identifies the majority of those who will require prolonged MV, the information is of little clinical use because the majority of those failing the DS in the first 10 days may still be extubated prior to the fourth week.

17.5 Conclusions and Answers to the Five Introductory Questions

In conclusion, successful removal of the mechanical ventilator at any time is associated with higher survival rates, which may be independent of severity of illness. During the first 10 days of MV, passing the DS is a predictor of survival and supports attempts at optimizing liberation from MV. Failure to pass the screen of weaning parameters is of little value prognostically, since up to 29% of such patients will survive their hospital stay. While physicians should always be motivated to remove ventilators as early as possible, the time during which the patient remains on MV *after* passing the DS presents a special opportunity to optimize care.

From their review of the literature on weaning, Dr. Cook and colleagues [1] concluded that the best answers to the five questions posed in the introduction of this chapter are as follows:

1. When should weaning be initiated?
   - The best answer on "when to start weaning" is to develop a protocol that begins testing soon after initiation of MV.
2. What criteria should be used to initiate the weaning process?
   - No weaning parameters have demonstrated reproducibly impressive positive and negative predictive values that would allow them to serve as stand-alone instruments in weaning. However, those with some predictive power include the f/V_T, the $P_{0.1}$/MIP, the CROP, and our daily screen of weaning parameters (see Table 17.2).
3. What are the most effective methods of weaning?
   - For step-wise reductions in MV, spontaneous breathing trials or pressure-support ventilation are superior to intermittent mandatory ventilation.
   - Early identification of readiness followed by extubation or extubation with noninvasive positive-pressure ventilation (NPPV) offers substantial benefits. NPPV must be studied in more diverse patient populations (e.g., those with acute and not chronic respiratory disease) prior to routine application in clinical weaning algorithms and protocols.
4. What are the optimal roles of non-physician HCPs in facilitating safe and expeditious weaning?
   - The implementation of nurse- or RCP-driven weaning protocols, regardless of what mode is employed, significantly expedites safe weaning.
   - Following cardiac surgery, rapid weaning protocols clearly allow early extubation, but impact on complications and cost is minimal.

5. What is the value of clinical practice algorithms and computers in expediting weaning?
   - Their value has been established in multiple RCTs and carries the strongest recommendation, since patient outcomes including length of stay, complications, and cost have all been improved. This recommendation includes protocolizing the delivery of sedative and analgesic medications, which are so frequently used in mechanically ventilated patients.
   - The role of computerized protocols has not been established.

17.6 References

1. Cook DJ, Meade MO, Guyatt GH, Griffith L, Booker L, for the McMaster Evidence-Based Practice Center (2000) Weaning from mechanical ventilation. Agency for Healthcare Research and Quality [Contract No. 290-97-0017, Task order number 2]
2. Weinberger SE, Weiss JW (1995) Weaning from ventilatory support. N Engl J Med 332: 388–389
3. Manthous CA, Schmidt GA, Hall JB (1998) Liberation from mechanical ventilation: a decade of progress. Chest 114:886–901
4. Hall JB, Wood LD (1987) Liberation of the patient from mechanical ventilation. JAMA 257:1621–1628
5. Esteban A, Frutos F, Tobin MJ, Alia I, Solsona JF, Valverdu I, et al (1995) A comparison of four methods of weaning patients from mechanical ventilation. N Engl J Med 332:345–350
6. Ely EW, Baker AM, Dunagan DP, Burke HL, Smith AC, Kelly PT, et al (1996) Effect on the duration of mechanical ventilation of identifying patients capable of breathing spontaneously. N Engl J Med 335:1864–1869
7. Esteban A, Alia I, Ibanez J, Benito S, Tobin MJ, The Spanish Lung Failure Collaborative Group (1994) Modes of mechanical ventilation and weaning. Chest 106:1188–1193
8. Brochard L, Rauss A, Benito S, Conti g, Mancebo J, Rekik N, et al (1994) Comparison of three methods of gradual withdrawal from ventilatory support during weaning from mechanical ventilation. Am J Respir Crit Care Med 150:896–903
9. Listello D, Sessler C (1994) Unplanned extubation: clinical predictors for reintubation. Chest 105:1496–1503
10. Tindol GA jr DiBenedetto RJ, Kosciuk L (1994) Unplanned extubations. Chest 105:1804–1807
11. Stroetz RW, Hubmayr RD (1995) Tidal volume maintenance during weaning with pressure support. Am J Respir Crit Care Med 152:1034–1040
12. Torres A, Gatell JM, Aznar E (1995) Re-intubation increases the risk of nosocomial pneumonia in patients needing mechanical ventilation. Am J Respir Crit Care Med 152:137–141
13. Wood KE, Flaten AL, Reedy JS, Coursin DB (1999) Use of a daily wean screen and weaning protocol for mechanically ventilated patients in a multidisciplinary tertiary critical care unit. Crit Care Med 27:A94–A94
14. Luce JM (1996) Reducing the use of mechanical ventilation. N Engl J Med 25:1916–1917
15. Kollef MH, Shapiro SD, Silver P, St.John RE, Prentice D, Sauer S et al (1997) A randomized, controlled trial of protocol-directed versus physician-directed weaning from mechanical ventilation. Crit Care Med 25:567–574
16. Cohen IL, Booth FV (1994) Cost containment and mechanical ventilation in the United States. New Horiz 2:283–290
17. Cohen IL (1994) Weaning from mechanical ventilation – the team approach and beyond. Intensive Care Med 20:317–318
18. Strickland JH jr, Hasson JH (1993) A computer-controlled ventilator weaning system: a clinical trial. Chest 103:1220–1226
19. Yang KL, Tobin MJ (1991) A prospective study of indexes predicting the outcome of trials of weaning from mechanical ventilation. N Engl J Med 324:1445–1450

20. Mohsenifar Z, Hay A, Hay J, Lewis JI, Loerner SK (1993) Gastric intramural pH as a predictor of success or failure in weaning patients from mechanical ventilation. Ann Intern Med 119:794–798

21. Gluck EH, Barkoviak MJ, Balk RA, Casey LC, Silver MR, Bone RC (1995) Medical effectiveness of esophageal balloon pressure manometry in weaning patients from mechanical ventilation. Crit Care Med 23:504–509

22. Shikora SA, Benotti PN, Johannigman JA (1994) The oxygen cost of breathing may predict weaning from mechanical ventilation better than the respiratory rate to tidal volume ratio. Arch Surg 129:269–274

23. Sassoon CS, Mahutte CK (1993) Airway occlusion pressure and breathing pattern as predictors of weaning outcome. Am Rev Respir Dis 148:860–866

24. Sassoon CSH, Te TT, Mahutte CK, Light RW (1987) Airway occlusion pressure: an important indicator for successful weaning in patients with chronic obstructive pulmonary disease. Am Rev Respir Dis 135:107–113

25. Gandia F, Blanco J (1992) Evaluation of indexes predicting the outcome of ventilator weaning and value of adding supplemental inspiratory load. Intensive Care Med 18: 327–333

26. Epstein SK (1995) Etiology of extubation failure and the predictive value of the rapid shallow breathing index. Am J Respir Crit Care Med 152:545–549

27. Capdevila XJ, Perrigault PF, Percy PJ, Roustan JP, d'Athis F (1995) Occlusion pressure and its ratio to maximum inspiratory pressure are useful predictors for successful extubation following T-piece weaning trial. Chest 108:482–489

28. Yang KL (1993) Inspiratory pressure/maximal inspiratory pressure ratio: a predictive index of weaning outcome. Intensive Care Med 19:204–208

29. Dojat M, Harf A, Touchard D, Laforest M, Lemaire F, Brochard L (1996) Evaluation of a knowledge-based system providing ventilatory management and decision for extubation. Am J Respir Crit Care Med 153:997–1004

30. Vassilakopoulos T, Zakynthinos S, Roussos C (1998) The tension-time index and the frequency/tidal volume ratio are the major pathophysiologic determinants of weaning failure and success. Am J Respir Crit Care Med 158:378–385

31. Vallverdu I, Calaf N, Subirana M, Net A, Benito S, Mancebo J (1999) Clinical characteristics, respiratory functional parameters, and outcome of a two-hour T-piece trial of patients weaning from mechanical ventilation. Am J Respir Crit Care Med 158:1855–1862

32. Bellemare F, Grassino A (1982) Effect of pressure and timing of contraction on human diaphragm fatigue. J Appl Physiol 53:1190–1195

33. Jaeschke RZ, Meade MO, Guyatt GH, Keenan SP, Cook DJ (1997) How to use diagnostic test articles in the intensive care unit: diagnosing weanability using f/Vt. Crit Care Med 25: 1514–1521

34. Ely EW, Bennett PA, Bowton DL, Murphy SM, Haponik EF (1999) Large scale implementation of a respiratory therapist-driven protocol for ventilator weaning. Am J Respir Crit Care Med 159:439–446

35. Epstein SK, Ciubotaru RL (1997) Influence of gender and endotracheal tube size on preextubation breathing pattern. Am J Respir Crit Care Med 154:1647–1652

36. Krieger BP, Isber J, Breitenbucher A, Throop G, Ershowsky P (1997) Serial measurements of the rapid-shallow-breathing index as a predictor of weaning outcome in elderly medical patients. Chest 112:1029–1034

37. Chatila W, Jacob B, Guaglionone D, Manthous CA (1996) The unassisted respiratory rate-tidal volume ratio accurately predicts weaning outcome. Am J Med 101:61–67

38. Esteban A, Alia I, Tobin M, Gil A, Gordo F, Vallverdu I, et al (1999) Effect of spontaneous breathing trial duration on outcome of attempts to discontinue mechanical ventilation. Am J Respir Crit Care Med 159:512–518

39. Esteban A, Alia I, Gordo F, Fernandez R, Solsona JF, Vallverdu I, et al (1997) Extubation outcome after spontaneous breathing trials with T-tube or pressure support ventilation. Am J Respir Crit Care Med 156:459–465

40. Brook AD, Ahrens TS, Schaiff R, Prentice D, Sherman G, Shannon W, et al (1999) Effect of a nursing implemented sedation protocol on the duration of mechanical ventilation. Crit Care Med 27:2609–2615
41. Kress JP, Pohlman AS, O'Connor MF, Hall JB (2000) Daily interruption of sedative infusions in critically ill patients undergoing mechanical ventilation. N Engl J Med 342:1471–1477
42. Inouye SK, van Dyck CH, Alessi CA, Balkin S, Siegal AP, Horowitz RI (1990) Clarifying confusion: the confusion assessment method. Ann Intern Med 113:941–948
43. Ely EW, Margolin R, Francis J, May L, Truman B, Wheeler A, et al (1999) Delirium in the ICU: measurement and outcomes. Am J Respir Crit Care Med 161:A506
44. Scheinhorn DJ, Chao DC, Stearn-Hassenpglug M, LaBree LD, Heltsley DJ (1997) Post-ICU mechanical ventilation. Treatment of 1123 patients at a regional weaning center. Chest 111:1654–1659
45. Scheinhorn DJ, Hassenpflug M, Artinian BM, LaBree L, Catlin JL (1995) Predictors of weaning after 6 weeks of mechanical ventilation. Chest 107:500–505
46. Make BJ, Hill NS, Goldberg AI, Bach JR, Criner G, Dunne PE, et al (1998) Mechanical ventilation beyond the intensive care unit: report of a consensus conference of the American College of Chest Physicians. Chest 113:289S–344S
47. Seneff MG, Zimmerman JE, Knaus WA, Wagner DP, Draper EA (1996) Predicting the duration of mechanical ventilation. The importance of disease and patient characteristics. Chest 110:469–479
48. Troche G, Moine P (1997) Is the duration of mechanical ventilation predictable? Chest 112:745–751
49. Ely EW, Baker AM, Evans GW, Haponik EF (1999) The prognostic significance of passing a daily screen of weaning parameters. Intensive Care Med 25:581–587
50. Sloane PJ, Gee MH, Gottleib JE, Albertine KH, Peters SP, Burns JR, et al (1992) A multicenter registry of patients with acute respiratory distress syndrome. Physiology and outcome. Am Rev Respir Dis 146:419–426
51. Marik P, Kaufman D (1995) Teaching medical students in the intensive care unit: building houses with no foundation. Crit Care Med 23:1933–1934
52. The Spanish Lung Failure Collaborative Group (1997)Timing and clinical outcomes of ventilated patients requiring tracheostomy. Am J Respir Crit Care Med 155:A404

18 Strategies for Implementation of Weaning Algorithms in the Clinical Arena

E.W. Ely

18.1 Introduction

A protocol that has been validated in an institution other than your own can at best be a guide, and during the implementation process must be modified in ways to "fit" your institutional needs and practices. It is the implementation process itself that is the focus of this chapter. What good is even the best tool if it is not implemented and subsequently used appropriately? Our patients deserve an algorithmic or protocolized approach to liberation from mechanical ventilation (MV) because we know that this enhances their timely removal from the ventilator and reduces complications and costs (see the previous chapter, entitled "The Importance of Clinical Algorithms to Facilitate Weaning and Extubation"). However, effectively incorporating the protocol into daily practice, continually updating or modifying it so that the protocol accommodates new data, and using good clinical judgment as part of the daily decision process will all be discussed in this chapter.

18.2 Implementation of a Protocol or an Algorithm

The ultimate success of any patient management protocol depends upon the level of institutional commitment to improving outcomes as well as upon the team's leadership, persistence, and consistency in implementation. Protocolized care has been advocated in many facets of medicine, but relinquishing control of the patient's management often creates resentment and frustration on the part of physicians. Even when the evidence clearly supports change, it is very difficult to get physicians to alter their management styles [1], and what is really required is a change of culture. In certain circles of physicians within some institutions, there may be a low "readiness to change", and these professionals may require either motivational intervention or consultation with respected opinion leaders [1, 2]. Important considerations that may increase the chances of successfully changing the behavior of health-care professionals include education, timely feedback, participation by physicians in the effort to change, administrative intervention, and even financial incentives and penalties [1]. Each of these factors has relevance to the implementation of new approaches to MV.

While our original protocol documented the vital contributions of nonphysician health-care professionals in the management of ventilated medical patients, it was conducted as a therapist-focused (or nurse-focused), rather than a therapist-driven (or nurse-driven) protocol (TDP). Other groups have stressed the importance of "weaning teams" [3] and TDPs [4, 5], but there are few data documenting the feasibility of and/or steps necessary in implementing such protocols on a large scale with monitoring of protocol compliance. We prospectively monitored the institution-wide implementation of our previously validated approach. Importantly, we made slight modifications and reintroduced the protocol without the daily supervision of a weaning team, physician, or RCP supervisor in order to test its feasibility as a TDP [6]. An example of a modification made to the original protocol prior to this large-scale implementation was that we no longer used only 120-min spontaneous breathing trials (SBTs), but advocated breathing trials as short as 30 min when the clinician felt that this was adequate, benefiting from recent data reported by Esteban et al. [7]. Lastly, we explored the challenges of modifying RCPs and physicians' practice styles in the "out-of-study" setting over a 1-year period.

A total of 1167 patients were enrolled in the protocol, and 9048 patient days of MV were appraised [6]. The mean age was 60.1 ± 16.9 (SD), and there were 605 men (56.7%) and 462 women (43.3%). The principal reasons for their respiratory failure were acute respiratory distress syndrome (14%), trauma (13%), chronic obstructive pulmonary disease (11%), complications related to general or cardiothoracic surgery (21%), congestive heart failure or myocardial infarction (12%), or other causes (29%). Compliance with the protocol was monitored closely, using a daily data collection tool that was included in the above-mentioned reference. RCP completion of the daily screening (DS) varied little on average throughout the year, with an overall completion above 95% (Fig. 18.1) ($p=0.35$). Correct interpretation of the DS was also high (95% overall correct) ($p=0.42$). Once the DS was completed and passed, the next step of the protocol was to assess the patient's

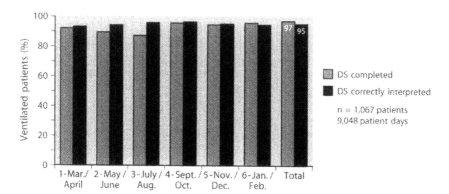

Fig. 18.1. Histogram showing completion and correct interpretation of daily screen (*DS*). This shows the percent of mechanically ventilated patients (*n*=1067 patients; 9048 patient-ventilator days) for whom the daily screen was completed and correct interpretation of the daily screen data by the respiratory care practitioners during each period of implementation. Total daily screen completion rate was 97% across the year of implementation with a 95% correct interpretation rate of the data within the daily screen ($p>0.35$). (From [6] with permission)

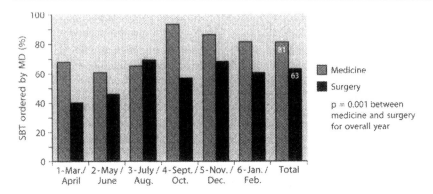

Fig. 18.2. Histogram showing the percent of time that physicians ordered spontaneous breathing trials. Once approached by respiratory care practitioners with data that their patients had passed the daily screen, the compliance rates with spontaneous breathing trials were 81% for medicine vs. 63% for surgery (p=0.001). (From [6] with permission)

ability to pass an SBT. Overall compliance rates in obtaining an SBT were initially low, but they increased in the fifth and sixth months and remained fairly stable thereafter. To determine whether the frequency of ordering SBTs differed in relation to physician specialty, we compared medical and surgical performance (Fig. 18.2). Across the year of implementation, SBTs were more often ordered on the medicine services (81% vs. 63%, p=0.001).

18.2.1 Discussion of Therapist-Driven Protocols

Experience has demonstrated the feasibility and challenges of implementing a previously validated protocol for discontinuation of MV. While TDPs were used relatively infrequently in respiratory care departments as recently as a decade ago, surveys conducted by the American Association of Respiratory Care [8, 9] have shown that up to 60% of participating hospitals were currently using TDPs, and one third of those had begun using TDPs during the previous year. Several editorials and overviews address the scope of TDPs, but few data have detailed the frequency of TDP use, implementation steps, or their impact upon ventilator weaning or management [4, 5, 10, 11]. We reintroduced a two-step process of DS and SBT assessments [12] in our institution as a TDP. The lack of an overseeing "study physician", use of an additional "readiness to wean" screen, and freedom of RCPs to make these adjustments represented other important differences from our original protocol. RCPs competently performed and interpreted the DS, and both RCPs and physicians improved their compliance rates in using SBT assessments in their patients who have recovered from respiratory failure. It became clear from this experience that a commitment to the implementation of the TDP was essential on the part of the hospital and its administration in order to ensure its success. The initial outlay of resources by the institution, including dedicated monitoring staff, computer support, and the time of RCPs to attend in-services, was key. Several practical barriers to protocol implementation also became apparent. Although some aspects of this experience are unique to our medical center, many observations have important implications for institutions currently dealing with the need for a more systematic approach to MV.

How to maximize the likelihood of success in achieving both a change of behavior and long-term protocol implementation:

- Identify the patient-care issue as a high priority item (e.g., ventilator weaning and timely extubation).
- Obtain baseline data (e.g., on lengths of stay and complication rates).
- Base the program on medical evidence, but also on reviews of other programs, and obtain local expert opinion.
- Acknowledge the need for a "change in culture" on the part of both physicians and non-physician health-care professionals.
- Work hard to attain "buy-in" and participation of key opinion leaders/physicians
- Establish a team including the hospital administration, respiratory care practitioners, nurses/nurse practitioners, potentially ethicists, and physicians
- As a team, establish goals and set objective definitions of success and failure.
- Structure a graded, staged implementation process which provides all of the following:
  - Education
  - Timely feedback
  - Compliance monitoring (particularly important and yet most often overlooked)
  - Tracking of appropriate outcomes (including cost) via daily data collection
- Avoid complicated plans aimed at perfection; rather remain practical and useful.
- Consider the entire process to be dynamic not fixed; incorporate innovative changes over time to respond to lessons learned.
- Avoid changing personnel too often.
- Avoid overly rigid interpretation of the "rules" of the protocol.
- Do not remove clinical judgment on the part of any team members.
- Acknowledge the need for and plan to have periodic refresher implementation processes to avoid the otherwise inevitable "regression to baseline".

18.2.2 Compliance with the Protocol

Other investigators have reported use of various weaning algorithms [13–15], but little published information about the details of compliance with such protocols exists. The first step of our approach involved the RCPs' morning assessment using the DS of weaning parameters. While the >95% compliance rates in collection of the DS data and correct interpretation are impressive (Fig. 18.1), they were achieved in a setting in which many RCPs had been involved in our original investigation. Therefore, they were familiar with how to conduct and calculate the measurements involved in the DS. The achievement of such high compliance in a group of 117 RCPs is comforting, but institutions in their initial phases of implementation should not underestimate the amount of work necessary to attain such success, especially with a large group of RCPs. Others have reported compliance rates of less than 40% during weaning protocol introduction [16]. Importantly, during a follow-up period in which regular reinforcements of all caregivers was discontinued, clinician behaviors manifested by DS and SBT compliance reverted to baseline levels prior to our educational interventions [17]. Thus, as with other behavioral modifications, continuous reinforcement is necessary to effect lasting change. The second step of the protocol involved performing SBTs in patients who had recovered from respiratory failure, as manifested by passing the DS. Initially, only 10% of patients who had passed their DS received an SBT, but significant improvement occurred over the first year of implementation. Both RCPs and physicians contributed to this initial low compliance rate, and each group showed significant improvements in their SBT compliance rates over time following educational interventions.

The increments in protocol compliance for both RCPs and physicians coincided with the period in which in-services to all members of these groups had been completed, and this underscores the importance of interventions directed toward all protocol participants. Increased general awareness of the protocol and support of its use by nurses and physicians might be expected to increase the likelihood of having RCPs being comfortable with and feeling compelled to adhere to the protocol maneuvers. Physician compliance with the SBTs is a slightly different matter. There were times when the physician made an appropriate clinical decision not to perform an SBT in a patient who passed a DS. For example, if the physician knew that the patient's chest X-ray had dramatically worsened or that the patient would be undergoing a surgical procedure later that day, it might be appropriate to forego an SBT. Therefore, lack of 100% compliance in Fig. 18.2 could, depending upon the circumstances, be referred to as "appropriate non-compliance".

18.3 Barriers to Protocol Compliance

With an RCP questionnaire, we identified six commonly cited barriers which warrant consideration. The first involved house-officer insecurity in advancing patients through the protocol without immediate input from their attending physicians. Even after support had been obtained from all of the participating attending physicians and in-servicing attendants and house officers, some unfamiliarity with and reservations about the protocol persisted. Some physicians among all specialties remained unaware of the importance and/or safety of weaning parameters and SBTs [12, 18], and their approaches to patients varied. It is also noteworthy that although no attending physician order was necessary for the RCPs to proceed with the DS, such an order was required for performance of an

SBT because of a lack of consensus on the part of attending physicians about making this step automatic. This represented a major barrier to improved compliance with this phase of the protocol and was a variation from the original investigation. At some centers in which RCPs are devoted to one unit, physicians might feel sufficiently comfortable to allow an automatic order for the SBT upon the patient's passing the DS, greatly facilitating timely progression through the protocol. The above points have given us two important tenants regarding implementation of a weaning algorithm: (a) One must work hard at the outset to attain consensus about the algorithm among the health-care professionals (nurses, RCPs, and physicians in both surgical and medical groups). (b) The team must grant reasonable autonomy to the nurses and RCPs who will be so instrumental in moving patients through the protocol.

Interestingly, while many RCPs expressed a desire for more autonomy and decision-making responsibilities, other RCPs reported reluctance to approach certain physician groups even when they were confident that patients were successfully passing the DS. As with many institutional changes, time proved beneficial, and improved protocol compliance was probably the cumulative result of a strategy including serial reinforcement of the goals of the program during its implementation, increased "team awareness" of the protocol, experience accrued from daily patient management, and communication at the bedside. Our investigation was not designed to define whether any single element of implementation was key to its success, nor did it separate the effects of time and simple diffusion upon adoption of any innovation.

18.3.1 Implementation Is an Ongoing Element of Protocolized Care

Implementation proved to be a dynamic process in which an initial plan was modified based upon the prospective monitoring of compliance with its components and feedback from all participating groups of caregivers. Alternative approaches might have more effectively promoted use of SBTs; the components and sequencing of our program were designed specifically for unique aspects of our ICU structure and staffing and would be expected to vary among institutions. Varying sizes and administrative structures of both academic and community medical centers might be expected to have intrinsic challenges in implementation of this and other protocols. Differences in the number of RCPs and RCP experience could make dramatic differences in the results presented in this investigation. Protocol implementation (and acceptance) might be considerably easier in smaller, self-contained units with fewer staff and more direct communication channels. As in other circumstances in which new care modalities are introduced, obtaining the "buy-in" of key physicians, RCPs, and nurses (i.e., the opinion leaders) is a major element of successful protocol implementation [1, 19] and was a factor in our experience.

Avoiding personnel changes as much as possible is also desirable: Devoting the same therapists to a unit who are knowledgeable of the protocol and who interact with the physicians and nurses in a comfortable and consistent manner appears helpful [3]. It is also apparent that overly rigid interpretation of the "rules" of the protocol seems counterproductive (see Chap. 17). For example, determining on consecutive days that a patient failed the DS because the PaO_2/FiO_2 ratio was 198 (rather than being >200) or their f/V_T was 107 (rather than being <105) is felt to be inappropriate because some patients do not fit within the confines of specified "cutoffs" or thresholds of the DS [18, 20–22]. Continuing to advance patients through the protocol at this point and proceeding to an SBT may be successful in many of these circumstances. We believe that active dialogue among participants in care can effectively identify these situations, and that the protocol should not be implemented in ways that compromise clinical judgment. Lastly, future randomized investigations might compare outcomes and cost-effectiveness of patient management strategies that are therapist-driven with those of a dedicated weaning team.

The availability of a protocol validated to result in better patient outcomes, increased safety, and cost savings does not ensure its immediate acceptance, even within the institution where it was designed. In addition, despite implementation, suboptimal compliance with this protocol may not improve outcome. Through large-scale implementation of our program, we found that it was essential to have an awareness of not only specific elements of MV and weaning, but also of general barriers to modifying health professionals' behaviors. Through graded steps every 2 months during the year of implementation, we observed improvements in protocol compliance and remarkable consistency (>95%) on the part of RCPs in obtaining and interpreting the DS of weaning parameters. Important barriers to obtaining SBTs were identified and addressed, and RCP and physician performance in proceeding to SBTs improved. Through diligence and with the passage of time, an ongoing change of culture can be achieved which allows protocol implementation and appropriate modification of bedside behavior of both physicians and RCPs. However, when this vigorous reinforcement through educational intervention was discontinued, recidivism to the previous baseline level of performance was observed.

18.4 Subgroups of Patients

There is little doubt that nuances in patient management are necessary and should be determined at the beside on a case-by-case basis, but little is known about how approaches to MV discontinuation should be modified in the presence of circumstances which might reduce physiological reserve or increase risks. Many physicians feel that different patient groups should be managed altogether differently. Some groups of patients who might require modified strategies include persons with COPD, ischemic heart disease, congestive heart failure, (CHF), ARDS, general surgery, trauma, neurosurgery, and perhaps the elderly. In our investigation of primarily medical patients [5], neither increased complication rates nor prolonged MV were found among those within any of these diagnostic groups (including persons with acute myocardial infarction or COPD). The following discussion will outline the literature concerning these subgroups and whether particular adjustments in weaning protocols in these groups merits further consideration.

18.4.1 Chronic Obstructive Pulmonary Disease

While numerous investigations have been performed to help predict the need for MV in patients with COPD [23–25] and to estimate the likelihood of survival [26–29], we suspect that many physicians are unaware that the majority of COPD patients who require MV actually survive, and that their mortality is not necessarily increased over that of other medical patients requiring such support. Our COPD patients' survival (75%) was comparable to that in the published literature [25–27, 30] and to that of patients with other causes of respiratory failure. In a recent multivariate analysis [26], the need for MV in COPD patients did not influence short-term or long-term outcome after adjusting for severity of illness. Rather, development of nonrespiratory organ dysfunction was the largest determinant of survival and accounted for 60% of the power of this prediction.

In our ICUs, the predictive characteristics of the DS worked as well for COPD patients as for persons with other diagnoses [31]. Others have reported that conventional weaning criteria may be inadequate for COPD patients [32]. While airway occlusion pressure at 0.1 s (i.e., $P_{0.1}$) has been shown repeatedly to be especially worthwhile in COPD patients [32–35], it has been neither widely accepted nor applied generally due to technical demands and high inter- and intraindividual variability of this measure. As newer mechanical ventilators begin to include the $P_{0.1}$ into their software, more clinicians may examine the incorporation of this parameter into weaning protocols for COPD patients.

With the advent of noninvasive positive pressure ventilation (NPPV) [30, 36], many have considered using PSV or bi-level positive airway pressure (BIPAP) as an aid in weaning from MV or as a means of avoiding MV altogether. SBTs may have important roles in this strategy. A recent multicenter RCT carried out by Nava et al. [37] investigated the use of a weaning protocol incorporating noninvasive PSV after extubation in patients with respiratory failure due to COPD. While this investigation is addressed in another chapter, we would like to discuss it briefly here, as it applies to implementation within this subgroup of patients. At 48 h after intubation, a T-piece weaning trial (i.e., SBT) was attempted in 50 patients. If this failed, two methods of weaning were compared: (a) extubation and application of NPPV (i.e., BIPAP) by a face mask vs. (b) further invasive PSV by endotracheal tube. The average PSV in the noninvasive group was 19 ± 2 cmH$_2$0, while the invasive group received 17.6 ± 2.1 cmH$_2$O. Importantly, both groups of COPD patients received at least two SBT attempts per day. The criteria to pass the SBTs were similar to those in our investigations (see Chap. 17) [6, 12], except that the duration of successful spontaneous breathing was 3 h and a pH >7.35 was required. Outcomes of this important investigation included reduced weaning time and ICU stay, fewer instances of nosocomial pneumonia, and improved 60-day survival rates [37].

18.4.2 Congestive Heart Failure and Myocardial Infarction Patients

Our original investigation included 73 medical and nonsurgical cardiac patients with significant co-morbidities [12], differing from other studies, which have included a surgical or mixed population or excluded patients with acute coronary disease. We subsequently enrolled 123 coronary patients with myocardial infarction (MI) and congestive heart failure, and 95 patients in the cardiothoracic surgical ICU [6]. The latter were enrolled only if they remained on MV for over 24 h, as they are routinely managed during the first day with a rapid "wean-to-extubation" protocol, and thus represented a select group. Cardiac surgical patients often have many aspects of their care (especially weaning from MV), directed by non-physicians under protocol guidance [11, 38]. Importantly, none of these nearly 300 patients with cardiac diseases had a higher rate of detectable complications, suggesting that broad application of this strategy to cardiac patients is safe and effective. While others have shown that some patients have electrocardiographic changes consistent with ischemia during weaning trials [39], there have been no prospective studies documenting clinically important ischemic events resulting from management by a weaning protocol. Until such investigations are performed, bedside clinical judgment must remain an important component in individual cases. Using the above experience of safety, however, intensivists and surgeons must take care to avoid delaying extubation unnecessarily and realize that even cardiothoracic surgical patients (when not able to wean rapidly the first day) may benefit from enrollment in standard weaning protocols.

18.4.3 Acute Respiratory Distress Syndrome (ARDS) and Acute Lung Injury (ALI)

The recently completed ARDS/ALI randomized investigation sponsored by the NHLBI documented that ventilating a patient using a protocol that dictates a tidal volume of 6 ml/kg ideal body weight and maintains a plateau pressure of less than 30 cmH$_2$O can reduce mortality by 25% and increase by 2 days the amount of time alive and off the ventilator at the 28-day mark ($p=0.007$) [40]. It is important to realize that this investigation incorporated a strict weaning algorithm in order to standardize the approach to liberation after the patients had recovered sufficiently from ALI. In fact, compliance with the various facets of the network protocol was 80% or better across the ten participating centers. Such impressive compliance within the context of an investigation should set the standard for all ICUs that seek the same magnitude of improvement in their patients' outcomes after adopting the ARDS-network protocol.

18.4.4 Neurosurgical Patients

Recognizing the vastly different neuromuscular and cardiopulmonary status of neurosurgical patients receiving MV, we have begun a series of investigations in this patient population [41, 42]. In our initial attempts at protocolizing the care of these patients, compliance on the part of the neurosurgeons with extubation after a patient had passed an SBT presented a particularly interesting dilemma. The most common reason cited for not extubating a spontaneously breathing patient was a depressed mental status. Moreover, an association was found between the Glasgow Coma Scale (GCS) and the need for reintubation ($p=0.0001$) [42], a finding that others have seen as well [43]. Of 109 extubation attempts, only 53% occurred without any complications or reintubations. Multivariate analysis demonstrated that GCS ($p<0.0001$) and P/F ratio ($p<0.0001$) were independent predictors of successful extubation. GCS >8 was associated with success in 67% of patients, while only 21% with a GCS <8 had successful extubation ($p<0.0001$) [42]. This observation supports the concerns of neurosurgeons regarding early liberation of patients from the ventilator. Future investigations of neurosurgical patients should appraise whether the coupling of mental status measures and GCS with DS- and SBT-based strategies can optimize the decision to extubate these patients.

Vallverdu et al. [35] studied weaning indices and MV liberation for 46 neurological patients, including those with ischemic stroke, intracerebral hemorrhage, subarachnoid hemorrhage, head trauma, encephalitis, metabolic encephalopathy, and brain tumor. While their average reintubation rate was 15%, 15 (33%) neurological patients needed reinstitution of invasive MV, while only 6% of the 171 other patients with acute respiratory failure and COPD required reintubation. The authors found that most predictors of weaning success lacked discriminatory ability in these patients. Interestingly, f/V_T and $P_{0.1}$ had their lowest accuracies in neurological patients (65% and 63%, respectively) and did not discriminate among weaning failure and success [35]. Only maximal inspiratory pressure (MIP, $p=0.05$) and expiratory pressure (MEP, $p=0.001$) were different among successfully extubated neurological patients. In this group, the ability to cough and clear secretions, objectively reflected by the MEP, may help in clinical decision-making. Since the need for reintubation was neither clinically nor physiologically suspected, the authors concluded that other tools need to be developed and prospectively validated to determine the optimum time to liberate patients with mental status changes and neurological impairment.

18.4.5 Elderly Patients

The number of adults 85 years and older is currently estimated to be about 4 million and is expected to double by the year 2030 [44]. Age has been considered an important prognostic indicator of hospital outcome [45, 46], but many prior investigations of MV have been limited by their retrospective design and the absence of adjustment for confounding factors such as severity of illness [47–49]. The diversity of the design (mostly retrospective investigations) and conclusions of studies about MV in the elderly has fueled the controversy over whether age has an independent impact upon the outcomes of patients treated with MV [50]. Data from the SUPPORT investigators have shown that age (especially above 70–75 years) has great importance for the intensity of care given to patients [51–53]. Once the decision has been made to utilize mechanical ventilation in the care of critically ill elderly patients, modifications in the weaning and liberation of elderly patients may be necessary, and this remains a point of growing interest in the pulmonary and critical care community.

In our prospectively followed cohort of 300 mechanically ventilated patients, we found that patients >75 years of age remained on MV a median of 4 days (interquartile ranges, 2–9) vs 6 days (3–11) for patients <75 years old ($p=0.14$)

[54]. Using the time it took to pass a daily screen of weaning parameters as a marker of recovery from respiratory failure, elderly patients passed the daily screen earlier than younger patients [risk ratio 1.58 (95% confidence interval, 1.13–2.22), $p=0.03$] (Fig. 18.3). The ICU cost of care was lower [\$12,822 (\$9821–\$26,313) vs \$19,316 (\$9699–\$39,950)] for older patients ($p=0.03$). In-hospital mortality was 38% among the elderly versus 39% among younger patients ($p=0.98$), and Cox proportional-hazards analysis confirmed there was no difference in survival between the two groups (relative risk for older patients = 0.82, 95% confidence interval 0.52–1.29). We found these data counterintuitive, especially the comparable time to recovery and passing weaning parameters, and we have begun to study the weaning process in our elderly population [55–57].

Kollef and colleagues [58] reported that women patients had a longer duration of MV ($p=0.056$), but we detected no gender differences in the rate of recovery of respiratory failure or length of time on MV. Because of differences in access to health care among women [59], and differences among physicians in their practice styles (including the vigor of their approaches to liberation from the ventilator), further prospective analyses of gender differences in outcomes from MV are needed. We believe that the care of elderly women will represent a major future priority of critical care medicine. Gender, associated body dimensions, and age are appropriate considerations that may affect not only outcome from MV but also objective measures of readiness to discontinue MV. Female gender, smaller endotracheal tube size (<7 mm), and older age have been associated with an elevated f/V_T ratio [21, 22], and it may be appropriate to adjust the "passing" threshold for this measurement in these instances to avoid erroneously regarding a patient as still requiring MV (Fig. 18.4).

In view of current uncertainties in physician decision-making regarding the use of MV in the elderly, major pitfalls should be recognized and avoided. These include the premature application of predictive equations [60] or anecdotal expe-

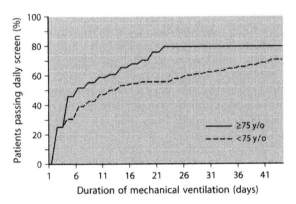

Fig. 18.3. Kaplan-Meier analysis of the rate of recovery of respiratory failure by age. This analysis used the percent of patients passing a daily screen of weaning parameters as a surrogate marker of "recovery". The distribution of times until passing the daily screen suggested that patients >75 years of age achieved this recovery milestone earlier than those less than 75 years old (risk ratio 1.58, 95% confidence interval 1.13–2.22, $p=0.03$). (From [53] with permission)

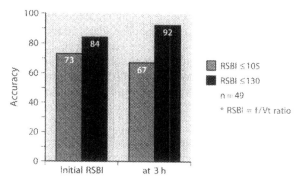

Fig. 18.4. Accuracy of rapid shallow breathing index in elderly. Histogram shows that in this group of elderly patients (>70 years old) the threshold for the rapid shallow breathing index (i.e., f/V_T) of 130 yielded a higher accuracy in predicting successful extubation than the conventional threshold of 105. Furthermore, measuring the index at 3 h enhanced the accuracy beyond that of measurements taken at the onset of spontaneous breathing. (From [22] with permission)

riences. Further prospective investigations are needed in order to define "physiological age" and to determine whether or not it is truly more important than chronological age [61, 62]. In the absence of validated measures of "physiological age," the current observations suggest that an over-reliance on chronological age is inappropriate. By using multivariate analysis to adjust for severity of illness and other variables, we found that the elderly (>75 years) spent an amount of time on the mechanical ventilator comparable to that of younger patients but had a lower cost of ICU and in-hospital care. Accordingly, the decision to use MV should not be based upon age alone, and the appropriate use of ventilatory support in the elderly requires further prospective evaluation.

18.5 Conclusions

In this chapter, many facets of the implementation process and individualization of protocols for different patient types and institutional needs have been discussed. Throughout these various settings, there remain common threads which all health-care professionals and organizations should follow in order to achieve success and optimize the use of MV. Some of the most frequent pitfalls of implementation are inadequate tracking of baseline patient outcomes and not measuring compliance with protocol procedures. Ongoing educational in-services and feedback from key "opinion leader" physicians within your institution is fundamental. The institution must also avoid changing personnel too often, and should attempt to have dedicated RCPs within each ICU if at all possible rather than rotating RCPs throughout the entire hospital (which is what we had to deal with). The dedicated personnel will help to achieve superior familiarity with the protocol and develop better relationships between physicians, nurses, and RCPs. It is imperative that protocols not be put in place to supplant clinical judgment. Protocols are meant as guides for patient management, not as a set of rules "engraved in stone". Likewise, protocols should not be viewed as static constructs, but rather as dynamic tools which evolve and are molded to accommodate new data and/or health-care professionals' preferences. Espousing these attitudes and incorporating new information as it becomes available will increase protocol acceptance by otherwise skeptical physicians, nurses, and respiratory care practitioners.

18.6 References

1. Greco PJ, Eisenberg JM (1993) Changing physicians' practices. N Engl J Med 329:1271–1273
2. Main DS, Cohen SJ, DiClemente CC (1995) Measuring physician readiness to change cancer screening: preliminary results. Am J Prev Med 11:54–58
3. Cohen IL (1994) Weaning from mechanical ventilation – the team approach and beyond. Intensive Care Med 20:317–318
4. Stoller JK (1994) Why therapist-driven protocols? Respir Care 39:706–708
5. Weber K, Milligan S (1994) Therapist-driven protocols: the state of the art. Respir Care 39:746–755
6. Ely EW, Bennett PA, Bowton DL, Murphy SM, Haponik EF (1999) Large-scale implementation of a respiratory therapist-driven protocol for ventilator weaning. Am J Respir Crit Care Med 159:439–446
7. Esteban A, Alia I, Tobin M, Gil A, Gordo F, Vallverdu I, et al (1999) Effect of spontaneous breathing trial duration on outcome of attempts to discontinue mechanical ventilation. Am J Respir Crit Care Med 159:512–518
8. Jacobs J (1994) How are we doing with operational restructuring and therapist-driven protocols? Am Assoc Respir Care Times 18:66–69
9. Tietsort J (1998) Benchmarking report on use of TDPs. Respir Care Manager 7:1–12
10. Shrake KL, Scaggs JE, England KR, Henkle JQ, Eagleton LE (1994) Benefits associated with a respiratory care assessment-treatment program: results of a pilot study. Respir Care 39:715–724
11. Wood G, MacLeod B, Moffatt S (1995) Weaning from mechanical ventilation: physician-directed vs a respiratory-therapist-directed protocol. Respir Care 40:219–224
12. Ely EW, Baker AM, Dunagan DP, Burke HL, Smith AC, Kelly PT, et al (1996) Effect on the duration of mechanical ventilation of identifying patients capable of breathing spontaneously. N Engl J Med 335:1864–1869
13. Saura P, Blanch L, Mestre J, Valles J, Artigas A, Fernandez R (1996) Clinical consequences of the implementation of a weaning protocol. Intensive Care Med 22:1052–1056
14. Burns SM, Marshall M, Burns JE, Ryan B, Wilmoth D, Carpenter R, et al (1998) Design, testing, and results of an outcomes-managed approach to patients requiring prolonged mechanical ventilation. Am J Crit Care 7:45–57
15. Djunaedi H, Cardinal P, Greffe-Laliberte G, Jones G, McMath B, Snell CC (1987) Does a ventilatory management protocol improve the care of ventilated patients? Respir Care 42:604–610
16. Schriefer J (1993) Reducing the length of stay for post-operative open heart surgical patients. Qual Connect 2:8–9
17. Bowton D, Ely EW, Bennett PA, Florance A, Haponik EF (1999) Successful implementation of a weaning protocol requires continued reinforcement. Am J Respir Crit Care Med 159:A83
18. Jaeschke RZ, Meade MO, Guyatt GH, Keenan SP, Cook DJ (1997) How to use diagnostic test articles in the intensive care unit: diagnosing weanability using f/Vt. Crit Care Med 25:1514–1521
19. Soumerai SB, McLaughlin TJ, Gurwitz JH, Guadagnoli E, Hauptman PJ, Borbas C, et al (1998) Effect of local medical opinion leaders on quality of care for acute mycradial infarction. A randomized controlled trial. JAMA 279:1358–1363
20. Epstein SK (1995) Etiology of extubation failure and the predictive value of the rapid shallow breathing index. Am J Respir Crit Care Med 152:545–549

21. Epstein SK, Ciubotaru RL (1997) Influence of gender and endotracheal tube size on preextubation breathing pattern. Am J Respir Crit Care Med 154:1647–1652
22. Krieger BP, Isber J, Breitenbucher A, Throop G, Ershowsky P (1997) Serial measurements of the rapid-shallow-breathing index as a predictor of weaning outcome in elderly medical patients. Chest 112:1029–1034
23. Vitacca M, Clini E, Porta R, Foglio K, Ambrosino N (1996) Acute exacerbations in patients with COPD: predictors of need for mechanical ventilation. Eur Respir J 9:1487–1493
24. Jeffrey AA, Warren PM, Flenley DC (1992) Acute hypercapnic respiratory failure in patients with chronic obstructive lung disease: risk factors and use of guidelines for management. Thorax 47:34–40
25. Moran JL, Green JM, Homan SD, Leeson RJ, Leppard PI (1998) Acute exacerbations of chronic obstructive pulmonary disease and mechanical ventilation: a reevaluation. Crit Care Med 26:71–78
26. Seneff MG, Wagner DP, Wagner RP, Zimmermann JE, Knaus WA (1995) Hospital and 1-year survival of patients admitted to intensive care units with acute exacerbation of chronic obstructive pulmonary disease. JAMA 274:1852–1857
27. Hudson LD (1989) Survival data in patients with acute and chronic lung disease requiring mechanical ventilation. Am Rev Respir Dis 140:S19–S24
28. Menzies R, Gibbons W, Goldberg P (1989) Determinants of weaning and survival among patients with COPD who require mechanical ventilation for acute respiratory failure. Chest 95:398–405
29. Anthonisen NR (1989) Prognosis in chronic obstructive pulmonary disease: results from multicenter clinical trials. Am Rev Respir Dis 140:S95–S99
30. Brochard L, Mancebo J, Wysocki M, Lofaso F, Conti g, Rauss A, et al (1995) Noninvasive ventilation for acute exacerbations of chronic obstructive pulmonary disease. N Engl J Med 333:817–822
31. Ely EW, Baker AM, Evans GW, Haponik EF (2000) The cost of respiratory care in mechanically ventilated patients with chronic obstructive pulmonary disease. Crit Care Med 28:408–413
32. Conti G, DeBlasi R, Pelaia P, Benito S, Rocco M, Antonelli M, et al (1992) Early prediction of successful weaning during pressure support ventilation in chronic obstructive pulmonary disease patients. Crit Care Med 29:366–371
33. Sassoon CSH, Te TT, Mahutte CK, Light RW A(1987) irway occlusion pressure: an important indicator for successful weaning in patients with chronic obstructive pulmonary disease. Am Rev Respir Dis 135:107–113
34. Sassoon CSH, Light RW, Lodia R, Sieck GC, Mahutte CK (1991) Pressure-time product during continuous positive airway pressure, pressure support ventilation, and T-piece during weaning from mechanical ventilation. Am Rev Respir Dis 143:469–475
35. Vallverdu I, Calaf N, Subirana M, Net A, Benito S, Mancebo J (1999) Clinical characteristics, respiratory functional parameters, and outcome of a two-hour T-piece trial of patients weaning from mechanical ventilation. Am J Respir Crit Care Med 158:1855–1862
36. Antonelli M, Conti g, Rocco M, Bufi M, DeBlasi RA, Vivino G, et al (1998) A comparison of noninvasive positive-pressure ventilation and conventional mechanical ventilation in patients with acute respiratory failure. N Engl J Med 339:429–435
37. Nava S, Ambrosino N, Clini E, Prato M, Orlando GVM, Brigada P, et al (1998) Noninvasive mechanical ventilation in the weaning of patients with respiratory failure due to chronic obstructive pulmonary disease: a randomized controlled trial. Ann Intern Med 128: 721–728
38. Kollef MH, Horst HM, Prang L, Brock WA (1998) Reducing the duration of mechanical ventilation: three examples of change in the intensive care unit. New Horizons 6:52–60
39. Chatila W, Ani S, Guaglianone D, Jacob B, Amoateng-Adjepong Y, Manthous CA (1996) Cardiac ischemia during weaning from mechanical ventilation. Chest 109:1577–1583
40. The Acute Respiratory Distress Syndrome Network (2000) Ventilation with lower tidal volumes as compared with traditional tidal volumes for acute lung injury and the acute respiratory distress syndrome. N Engl J Med 342: 1301–1308

41. Ely EW, Namen AM, Tatter S, Lucia MA, Smith AC, Landry S, et al (1999) Impact of a ventilator weaning protocol in neurosurgical patients: a randomized, controlled trial. Am J Respir Crit Care Med 159:A371
42. Namen AM, Ely EW, Tatter S, Case D, Lucia MA, Smith A, et al (2001) Predictors of successful extubation in neurosurgical patients. Am J Respir Crit Care Med 163:654–658
43. Chevron V, Menard J, Richard J, Girault C, Leroy J, Bonomarchand G (1998) Unplanned extubation: risk factors of development and predictive criteria for reintubation. Crit Care Med 26:1049–1053
44. Hobbs F, Damon BL, Taeuber CM (1996) Sixty-five plus in the United States. U.S. Department of Commerce, Economics, and Statistics Administration, Bureau of the Census, Washington, DC
45. Sage WM, Hurst CR, Silverman JF, Bortz WM (1987) Intensive care for the elderly: outcome of elective and nonelective admissions. J Am Geriatr Soc 35:312–318
46. Knaus WA, Draper EA, Wagner DP, Zimmerman JE (1986) An evaluation of outcome from intensive care in major medical centers. Ann Intern Med 104:410–418
47. Cohen IL, Lambrinos J (1995) Investigating the impact of age on outcome of mechanical ventilation using a population of 41,848 patients from a statewide database. Chest 107:1673–1680
48. Kurek CJ, Cohen IL, Lambrinos J, Minatoya K, Booth FV, Chalfin DB (1997) Clinical and economic outcome of patients undergoing tracheostomy for prolonged mechanical ventilation in New York state during 1993: analysis of 6,353 cases under diagnosis-related group 483. Crit Care Med 25:983–988
49. Kurek CJ, Dewar D, Lambrinos J, Booth FV, Cohen IL (1998) Clinical and economic outcome of mechanically ventilated patients in New York State during 1993. Chest 114:214–222
50. Chelluri L, Grenvik A, Silverstein M (1995) Intensive care for critically ill elderly: mortality, costs, and quality of life. Review of the literature. Arch Intern Med 155:1013–1022
51. Hamel MB, Philips RS, Teno JM, Lynn J, Galanos AN, Davis RB, et al (1996) Seriously ill hospitalized adults: do we spend less on older patients? J Am Geriatr Soc 44:1043–1048
52. Hakim RB, Teno JM, Harrell FE, Knaus WA, Wenger NS, Phillips RS, et al (1996) Factors associated with do-not-resuscitate orders: patients' preferences, prognoses, and physicians' judgments. SUPPORT Investigators. The Study to Understand Prognoses and Preferences for Outcome and Risks of Treatments. Ann Intern Med 125:284–293
53. Hamel MB, Teno JM, Goldman L, Lynn J, Davis RB, Galanos AN, et al (1999) Patient age and decisions to withhold life-sustaining treatments from seriously ill, hospitalized adults. Ann Intern Med 130:116–125
54. Ely EW, Evans GW, Haponik EF (1999) Mechanical ventilation in a cohort of elderly patients admitted to an intensive care unit. Ann Intern Med 131:96–104
55. Ely EW, Margolin R, Francis J, May L, Truman B, Wheeler A, et al (2000) Delirium in the ICU: measurement and outcomes. Am J Respir Crit Care Med 161:A506
56. Esteban A, Anzueto A, Alia I, Ely EW, Frutos F, Brochard L, et al (2000) The effect of age on outcome from mechanical ventilation. Am J Respir Crit Care Med 161:A385
57. Ely EW, Wheeler A, Thompson T, Steinberg KP, Ancukiewicz M, Bernard G (2000) Age is an independent predictor of outcomes in ARDS. Am J Respir Crit Care Med 161:A210
58. Kollef MH, O'Brien JD, Silver P (1997) The impact of gender on outcome from mechanical ventilation. Chest 111:434–441
59. Yuen EJ, Gonnella JS, Louis DZ, Epstein KR, Howell SL, Markson LE (1995) Severity-adjusted differences in hospital utilization by gender. Am J Med Qual 10:76–80
60. Cohen IL, Lambrinos J, Fein IA (1993) Mechanical ventilation for the elderly patient in intensive care. Incremental changes and benefits. JAMA 269:1025–1029
61. Boult C, Dowd B, McCaffrey D, Boult L, Hernandez R, Krulewitch H (1993) Screening elders for risk of hospital admission. J Am Geriatr Soc 41:811–817
62. Goldberg AI (1988) Life-sustaining technology and the elderly. Prolonged mechanical ventilation factors influencing the treatment decision. Chest 94:1277–1282

19 The Role of Muscle Training and Rehabilitation During Weaning

G.C. Piaggi, E. De Mattia, and S. Nava

The intensive care unit is a very different environment from the rehabilitative centers or services where pulmonary rehabilitation is usually performed. Indeed, whereas in the former setting most patients are desperately ill or recovering from an acute episode [1], in the latter the patients usually have chronic stable disease and are often treated as outpatients. One of the most common reasons for admission to an ICU is a severe episode of acute respiratory failure due either to an exacerbation of chronic pulmonary disease or its aggravation after a surgical procedure, trauma, or medical complications. Weaning from mechanical ventilation is often a major clinical problem in the subset of patients affected by COPD or chronic restrictive diseases [2]. These patients usually report, at admission to the ICU, leading a sedentary life before the acute episode; the evolution of the disease is characterized by a progressive decline, not only in respiratory function (e.g., FEV_1), but also in the functional status [3], due to the effects of lack of exercise, drug administration (e.g., steroids) [4], malnutrition [5] and, later on, gas-exchange abnormalities. Together with specific vital organ support, such as mechanical ventilation, patients admitted to an ICU may require other complex and integrated interventions in order to maintain the spared function and to prevent further damage [6]. These interventions include nutritional and psychological support, counseling, nursing, prevention (e.g., to preserve skin integrity), and in particular a complete rehabilitation program that may range from simple help to maintain a correct posture to complete recovery of walking autonomy.

This chapter will deal with rehabilitation and respiratory muscle training in patients admitted to an ICU, with particular emphasis on the problem of weaning from mechanical ventilation.

19.1 What Is Pulmonary Rehabilitation?

Before going any further we need to define the specific goals of our rehabilitative treatment. There is general agreement that the term "rehabilitation" is reserved for a multidisciplinary intervention that includes the chest physician or the intensive care specialist as a coordinator; the respiratory, physical, and occupational therapist; the primary care nurse; the speech therapist; the psychologist and psychiatrist; the pharmacist; the dietician; the social worker and, last but not least, the patient's family or support system. The other essential key to the rehabilitation program is that the management of each patient be individualized. A recent official European definition of rehabilitation was given by the European Respiratory Society Task Force Position Paper [7]: "Pulmonary rehabilitation is a process which systematically uses scientifically based diagnostic management and evaluation options to achieve the optimal daily functioning and health-related quality of life of individual patients suffering from impairment and disability due to chronic respiratory disease, as measured by clinically and/or physiologically relevant outcome measures." The American Thoracic Society [8] adopted the following definition: "…a multidisciplinary program of care for patients with chronic respiratory impairment that is individually tailored and designed to optimize physical and social performance and autonomy". These "broad" definitions, while giving a panoramic view of what should be achieved, do not enter into the specific details of how. Thus pulmonary rehabilitation may vary, according to different environments, from simple passive mobilization of a patient to more complex interventions, such as weaning from mechanical ventilation. One thing that is clear, however, from these official statements is that the common idea that there is no hope for improvement in patients with chronic diseases, especially if recovering from an episode of acute respiratory failure, is no longer acceptable, either clinically or scientifically.

19.2 Who Is in Charge of the Rehabilitation Program?

As stated before, besides the coordinating figure, the main professional group involved in the program comprises the respiratory therapists. Their professional names, specific tasks, educational profile, and autonomy vary, unfortunately, according to the different environment in which rehabilitation is performed. For example, Kida et al. [9] published a survey about pulmonary rehabilitation in which it was clear that while almost all rehabilitation teams in North America are composed of both respiratory therapists and physiotherapists, most European institutions have only one of the two professional figures. In this confused and fragmented setting it is not surprising that single professional associations may have difficulties in producing official recommendations for staffing and service delivery in ICU rehabilitation. Even more recently, Norrenberg and Vincent [10] reported that 29% of physiotherapists working in an ICU have post-graduate specialization in critical care and 43% in respiratory therapy, which means that 28% do not belong to any specific category. Interestingly enough, 25% of the ICUs do not have physiotherapists who work exclusively in them, and 48% have no more than two such physiotherapists, suggesting that most, if not all, ICUs lack an autonomous physiotherapy service, having to depend on their hospital's physical therapy department. The time has come for a clear differentiation, especially in Europe, between the definition and tasks of physiotherapists, involved mainly in "nonspecific" rehabilitation programs (e.g., walking, limb muscle strengthening, correction of posture), and respiratory therapists, involved mainly in "specific" programs (e.g., respiratory muscle training, secretion removal, breathing exercises, assistance with noninvasive mechanical ventilation, weaning from ventilation).

19.3 Aims of Rehabilitation

The general aims of an ICU respiratory rehabilitation program are to apply advanced, cost-effective therapeutic modalities to save and eventually to improve the remaining function, to decrease the patient's dependency (i.e., on the ventilator), and to prevent the need for further hospitalization – in brief, to improve the patient's measured quality of life.

19.3.1 Prevention of Prolonged Bed Rest

The earlier the rehabilitation program of a ventilated patient is started, the greater is its effect, since later consequences such as limited mobility or, even worse, total dependency on a ventilator, may make the high costs spent on taking care of the patient futile [11]. As illustrated in Fig. 19.1, the physiological changes caused by inactivity involve skeletal muscle, cardiovascular and respiratory functions, body and blood composition, and the central nervous and endocrine systems. During a period of inactivity muscle mass declines and the potential efficiency of a muscle to perform aerobic exercise declines. Skeletal muscles are composed of two major fiber types. Type I fibers are involved mainly in aerobic activity, while type II fibers have a lower capacity for this activity. Deconditioning causes a distinct transformation of subtypes of type II fibers: type IIa fibers convert to type IIb fibers [12], the former having a higher aero-

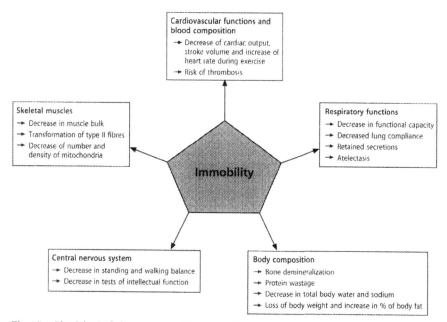

Fig. 19.1. Physiological changes caused by inactivity

bic capacity. Moreover, during immobility, the number and density of mitochondria decrease. The cardiovascular response to exercise is also dramatically altered after a period of bed rest, since there is a decrease in cardiac output and stroke volume during maximal exercise and an increase in heart rate during submaximal exercise [13–17]. Indeed, of particular importance for bed-ridden patients is that the ability of the system to adjust to changing posture, such as moving from the supine to the sitting position, is impaired [18, 19]. In postoperative patients, if early rehabilitation (i.e., the application of positive end-expiratory pressure) is not started, the decrease in functional residual capacity and lung compliance may lead to atelectasis, retained secretions, and in some cases pneumonia, which if occurring in ventilated patients may dramatically increase the probability of death.

Immobility also leads to clinically significant bone demineralization, together with protein wastage [18] and a decrease in total body water and sodium [20]. There is generally a loss of body weight and an increase in the percentage of body fat. Deterioration of central nervous system function results in a decreased capacity to maintain the standing position and to walk; the performance of tests of intellectual function may also be impaired, and disorientation may occur [21].

The first goals of rehabilitation in these patients are therefore targeted to all the procedures aimed at obtaining early mobilization. Maintenance of correct posture and passive mobilization of legs and arms are the preliminary steps, followed by active sitting up in bed and thereafter sitting in a chair. It is also clear that physical therapy per se may not be enough to obtain satisfactory outcomes for our ICU patients, so comprehensive interventions are mandatory in these first steps of treatment. Correction of electrolyte disturbances, nutritional and psychological support, and a balanced use of cardiovascular drugs may also help to improve the clinical picture.

19.3.2 Training of the Skeletal Muscle

Specific training of the upper and lower limbs with the classical rehabilitation techniques such as arm ergometry or bicycle training is, for obvious reasons, very seldom performed in the ICU. Skeletal muscle strength and endurance performances are impaired not only as a consequence of bed rest but also as a direct effect of hypercapnia, hypoxia, malnutrition, treatment with corticosteroids or other agents, and hemodynamic instability. The possible need for heavy sedation or curarization during the first few days of ventilation may also lead to generalized myopathy [22]. Training is nevertheless an important aspect of caring for these patients, since one of the rehabilitative end points in the ICU is defined as a return of a muscle strength that allows basic activities of daily life (e.g., washing, combing hair, cooking) and the ability to walk 20–50 m independently. After the first few days aimed at mobilizing the patients, they may undergo sessions aimed at passively and actively training the lower and upper extremities, such as lifting light weights or pushing against a resistance. Any patient able to walk at one point in time can start directly with progressive walking retraining, aided by a rolling platform walker or by the therapist, if needed. When a patient cannot be weaned from the ventilator, a portable resistor can be used to decrease the work of breathing during walking. As soon as possible, it is useful to monitor the patient's outcome using dyspnea scales (VAS, the Borg scale, etc.) and exercise tolerance tests (6-min walked distance). Patients who successfully regain complete autonomy and are therefore discharged from the ICU to a medical ward should not be "abandoned", but should be included in training programs with cyclette, treadmill, and ergometry for the upper extremities. The usefulness of gradual retraining has recently been assessed in COPD patients recovering from an acute episode of hypercapnic respiratory failure [23], most of whom were admitted to the respiratory ICU while still being ventilated. The patients enrolled for complete skeletal and respiratory muscle training, including lifting weights, climbing stairs, and pedaling on a bicycle, showed a significant improvement in exercise capacity and in breathlessness compared with the control group undergoing simple ground-based walking. From a physiological point of view, there are different types of training that modify the structure and function of the muscle. *Endurance training* is characterized by low-tension contractions with frequent repetitions; *force training* consists of high-tension contractions with fewer repetitions, while *coordination training* is aimed at improving performance of a more complex task. Endurance training will increase the proportion of oxidative fibers, force training will increase muscle fiber size and protein content, while coordination training will improve neural aspects of recruitment patterns [24].

Two aspects of training are basic: threshold and specificity. If the training threshold is too low, there will be no change in the muscle; if it is too high, there will be fiber damage and muscle degenerative changes. Specificity of training means that training produces an increase in VO_2max only in the specific muscles in use.

19.3.3 Respiratory Muscle Training

Like the other skeletal muscles, the ventilatory pump may be profoundly altered by the effects of bed rest and of the disease itself and any co-morbid conditions. Indeed, the "abuse" of controlled mechanical ventilation in the ICU may lead to the development of selective diaphragmatic atrophy after only 48 h, as shown in a laboratory study performed on rats [25]. The weakness of the respiratory muscle and, in particular, an imbalance between the load the respiratory system has to face and its capacity is, together with the cardiovascular impairment, the major determinant of weaning failure in ventilated patients. The rationale for respiratory muscle training in the ICU is nevertheless controversial. Patients affected by COPD, for example, are not likely to benefit much from this specific treatment. Chronic airflow obstruction is always present, at least in the end-stage of the disease, leading to acute respiratory failure by pulmonary hyperinflation [26]. It has been shown that the impaired inotropic effect of the diaphragm in these patients is due to the altered geometric shape of the diaphragm dome, rather than to muscle atrophy. As a matter of fact, Similowski et al. [27] demonstrated how the diaphragm of patients with COPD was as good as that of normal subjects in generating pressure in response to bilateral phrenic nerve stimulation, at the same lung volumes. Their conclusions were quite strongly against the use of inspiratory muscle training, since "the absence of central inhibition and the absence of evidence of chronic fatigue cast doubts on the need to treat such patients with interventions intended to improve the contractility of the diaphragm". More recently, Levine and co-workers [28] added support to this statement when they showed, after having obtained diaphragmatic biopsy specimens from six patients with severe COPD, that the disease increases the slow-twitch characteristics of the muscle fibers as an adaptive mechanism which increases resistance to fatigue. Does this mean that respiratory muscle training in the ICU should be definitively abandoned? We do not think so. We must say that the above-mentioned studies were performed in patients with severe, but probably (although this was not clearly stated in either paper) normocapnic COPD, likely to have a different histological picture from that of critically ill patients. Nevertheless, there is an urgent need for controlled studies, even in stable patients, for whom the clinical role of respiratory muscle training has not yet been defined. In particular, only about 50% of the studies reported clear, significant benefits on maximal inspiratory pressure, while more than 70% described an improvement in the endurance time [29–34]. Extrapolating these results to ICU patients, it is interesting to note that the above-mentioned changes were observed after a mean duration of 7 weeks; such prolonged training is unlikely to be feasible in the ICU. The load, frequency, and intensity of training should also be scientifically specified since, if it is true that during the training exercises the pressure generated per breath should be at least 30% of the maximum generated in order to achieve significant improvement, it should also be kept in mind that high resistances may induce structural changes in the diaphragm. It has been shown in animals trained for 4 days (2 h/day) that this protocol induces diaphragm membrane damage, sarcomere disruption, and damage to predominantly type I fibers [35]. Muscle training does not, however, necessarily mean performing loading breathing, since in ICU patients, potentiation of the expiratory muscles may be nonspecifically obtained with cough exercises, which, by reinforcing the abdominal muscles, may also improve clearance of the airways. Despite COPD patients being by far the most likely to experience weaning problems, inspiratory muscle training may also have a rationale in other kinds of pathologies. In a larger, but also uncontrolled study, Aldrich et al. [36] recruited 30 patients, some of whom were affected by neuromuscular disorders, who had been in stable chronic respiratory failure for at least 3 weeks and who had failed repeated weaning attempts. They provided a mean of five weekly inspiratory training sessions of spontaneous breathing through an adjustable nonlinear resistor, with gradually increasing duration and resistance. The authors concluded that inspiratory muscle training could improve respiratory muscle strength and endurance in patients with respiratory failure, and could allow many of them to be weaned from mechanical ventilation. These findings may not be applicable to most patients recovering from respiratory failure, however, because the study was uncontrolled and selective.

Furthermore, Braun et al. [37] noted, in patients with chronic failure, that an inspiratory muscle pressure of about 20 cmH$_2$O led to CO$_2$ retention upon weaning because of development of fatigue. Another interesting potential role of inspiratory muscle training may be its use in preventing steroid-induced myopathy. In fact, Weiner et al. [38] showed, in a randomized-controlled trial, that the inotropic and endurance capacities of inspiratory muscles were spared from the damage due to 2 weeks' administration of this drug only in the group of patients undergoing specific training.

19.3.4 Aiding the Removal of Secretions

Clearance of secretions and airway humidification are primary goals of respiratory therapists working in the ICU. This is particularly true for elderly and malnourished patients with respiratory muscle weakness, but also holds for post-surgical patients. Pulmonary complications following open heart surgery or thoracotomy are well-known; they are due mainly to a reduction in functional residual capacity, which leads to collapse of peripheral airways in dependent lung regions [39]. There may be dysfunction and reflex inhibition of the diaphragm, leading to insufficient cough and accumulation of secretion. The principal techniques of secretion removal are directed cough, postural drainage, forced expiratory technique, and autogenic drainage, among others. Despite the fact that all these techniques seem to be clinically very useful, there are no controlled studies performed in the ICU that clearly specify which patients may benefit more and what maneuvers may be more efficient. Concerning the problem of prevention of post-surgical atelectasis, continuous positive airway pressure (CPAP) by mask has been shown to be effective in reducing the frequency of this complication by increasing intrapulmonary pressure, so that the closed alveoli may be reopened.

19.3.5 Assistance During Mechanical Ventilation and Weaning

The strategy of a respiratory therapist-driven protocol during mechanical ventilation [40–42], and in particular in the weaning process, is illustrated in more detail in another chapter. A therapist-driven protocol (TDP) is a consensus of medical knowledge and opinion that is summarized into a care plan or algorithm with changes in therapy directed by changes in objectively measurable patient variables. It is important to stress the specific roles of the respiratory therapists in this procedure. With the institution of a TDP the interaction between the therapist and the nurse regarding the indications for arterial blood gas and maximal inspiratory pressure (MIP) measurements, bronchial secretions, suctioning procedures, and number of hours without mechanical ventilation (MV) causes a significant change in the ordering behaviors of the nursing and medical staff. The team for a TDP usually consists of a physician, the patient, the family, a nurse, and a respiratory therapist. The daily plan of a TDP consists in recording functional activities early in the morning, followed by a rest period before initiation of the weaning process in the optimal position, i.e., sitting upright in bed or sitting upright in a chair. The plan for a TDP also addresses prevention and improvement of the deleterious effects of bed rest, communication, emotional support, psychological well-being, and function. Initial evaluation includes assessment of the patient and ventilator status and patient-ventilator synchrony. This evaluation is performed routinely every 2 h and with each ventilator setting change. The aid of respiratory therapists is also very important during the application of noninvasive mechanical ventilation. One of the keys to NPPV success is the continuous monitoring, preparation, and nursing of patients. For this reason, in the first phases of treatment, the constant presence of the respiratory therapist and the nurse is necessary to ensure correct positioning of the mask, to reassure the patient, to aspirate bronchial secretions, and to evaluate the patient's subjective and objective compliance and tolerance (Table 19.1).

Mask (or interface) selection is critical for successful application of NPPV. To avoid ulceration of the nasal bridge, strap tension should be kept at a minimum at all times; if ulceration should occur, artificial skin may be useful. However, as for invasive mechanical ventilation, a large variability of tasks performed is evident between North America and Europe. For example, it was reported that fewer than 50% of therapists usually supervise and implement noninvasive mechanical ventilation and that, mainly because of legal and insurance problems, this procedure differs according to different environments [10]. Thus, in a "European" paper [43] it was stated that "respiratory therapists are essential in the preparation of vents, in coaching the patients and in positioning of the interfaces," while the authors of a study performed in the USA [44] reported that respiratory therapists were involved in the same tasks just listed, but that they also "adjust the vent at the beginning, adjust FiO_2, perform ABG, set alarms and evaluate patient tolerance and clinical benefit from NIMV, making all necessary adjustment. [.....] must remain in close communication with the medical doctor, to report any variation in vital parameters."

Does all this mean that we (Europeans) have everything to learn from the North American experience and nothing to give? We firmly believe that the professional skill and theoretical preparation of physiotherapists on the two continents are comparable. Above all, we urgently need to solve our professional "political" problems. It is time, in the name of the fledgling European Community, to

Table 19.1. NPPV monitoring

Objective parameters	Subjective parameters
Vigilant state	Dyspnea
Respiratory rate	Discomfort
Heart rate	Pain
Arterial pressure	
Utilization of abdominal and accessory muscles	
Bronchial secretions	
Leaks from the mask	
Skin ulcerations	

increase links between our universities in order to produce common educational pathways, and especially to break down the barriers between the different professional associations that each consider physiotherapists their unique property. On their part, physiotherapists should become autonomous professionals, with a common European roster, and should be able to decide immediately after starting university, or after 1 or 2 years of a generic educational pathway, the specialization they want to practice, exactly as physicians do. Physicians must provide physiotherapists with strong support but also allow them autonomy. Hospitals should guarantee autonomous services within the hospital for physiotherapists, respiratory therapists, and occupational therapists.

19.4 References

1. Bishop KL (1996) Pulmonary rehabilitation in the intensive care unit. In: Fishman AP (ed) Pulmonary rehabilitation. Marcel Dekker, New York, pp 725–738
2. Troche G, Moine P (1997) Is the duration of mechanical ventilation predictable? Chest 112:745–751
3. Connors AF jr, Dawson NV, Thomas C, Harrell FE jr, Desbiens N, et al (1996) Outcomes following acute exacerbation of severe chronic obstructive lung disease. Am J Respir Crit Care Med 154:959–967
4. Nava S, Gayan-Ramirez G, Rollier H, Bisschop A, Dom R, de Bock V, Decramer M (1996) Effects of acute steroid administration on ventilatory and peripheral muscles in rats. Am J Respir Crit Care Med 153:1888–1896
5. Wilson DO, Rogers RM, Wright EC, Anthonisen NR (1989) Body weight in chronic obstructive pulmonary disease. The National Institutes of Health Intermittent Positive-Pressure Breathing Trial. Am Rev Respir Dis 139:1435–1438
6. Adam S, Forrest S (1999) ABC of intensive care – other supportive care. BMJ 319: 175–178
7. Donner CF, Muir JF and the Rehabilitation and Chronic Care Scientific Group of the European Respiratory Society (1997) Position paper. Selection criteria and programmes for pulmonary rehabilitation in COPD patients. Eur Respir J 10:744–757
8. American Thoracic Society (1999) Official statement. Pulmonary rehabilitation 1999. Am J Respir Crit Care Med 159:1666–1682
9. Kida K, Jinno S, Nomura K, Yamada K, Katsura H, Kudoh S Pulmonary rehabilitation program survey in North America, Europe and Tokyo. J Cardiopulmonary Rehabil 1998 18:301–308
10. Norremberg M, Vincent JL (2001) A profile of European intensive care unit physiotherapists. Intensive Care Med (in press)
11. Casaburi R (1996) Deconditioning. In: Fishman AP (ed) Pulmonary rehabilitation. Marcel Dekker, New York, pp 213–230
12. Coyle EF, Martin WH, Bloomfield SA, Lowry OH, Holloszy JO (1985) Effects of detraining on response to submaximal exercise. J Appl Physiol 59:853–859
13. DeBusk RF, Convertino VA, Hung J, Goldwater D (1983) Exercise conditioning in middle-aged men after 10 days of bed rest. Circulation 68:245–250
14. Hung J, Goldwater D, Convertino VA, McKillop JH, Goris ML, DeBusk RF (1983) Mechanism for decreased exercise capacity after bed rest in normal middle-aged men. Am J Cardiol 51:344–348
15. Saltin B, Blomqvist G, Mitchell JH, Johnson RL, Wildenthal K, Chapman CB (1968) Response to exercise after bed rest and after training. Circulation 38 [Suppl 7]: 1–78
16. Martin WH, Coyle EF, Bloomfield SA, Eshani AA (1986) Effects of physical deconditioning after intense endurance training on left ventricular dimension and stroke volume. J Am Coll Cardiol 7:982–989

17. Ehsani AA, Hagberg JM, Hiskson RC (1978) Rapid changes in left ventricular dimensions and mass in response to physical conditioning and deconditioning. Am J Cardiol 42:52–56
18. Deitrick JE, Whedon GD, Shorr E (1948) Effects of immobilization upon various metabolic and physiologic functions of normal men. Am J Med 4:3–36
19. Fareeduddin K, Abelmann WH (1969) Impaired orthostatic tolerance after bed rest in patients with myocardial infarction. N Engl J Med 280:345–350
20. Bortz WM (1982) Disuse and aging. JAMA 248:1203–1208
21. Downs F (1974) Bed rest and sensory disturbances. Am J Nurs 74:434–438
22. Berek K, Margreiter J, Willeit J, Berek A, Schmutzard E, Mutz NJ (1996) Polyneuropathies in critically ill patients: a prospective evaluation. Intensive Care Med 22:849–855
23. Nava S (1998) Rehabilitation of patients admitted to a respiratory intensive care unit. Arch Phys Med Rehabil 79:849–854
24. Grassino A (1984) A rationale for training respiratory muscles. Int Rehabil Med 6: 175–178
25. Le Bourdelles G, Vires N, Bockzowki J, Seta N, Pavlovic D, Aubier M (1994) Effects of mechanical ventilation on diaphragmatic contractile properties in rats. Am J Respir Crit Care Med 149:1539–1544
26. Hubmayr RD, Litchy WJ, Gay PC, Nelson SB (1989) Transdiaphragmatic twitch pressure: effects of lung volume and chest wall shape. Am Rev Respir Dis 139:647–652
27. Similowski T, Yan S, Gauthier AP, Macklem PT, Bellemare F (1991) Contractile properties of the human diaphragm during chronic hyperinflation. N Engl J Med 325:917–923
28. Levine S, Kaiser L, Leferovich J, Tikunov B (1997) Cellular adaptations in the diaphragm in chronic obstructive pulmonary disease. N Engl J Med 337:1799–1806
29. Chen H, Dukes R, Martin BJ (1985) Inspiratory muscle training in patients with chronic obstructive pulmonary disease. Am Rev Respir Dis 131:251–255
30. McKeon JL, Dent A, Turner J, et al (1986) The effect of inspiratory resistive training on exercise capacity in optimally treated patients with severe chronic airflow limitation. Aust N Z J Med 16:648–652
31. Falk P, Eriksen A, Kolliker K, Andersen J (1985) Relieving dyspnea with the inexpensive and simple method in patients with severe chronic airflow limitation. Eur J Respir Dis 66:181–186
32. Pardy RL, Rivington RN, Despas PJ, Macklem PT (1981) Inspiratory muscle training compared with physiotherapy in patients with chronic airflow limitation. Am Rev Respir Dis 123:421–425
33. Andersen JB, Falk P (1984) Clinical experience with inspiratory resistive breathing training. Int Rehab Med 6:183–185
34. Sonne LJ, Davis JA (1982) Increased exercise performance in patients with severe COPD following inspiratory resistive training. Chest 81:436–438
35. Zhu E, Petrof BJ, Gea J, Comtois N, Grassino A (1997) Diaphragm muscle fiber injury after inspiratory resistive breathing. Am J Respir Crit Care Med 155:1110–1116
36. Aldrich TK, Uhrlass RM (1987) Weaning from mechanical ventilation: successful use of modified inspiratory resistive training in muscular dystrophy. Crit Care Med 15:427–429
37. Braun N, Faulkner J, Hughes R, et al (1984) When should respiratory muscles be exercised? Chest 84: 76–83
38. Weiner P, Azgady Y, Weiner M (1995) Inspiratory muscle training during treatment with corticosteroids in humans. Chest 107:1041–1044
39. Ingwersen UM, Larsen KR, Bertelsen MT, Kiil-Nielsen K, Laub M, Sandermann J, Bach K, Hansen H (1993) Three different mask physiotherapy regimens for prevention of post-operative pulmonary complications after heart and pulmonary surgery. Intensive Care Med 19:294–298
40. Durbin C (1996) Therapist-driven protocols in adult intensive care unit patients. In: Stoller JK, Kester L (eds) Therapist-driven protocols. Saunders, Philadelphia
41. Ely EW, Baker AM, Dunagan DP, Burke HR, Smith AC, Kelly PT, Johnson MM, Browder RW, Bowton DL, Haponik EF (1996) Effect of the duration of mechanical ventilation of identifying patients capable of breathing spontaneously. N Engl J Med 335:1864–1869

42. Kollef MH, Shapiro SD, Silver P, St.John RE, Prentice D, Sauer S, Ahrens TS, Shannon W, Baker-Clinkscale D (1997) A randomized, controlled trial of protocol-directed versus physician-directed weaning from mechanical ventilation. Crit Care Med 25:567–574
43. Nava S, Evangelisti I, Rampulla C, Compagnoni ML, Fracchia C, Rubini F (1997) Human and financial costs of non-invasive mechanical ventilation in patients affected by chronic obstructive pulmonary disease and acute respiratory failure. Chest 111:1631–68
44. Wood KA, Lewis L, Von Harz B, Kollef MH (1998) The use of noninvasive positive pressure ventilation in the emergency department. Results of a randomized clinical trial. Chest 113:1339–1346

20 The Role of Noninvasive Mechanical Ventilation in Facilitating Weaning and Extubation

S. Nava and S. Karakurt

As correctly stated recently, "the physician should distinguish between liberation (no need for the ventilator) and extubation (no need for endotracheal tube)," so that after a patient has successfully undergone a trial of unassisted breathing, a second judgment must be made about whether the artificial airway is still required [1]. The term "weaning success" should, in our opinion, be used only after both of the two conditions have been met. Another crucial point in the definition of weaning success, never systematically addressed, is the minimum time a patient must remain disconnected from a ventilator in order to be considered "weaned". If we considered weaning from mechanical ventilation purely as a matter of numbers, we could easily conclude that it is not a major clinical problem, since about 75%–80% of patients admitted to an ICU and mechanically ventilated because of acute respiratory failure resume spontaneous breathing quite easily [2, 3]. The presence of a respiratory disorder is, however, strongly associated with mechanical ventilation lasting longer than 15 days [4]. Once these chronically ill patients have recovered from the most acute phase of their critical illness, they are still likely to require intensive nursing and/or physiotherapy for several weeks before they can be weaned [5]. In one study these "chronically critically ill" patients, representing only 3% of the total number of patients admitted to the ICUs, used almost 40% of the total patient days of care [6]. Endotracheal intubation and invasive mechanical ventilation are often accompanied by complications that carry their own morbidity and mortality. Long-term sequelae may develop after complications directly related to intubation, while the possible need for heavy sedation or curarization during the first few days of ventilation may lead to generalized myopathy [7]. The "abuse" of controlled mechanical ventilation may also carry the risk of development of selective diaphragmatic atrophy after only 48 h, as shown in a laboratory study performed on rats [8]. Infective complications are also important. Torres and co-workers [9] considered the correlation between several risk factors and the development of nosocomial pneumonia; presence of chronic airway obstruction and an endotracheal tube in situ for more than 3 days were significantly associated with an increased risk of nosocomial pneumonia. Nosocomial pneumonia is responsible for longer hospital stay as well as for an increase in mortality. All these complications, due directly or indirectly to invasive mechanical ventilation, may explain why the so-called difficult-to-wean patients have such a poor prognosis. It is therefore essential to reach one of these goals: (a) to avoid intubation and, if it is needed, (b) to reduce the duration of invasive ventilation, and (c) to make weaning as "delicate" as possible, especially for the most "sensitive" populations such as COPD patients. Avoiding intubation by using noninvasive mechanical support is not always possible in these patients. Brochard et al. [10] demonstrated that, compared with medical therapy, noninvasive mechanical ventilation was able to reduce the occurrence of intubation significantly; on the other hand, they also showed that it could be applied for only about 30% of the COPD patients admitted to the ICU. As a matter of fact, in France, one of the countries where noninvasive ventilatory support is most popular, only 20% of all patients are ventilated "nonconventionally".

As far as weaning is concerned, one proposed technique seems to have advantages over the others, especially in COPD patients [11, 12]. Several studies have recently been performed to assess the use of noninvasive ventilation in an attempt to shorten the time of intubation, thereby making weaning as "delicate" as possible. Noninvasive mechanical ventilation has been used in the weaning process since the early 1990s, but none of the studies examining its use was controlled and/or randomized, and it had usually been performed after the patients had been tracheotomized [13–15]. The technique was first used in the Royal Brompton Hospital in London, UK, where Udwadia and co-workers [13] studied 22 consecutive patients referred to their hospital for weaning difficulties. Nine patients had chest wall defects, six had neuromuscular disorders, and seven had primary cardiac disease. Most of the patients had hypercapnic respiratory insufficiency. All of them had undergone at least one conventional weaning attempt, including the use of pressure-support ventilation. The decision to attempt weaning through noninvasive ventilation was made only if the patients met the following criteria: (a) intact bulbar function with preserved cough reflex, (b) minimal airway secretion, (c) ability to breathe spontaneously for 10–15 min, (d) low requirement of oxygen supplementation, (e) cardiac stability, and (f) functioning gastrointestinal tract. Weaning was performed using either volume-cycled ventilation or pressure-support ventilation plus CPAP; mechanical ventilation was continued for 16–20 h a day during the first few days and was then gradually decreased to nocturnal use, depending on the rate of progress of the individual patient. Twenty of the 22 patients were successfully established on noninvasive ventilation, and all of these were transferred from the ICU to a step-down unit or a general ward. Only two patients did not tolerate noninvasive ventilation, and it is noteworthy that both were affected by "pure" hypoxemic respiratory failure due to pulmonary fibrosis after ARDS and cryptogenic pulmonary fibrosis. Weaning from invasive mechanical ventilation was successful in all the 20 patients, although after discharge from hospital two patients died of complications, after having been reintubated. Follow-ups (median 21 months) showed that 16 patients were still alive and well. This study has the scientific limitation of being neither randomized nor controlled, but it was extremely important from a clinical point of view because it was the first to describe the feasibility and utility of this method of weaning. Indeed, it clearly demonstrated that the technique is possible only in a selected population of patients, based not only on the disease (failure of the two patients with pulmonary fibrosis), but also on the clinical status and stability of the patients (see the exclusion criteria).

The same year (1992), Goodemberger et al. [14] published the case reports of two patients affected by neuromuscular diseases in whom nocturnal invasive ventilation was fully substituted by nighttime noninvasive ventilation through a nasal mask, allowing the tracheostomy to be removed.

Restrick and co-workers [15], at the London Chest Hospital, reported later on their experience of weaning patients through noninvasive ventilation. They enrolled 14 patients, eight of whom had COPD and four of whom had restrictive disease. Besides having different diseases, the patients were also at different points in the weaning process, making interpretation of the data somewhat difficult. Restrick et al. did show, however, that 13/14 patients were successfully weaned with the new technique, while only one patient died in the ICU. The most striking result reported in this paper was that in 5/14 patients the trial with noninvasive ventilation was started within a week of intubation, and that in three of them it was performed within the first 24 h. This experience introduced the idea that the switch from intubation to noninvasive ventilation could be carried out earlier than normal, even in patients considered by the attending physician to be "individuals in whom weaning from ventilation was predicted to be difficult".

Interestingly enough, this technique was first developed and tested in Europe where, at the time, legal and ethical issues were perhaps less in the forefront than in the United States. It is not surprising, therefore, that the two randomized trials of noninvasive mechanical ventilation were carried out in Europe [16, 17]. After intubation due to emergency situations, the patients of both studies were conventionally ventilated for a period ranging from 2 to 6 days and were then randomized to follow a standard weaning process with invasive PSV or one with noninvasive PSV, once they had failed a traditional T-piece trial. Both studies reported that the duration of invasive mechanical ventilation was significantly shorter with noninvasive PSV, but only the Italian study demonstrated a positive effect also on 3-month survival, probably related to the lower rate of pneumonia in patients receiving noninvasive ventilation. Nava et al. [16] found that by 60 days 22/25 (88%) patients ventilated noninvasively had been successfully weaned vs 17/25 (68%) patients ventilated invasively. Mean duration of their mechanical ventilation was significantly different, being 10 ± 6 days vs 16 ± 11, respectively. The probability of success (survival and weaning) during ventilation was found to be significantly higher in the noninvasively ventilated group. ICU stay was significantly shorter in this group (15 ± 5 days vs 24 ± 13). Survival rates at 60 days were also statistically different (92% for noninvasively ventilated group vs 72% for the invasively ventilated group). Interestingly, in the paper by Girault et al. [17] the "total" duration of mechanical ventilation was longer in the noninvasively ventilated group. This apparently contradictory result may be explained by the different definition of weaning in the two studies. In the Italian study weaning was defined as an "all-or-none" phenomenon" to make a real comparison with extubation, while the French study reflected a more clinical attitude of ventilating the patients, once extubated, for a few hours a day to provide them with further ventilatory support, even in the absence of any sign of post-extubation failure. Before going any further, we would like to repeat and emphasize that all the studies, and therefore all the conclusions drawn from them, are related to selected populations of patients affected mainly by acute-on-chronic, or hypercapnic, respiratory failure, who had been meticulously selected, since at the time of extubation they were hemodynamically stable, with an acceptable SaO_2, without fever or any sensorial impairment, and had at least a weak cough reflex so that clearing of the airway was possible. Theoretically, noninvasive mechanical ventilation should be reappraised as a weaning technique in COPD only after an initial attempt with the same mode has failed. There are four main reasons for failure of NIMV during an episode of acute respiratory failure in COPD patients: (a) lack of cooperation, (b) excessive secretions, (c) severe strength-load imbalance, and (d) hemodynamic instability. Most, if not all, of these problems may be swiftly corrected by protection of the airways and proper medical therapy. Without large-scale studies it is difficult to quantify how many COPD patients admitted to ICUs and intubated could successfully undergo this technique of weaning, but probably about 30%–35% of the patients affected by COPD are unlikely to benefit from this technique. Figure 1 is a proposed flow diagram of patients with acute hypercapnic respiratory failure entering an ICU or an intermediate care unit. While this appears to be the current situation for patients with hypercapnic respiratory failure, further studies are clearly needed to assess the feasibility of the technique in other forms of respiratory failure, such as ARDS, post-surgical complications, or cardiac impairment, particularly since some preliminary results appear promising [18].

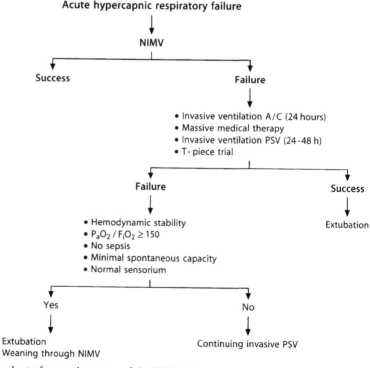

Fig. 20.1. Flow chart of a weaning approach in COPD patients

The only study so far on patients affected by hypoxemic respiratory failure was recently performed by Gregoretti and co-workers [18]. The primary aim of their study was to compare blood gases, tidal volume, and respiratory rate at equal pressure values delivered invasively or noninvasively, but some important clinical data were obtained from the follow-up. Twenty-two trauma patients underwent a T-piece trial of at least 15 min after a median period of 4 ± 2 days of invasive ventilation and were then switched to noninvasive ventilation. Nine patients (41%) were reintubated after about 2 days because of clinical deterioration, intolerance to the mask, or inability to clear the airways, and six of them died while still being ventilated. Despite the fact that this study was not controlled and not specifically aimed at assessing the feasibility of using noninvasive ventilation as a weaning strategy, it was the first study to show that this approach could be used in patients other than those with COPD or restrictive thoracic disease. The probability of success was lower than in these latter groups, however, once again highlighting the possible important difference in outcome according to the underlying pathology.

As shown in Table 20.1 [11, 19–32], which reports data from the past 30 years, post-extubation failure remains one of the major clinical problems in ICUs. It was recently reported that the incidence of post-extubation failure in patients ventilated in ICUs is relatively high, and that the prognosis of these patients is very poor since their hospital mortality exceeds 30%–40%, with the cause of extubation failure (i.e., non-airway problems) and the time to reintubation being independent predictors of outcome [30]. Since clinical evidence suggests that the act of reintubation itself is an insufficient explanation for the high mortality, it has been claimed that the clinical deterioration occurring during the period of

Table 20.1. Incidence of failed extubation

Reference	Incidence (%)
Sahn and Lakshminarayan [19]	17
Hilberman et al. [20]	18
Tahvanainen et al. [21]	19
DeHaven et al. [22]	6
Demling et al. [23]	6
Krieger et al. [24]	10
Sassoon and Mahutte [25]	12
Mohsenifar et al. [26]	14
Lee et al. [27]	17
Brochard et al. [11]	23
Torres et al. [28]	23
Esteban et al. [12]	16
Epstein et al. [29]	14
Epstein and Ciubotaru [30]	12
Vallverdu et al. [31]	12
Esteban et al. [32]	10
Total	17.7

unsupported ventilation allows the development of multiple organ failure, which leads to a poor prognosis. This period of unsupported ventilation may in some cases be unduly protracted, because physicians avoid new intubation due to the severity of the disease, considering the patient to have a very poor chance of survival, or because of concerns about worsening the patient's clinical status as a result of the well-known complications associated with intubation. Although we must bear in mind the importance of this time factor, early institution of a noninvasive form of mechanical ventilation in those patients who show signs of "incipient" respiratory failure, or even the sequential use of this technique right from the time of extubation, may be attractive strategies that deserve future study. A historically controlled study [33] demonstrated that the use of noninvasive ventilation to treat post-extubation failure significantly reduced the need for endotracheal intubation, the mean duration of ventilatory assistance, and the duration of ICU stay, while it did not have statistically significant effects on mortality (however, mortality was three times higher in the group treated conventionally, suggesting that a study on a larger group of patients might show a significant difference in survival). Interestingly, this study also demonstrated a lower incidence of pneumonia in the group treated noninvasively (7% vs 20%). A more recent, uncontrolled study [34] by Kilger et al. also investigated the effects of noninvasive ventilation in treating acute respiratory insufficiency occurring after early extubation in non-COPD patients. Only 2/15 patients needed to be re-intubated, since noninvasive ventilation significantly improved gas exchange and breathing pattern, decreased intrapulmonary shunt fraction, and reduced the work of breathing. Randomized, controlled studies are therefore needed to confirm the feasibility and utility of noninvasive ventilation after extubation has been performed.

Another important field of application for noninvasive ventilation is during unplanned extubation, which occurs in 3%–13% of intubated patients, but no data are available at present [35].

20.1 References

1. Manthous C, Schmidt GA, Hall J (1998) Liberation from mechanical ventilation. A decade of progress. Chest 114:886–901
2. Goldstone J, Moxham J (1991) Weaning from mechanical ventilation. Thorax 46:56–62
3. Lemaire F (1993) Difficult weaning. Intensive Care Med 19:S69–S73
4. Troche G, Moine P (1997) Is the duration of mechanical ventilation predictable? Chest 112:745–751
5. Nava S (1998) Rehabilitation of patients admitted to a respiratory intensive care unit. Arch Phys Med Rehabil 79:849–854
6. Wagner DP (1989) Economics of prolonged mechanical ventilation. Am Rev Respir Dis 140:514–518
7. Kollef MH, Levy NT, Ahrens TS, Schaiff R, Prentice D, Sherman G (1998) The use of continuous i.v. sedation is associated with prolongation of mechanical ventilation. Chest 114:541–548
8. Le Bourdelles G, Vires N, Bockzowki J, Seta N, Pavlovic D, Aubier M (1994) Effects of mechanical ventilation on diaphragmatic contractile properties in rats. Am J Respir Crit Care Med 149:1539–1544
9. Torres A, Aznar R, Gatell JM, Jimenez P, Gonzales J, Ferrer A, Celis R, Rodriguez-Roisin R (1990) Incidence, risk, and prognosis factors of nosocomial pneumonia in mechanically ventilated patients. Am Rev Respir Dis 142:523–528

10. Brochard L, Mancebo J, Wysocki M, Lofaso F, Conti G, Rauss A, Simonneau G, Benito S, Gasparetto A, Lemaire F, Isabey D, Harf A (1995) Noninvasive ventilation for acute exacerbations of chronic obstructive pulmonary disease. N Engl J Med 333:817–822

11. Brochard L, Rauss A, Benito S, Conti G, Mancebo J, Rekik N, Gasparetto A, Lemaire F (1994) Comparison of three methods of gradual withdrawal from ventilatory support during weaning from mechanical ventilation. Am J Respir Crit Care Med 150:896–903

12. Esteban A, Frutos F, Tobin MJ, Alia I, Solsona JF, Valverdu' I, Macias S, Allegue JM, Blanco J, Carriedo D, Leon M, de la Cal MA, Taboada F, Gonzales de Velasco J, Palazon E, Carrizosa F, Tomas R, Suarez J, Goldwasser RS (1995) A comparison of four methods of weaning from mechanical ventilation. Spanish Lung Failure Collaborative Group. N Engl J Med 332:345–350

13. Udwadia ZF, Santis GK, Steven MH, Simonds AK (1992) Nasal ventilation to facilitate weaning in patients with chronic respiratory insufficiency. Thorax 47:715–718

14. Goodenberger DM, Couser J, May JJ (1992) Successful discontinuation of ventilation via tracheostomy by substitution of nasal positive pressure ventilation. Chest 102:1277–1279

15. Restrick LJ, Scott AD, Ward EM, Feneck RO, Cornwell WE, Wedzicha JA (1993) Nasal intermittent positive-pressure ventilation in weaning intubated patients with chronic respiratory disease from assisted intermittent, positive-pressure ventilation. Respir Med 87:199–204

16. Nava S, Ambrosino N, Clini E, Prato M, Orlando G, Vitacca M, Brigada P, Fracchia C, Rubini F (1998) Noninvasive mechanical ventilation in the weaning of patients with respiratory failure due to chronic obstructive pulmonary disease. A randomized, controlled trial. Ann Intern Med 128:721–728

17. Girault C, Daudenthun I, Chevron V, Tamion F, Leroy J, Bonmarchand G (1999) Noninvasive ventilation as a systematic extubation and weaning technique in acute-on-chronic respiratory failure. A prospective, randomized controlled study. Am J Respir Crit Care Med 160:86–92

18. Gregoretti C, Beltrame F, Lucangelo U, Burbi L, Conti G, Turello M, Gregori D (1998) Physiologic evaluation of non-invasive pressure support ventilation in trauma patients with acute respiratory failure. Intensive Care Med 24:785–790

19. Sahn SA, Lakshminarayan S (1973) Bedside criteria for discontinuation of mechanical ventilation. Chest 63: 1002–1005

20. Hilberman M, Dietrich HP, Martz K, Osborn JJ (1976) An analysis of potential physiological predictors of respiratory adequacy following cardiac surgery. J Thorac Cardiovasc Surg 71: 711–720

21. Tahvanainen J, Salmenpera M, Nikki P (1983) Extubation criteria after weaning from intermittent mandatory ventilation and continuous positive airway pressure. Crit Care Med 11: 702–707

22. DeHaven CB jr, Hurst JM, Branson RD (1986) Evaluation of two different extubation criteria: attributes contributing to success. Crit Care Med 14: 92–95

23. Demling RH, Read T, Lind LJ, Flanagan HL (1988) Incidence and morbidity of extubation failure in surgical intensive care patients. Crit Care Med 16: 573–577

24. Krieger BP, Ershowsky PF, Becker DA, Gazeroglu HB (1989) Evaluation of conventional criteria for predicting successful weaning from mechanical ventilatory support in elderly patients. Crit Care Med 17: 858–861

25. Sassoon CS, Mahutte CK (1993) Airway occlusion pressure and breathing pattern as predictors of weaning outcome. Am Rev Respir Dis 148: 860–866

26. Mohsenifar Z, Hay A, Hay J, Lewis ML, Koerner SK (1993) Gastric intramural pH as a predictor of success or failure in weaning patients from mechanical ventilation. Ann Intern Med 119: 794–798

27. Lee KH, Hui KP, Chan TP, Tan WC, Lim TK (1994) Rapid shallow breathing (frequency-tidal volume ratio) did not predict extubation outcome. Chest 105: 540–543

28. Torres A, Gatell JM, Aznar E, el-Ebiary M, Puig de la Bellacasa J, Gonzalez J, Ferrer M, Rodriguez-Roisin R (1995) Re-intubation increases the risk of nosocomial pneumonia in patients needing mechanical ventilation. Am J Crit Care Med 152: 137–141

29. Epstein SK, Ciubotaru RL, Wong JB (1997) Effect of extubation on the outcome of mechanical ventilation. Chest 112: 186–192
30. Espstein SK. Ciubotaru RL (1998) Independent effects of etiology of failure and time to reintubation on outcome for patients failing extubation. Am J Respir Crit Care Med 158:489–493
31. Vallverdu I, Calaf N, Subirana M, Net A, Benito S, Mancebo J (1998) Clinical characteristics, respiratory functional parameters and outcome of a two-hour T-piece trial in patients weaning from mechanical ventilation. Am J Crit Care Med 158: 1855–1862
32. Esteban A, Alia I, Tobin MJ, Gil A, Gordo F, Vallverdu I, Blanch L, Vazquez A, Bonet A, de Pablo R, Torres A, de la Cal MA, Macias S (1999) Effects of spontaneous breathing trial duration on outcome of discontinue mechanical ventilation. Spanish Lung Failure Collaborative Group. Am J Crit Care Med 159: 512–518
33. Hilbert G, Gruson D, Portel L, Gbikpi-Benissan G, Cardinaud JP (1998) Noninvasive pressure support ventilation in COPD patients with postextubation hypercapnic respiratory insufficiency. Eur Respir J 11:1349–1353
34. Kilger E, Briegel J, Haller M, Frey L, Schelling G, Stoll C, Pichler B, Peter K (1999) Effects of noninvasive positive pressure ventilatory support in non-COPD patients with acute respiratory insufficiency after early extubation. Intensive Care Med 25:1374–1380
35. Chevron V, Menard JF, Richard JC, Girault C, Leroy J, Bonmarchand G (1998) Unplanned extubation: risk factors of development and predictive criteria for reintubation. Crit Care Med 26:1049–1053

21 Expanding Horizons of Noninvasive Ventilation

L. Brochard and J. Mancebo

Noninvasive ventilation (NIV) for acute respiratory failure has the potential to improve dyspnoea, to reduce the need for endotracheal intubation (ETI) and the number of complications associated with mechanical ventilation and intensive care unit (ICU) stay, and subsequently to reduce mortality (Brochard et al. 1990; Meduri et al. 1996).

Patients with hypercapnic forms of acute respiratory failure are more likely to benefit from this technique, but recent studies also showed that these results may be extended to selected forms of hypoxaemic respiratory failure. Most of these benefits are explained by the fact that ETI can be avoided by this procedure, which, as a consequence, means a reduction in ICU complications.

Knowledge of the benefits of and indications for NIV is important. It is also necessary to understand what can cause the failure of the technique in an individual ICU patient, and to estimate well the importance of the specific aspects of NIV. NIV is based on the absence of ETI and requires merely the same ventilator equipment as the standard approach, in combination with a device providing the interface between the patient and the ventilator, which in most instances is a nasal or facial mask. It has several specific features that constitute a new area of knowledge for everyone who wants to implement this technique in his/her own department.

21.1 Physiologic Effects and Mechanisms of Action of Noninvasive Ventilation in Acute Respiratory Failure

21.1.1 Breathing Pattern

The spontaneous breathing pattern of patients developing acute ventilatory failure markedly differs from normal and can result in respiratory acidosis. In patients with chronic obstructive pulmonary disease (COPD), rapid shallow breathing, i.e. small tidal volumes at a high respiratory frequency, is a typical feature of the acute exacerbation, resulting in alveolar hypoventilation despite preserved minute ventilation. This pattern can be modified by the use of NIV, which allows the patient to take deeper breaths with less effort. Although continuous positive airway pressure, used to counterbalance intrinsic positive end-expiratory pressure, can significantly reduce the patient's effort (Petrof et al. 1990; Smith and Marini 1988), it seems that the addition of positive inspiratory pressure, as delivered with pressure-support (PSV) or assist-control ventilation, is necessary to substantially alter the breathing pattern and improve CO_2 elimination. The reduction in respiratory rate and the increase in tidal volume under NIV are the best markers of the efficacy of the technique (Appendini et al. 1994; Brochard, et al. 1990).

21.1.2 Gas Exchange

In case of hypercapnic respiratory failure, improvement of arterial blood gas disturbances can be achieved with NIV. In patients with chronic CO_2 retention, $PaCO_2$ usually worsens under oxygen treatment; however, NIV improves oxygenation without any worsening in CO_2 retention (Warren et al. 1980). Improvement in $PaCO_2$ and pH can be more gradual with time than the effect on oxygenation (Brochard et al. 1995). A drop in $PaCO_2$ and a rise in pH towards normal values can also be observed rapidly within the first hour, and in this case, the 2-h response in blood gases can predict the success of the technique (Meduri et al. 1996). Indeed, a recent multicentre randomised trial by Plant et al. (Plant et al. 2000) showed that NIV led to a more rapid improvement in pH at 1 h ($p=0.02$), and to a greater fall in respiratory rate at 4 h ($p=0.03$) when compared with controls.

Diaz and co-workers investigated the effects of NIV on oxygenation in COPD patients with acute exacerbation (Diaz et al. 1997). Interestingly, improvement in the ventilation-perfusion relationship did not play any significant role, and attainment of an efficient breathing pattern was by far the most important mechanism to explain the improvement in oxygenation during NIV. The authors concluded that the main objective of NIV was improvement in alveolar ventilation, i.e. in tidal volume.

More recently, Jolliet et al. (Jolliet et al. 1999) have shown that breathing a mixture of helium:oxygen instead of nitrogen:oxygen, administered to decompensated COPD patients undergoing NIV with pressure support, is beneficial in terms of gas exchange and dyspnoea. Patients followed a crossover treatment during 45 min, at the end of which arterial blood gases and dyspnoea scores were measured. $PaCO_2$ decreased more with helium:oxygen than with nitrogen:oxygen at the same FiO_2: from 54±7 mmHg to 48±6 mmHg and from 55±8 mmHg to 52±6 mmHg, respectively ($p<0.05$). PaO_2 significantly increased with both mixtures, and the dyspnoea score decreased more with helium:oxygen than with nitrogen:oxygen, from 4.6±1.5 to 2.8±1.6 and from 4.5±1.4 to 3.7±1.6, respectively ($p<0.05$). No untoward hemodynamic effects were observed with any treatment.

21.1.3 Reduction in Respiratory Muscle Effort and Work of Breathing

In patients with acute exacerbation of COPD, several investigators have shown the efficacy of face mask PSV to reduce the patient's effort to breathe (Brochard et al. 1990; Nava et al. 1993; Nava et al. 1995). At baseline, the transdiaphragmatic pressure swings measured in these patients can be considerably higher than normal values, suggesting that they often develop a high percentage of their maximal capacity at each breath, a situation at high risk for respiratory muscle fatigue (Brochard et al. 1990). A substantial and constant reduction in the pressure swings was obtained under noninvasive PSV in all patients. Appendini and colleagues suggested that the combination of PSV and PEEP in patients with COPD is more efficient than each one alone in reducing diaphragmatic effort and steering the patient clear of a potential zone of fatigue (Appendini et al. 1994).

A recent investigation by Jaber et al. (Jaber et al. 2000) compared the effects on inspiratory muscle effort of NIV using nitrogen:oxygen vs NIV using helium:oxygen in ten acutely decompensated COPD patients. The authors observed that the use of helium:oxygen during NIV markedly enhanced the ability of standard NIV (using nitrogen:oxygen) to decrease a patient's effort to breathe (evaluated in terms of pressure-time product of the inspiratory muscles and work of breathing). $PaCO_2$ also exhibited significant reductions with helium:oxygen NIV when compared with standard NIV.

21.1.4 Hemodynamic Consequences

Usually, no major hemodynamic changes are observed in patients treated with NIV. PSV has usually no or little hemodynamic effect, except when PEEP is added (Diaz et al. 1997; Nava et al. 1993). Thorens and his colleagues showed that correction of arterial blood gas abnormalities was accompanied by a decrease in systolic and mean pulmonary arterial pressure and an increase in right ventricular ejection fraction, and that peripheral oedema subsequently decreased in all patients (Thorens et al. 1997). In the study by Diaz et al, cardiac output fell in patients under NIV, but with no change in mixed venous PO_2; this could reflect a decrease in oxygen demand under NIV, rather than a real impairment in cardiac function (Diaz et al. 1997).

21.2 Reasons for Failure of NIV to Improve Gas Exchange

The patient-ventilator interface is, in most instances, either a full face mask covering both the nose and the mouth, or a nasal mask, which is the device predominantly used for long-term ventilation. The first reason for failure is leakage around the mask, or through the mouth in case of nasal masks. Nasal masks, for instance, can be impossible to use with patients unable to close their mouth. Leaks through the mouth make the technique inefficient, can generate nasal congestion and increase nasal resistance, and induce patient-ventilator asynchrony (Carrey et al. 1990; Richards et al. 1996). A recent study of stable patients showed that facial masks were more efficient than nasal masks to increase tidal volume and reduce PCO_2 (Navalesi et al. 2000). Nasal masks were found to be slightly more comfortable. The leaks can also impede the ventilator in detecting the threshold for inspiratory flow to switch to expiration. Prolonged inspiratory time and major asynchrony may ensue (Calderini et al. 1999). Using a time-cycled mode as assist-pressure controlled ventilation may help to solve the problem.

Another cause of failure is the intolerance of the mask by the patient. This certainly depends on the equipment used, but also on the attention given by the caregiver to the procedure. This includes the use of dressings on the bridge of the nose, adapting the mask well to avoid or minimise leaks around the mask, and starting NIV smoothly. This requires some specific expertise, and at least two studies have shown that extra time for the respiratory therapist is needed in the first 6–8 h of treatment with NIV compared with a more conventional approach using invasive mechanical ventilation and ETI (Kramer et al. 1995; Nava et al. 1997b).

Another limitation of the technique may come from the risk of CO_2 rebreathing and of the equipment dead space. Some of the bi-level airway pressure devices used for home mechanical ventilation have been designed to force the exhaled gases to pass through holes placed on the inspiratory line, thanks to an expiratory bias flow, the level of which is dependent on the PEEP set on the ventilator. In case of low PEEP level and/or high minute ventilation, substantial rebreathing may occur (Ferguson and Gilmartin 1995; Lofaso et al. 1995, 1996). This may prevent ventilatory support from reducing $PaCO_2$ and may cause an increase in the patient's work of breathing. The use of nonrebreathing valves can reduce this problem. Large dead-space ventilation may also be favoured by the internal volume of the full face mask, by the heat and moisture exchanging filter, or by the connections placed between the patient and the ventilator.

The level of ventilatory support may also be insufficient. Usual settings use 5 cmH$_2$O of PEEP and 10–20 cmH$_2$O of pressure support. The ability of NIV to increase tidal volume may be limited, however, because high inspiratory pressures may increase leaks and/or create gastric insufflation.

21.3 Where to Perform NIV

Controversies exist about where NIV should be performed and whether it can be administered outside of the ICU. This seems to depend mainly on the local organisation and specific training of the personnel concerning the management of such patients. For instance, the study by Bott and colleagues demonstrated extremely positive results of NIV by treating patients in the emergency ward (Bott et al. 1993). By contrast, others did not find any benefit to the use of NIV in the emergency department (Wood et al. 1998). Several factors may have contributed to these results, including the type of patients. The delay in deciding on ETI therefore becomes a concern. Plant and his colleagues in the UK showed that extremely positive results could be obtained using NIV in the ward (Plant et al. 2000). Their results were obtained after implementing a strict educational program for the personnel. They showed that use of NIV for COPD patients admitted to the ward was able to decrease the need for intubation and the mortality of these patients. They suggested, however, that the more severe patients, with a pH below 7.30, should be treated with NIV in the ICU. Indeed, among patients with a pH<7.30 at admission, 42% in the control group and 36% in the NIV group were considered failures. However, among patients with a pH>7.30 at admission, 20% were considered failures in the control group and only 6% in the NIV group ($p=0.01$).

21.4 Mechanical Ventilators

Attention should be paid to the technical aspects of the ventilators (Bunbu-raphong et al. 1997; Lofaso et al. 1998). Several authors have compared portable ventilators and ICU ventilators with regard to their ability to give a fast response to a simulated patient's effort and to pressurise the airway. Interestingly, most of the newer small turbine ventilators performed as well or better than many of the ICU ventilators. Increased inspiratory flow demand modifies the response time of the ventilators, but most of them are able to reasonably meet the demand. The flow-triggering systems are usually preferable to the pressure-triggering systems (Aslanian et al. 1998; Nava et al. 1997a). These systems are also preferable for maintaining PEEP in case of leaks.

21.5 Ventilatory Modes

21.5.1 Continuous Positive Airway Pressure

CPAP has commonly been used to treat hypoxaemic patients who are able to breathe spontaneously. The beneficial effects of CPAP in hypoxaemic patients are due essentially to the increase in functional residual capacity induced by PEEP. This ventilatory technique is also indicated for patients with sleep apnoea or chronic obstructive lung disease, especially those with dynamic hyperinflation and auto-PEEP. However, few data exist to support the use of CPAP alone as an efficient way to deliver ventilator support to COPD patients (Goldberg et al. 1995; Miro et al. 1993). In most of the reports, gas exchange was often not modified by CPAP alone.

From the current literature, it is very difficult to accurately determine the impact of CPAP on mortality, morbidity, length of hospital stay, or even the need for ETI in most categories of patients with acute respiratory failure. Several physiologic studies showed a potential benefit of CPAP on cardiovascular function in patients with cardiogenic pulmonary oedema (Buda et al. 1979; Lenique et al. 1997). In addition, major reductions in the work of breathing can be observed (Lenique et al. 1997).

Several studies conducted by Räsänen et al. (Räsänen et al. 1985) and Lin et al. (Lin et al. 1995) had a specific design that essentially allowed showing a beneficial effect of CPAP on arterial oxygenation with a predetermined and fixed duration of CPAP. Bersten et al. (Bersten et al. 1991) studied 39 patients with cardiogenic pulmonary oedema presenting with hypoxaemia (mean PaO_2/FiO_2 between 136 and 138 mmHg) and acute hypercapnia (mean $PaCO_2$ between 58 and 64 mmHg), and compared continuous flow CPAP with PEEP 10 cmH_2O by face mask with the conventional therapy of oxygen given by mask. They found a significant improvement in PaO_2 and a significant decrease in $PaCO_2$ in patients treated with CPAP compared with those conventionally treated. Intubation and mechanical ventilation were needed in 35% of patients (7/20) in the conventional-treatment group within 3 h of study entry (the CPAP was administered for a total of 9±5 h). However, none of the 19 patients treated with CPAP required intubation. Mortality was similar in the two groups. A recent study confirmed the benefit of CPAP in patients with severe (hypercapnic) cardiogenic pulmonary oedema (L'Her et al. 1998).

A recent investigation by Delclaux et al. evaluated whether CPAP delivered by a face mask had physiologic benefit and would reduce the need for intubation and mechanical ventilation in patients suffering from pulmonary oedema and acute lung injury (Delclaux et al. 2000). One hundred and twenty-three patients with acute nonhypercapnic respiratory failure (PaO_2/FiO_2 ratio <300 mmHg) resulting from bilateral pulmonary oedema were randomised to receive either oxygen alone or oxygen plus CPAP. Randomisation was stratified on the existence of an underlying cardiopathy. After 1 h, both subjective response to treatment and PaO_2/FiO_2 ratio depicted a greater improvement with CPAP than with oxygen. However, no differences were found in the need for intubation and mechanical ventilation in the CPAP group versus the oxygen group (21/62 versus 24/61, $p=0.53$), in in-hospital mortality, or in length of the ICU stay. In addition, a higher number of complications occurred in the CPAP group. These results do not support the use of CPAP in the setting of acute nonhypercapnic respiratory failure such as acute lung injury.

Therefore, CPAP seems to be indicated mainly for acute pulmonary oedema of cardiac origin, especially when associated with hypercapnic respiratory failure. In this group of patients, the addition of PSV may also be beneficial (Hoffmann and Welte 1999; Rusterholtz et al. 1999), although great caution is necessary in the case of ischaemic heart disease; one study reported a high incidence of myocardial infarction with the latter technique (Mehta et al. 1997).

However, a recent randomised controlled trial (Masip et al. 2000) carried out in patients with ARF secondary to acute cardiogenic pulmonary oedema showed a decreased intubation rate, i.e. 5% (1/19), in those patients allocated to NIV (PSV+PEEP), compared with the control group (administration of oxygen by mask), which showed an intubation rate of 33% (6/18), $p=0.037$. In addition, the median resolution time (as assessed by clinical improvement + $SatpO_2>95\%$ + respiratory rate<30 breaths/min, was significantly lower in the NIV group compared with controls (30 min vs 105 min, $p=0.002$). Those patients who also were hypercapnic exhibited significant reductions in $PaCO_2$ only if they were allocated to the NIV group. No differences in mortality or length of hospital stay were noted between the two groups.

21.5.2 Noninvasive Negative Pressure Ventilation

Negative pressure ventilators were used in the early years of intensive care medicine to treat patients with acute respiratory failure of neuromuscular origin. In a very small number of centres, this technique has been kept to treat patients with acute-on-chronic respiratory failure (Corrado et al. 1992, 1996, 1998). Some reports suggest that, in experienced hands and in selected patients, it may have an efficacy comparable to that of standard invasive ventilation (Corrado et al. 1996). The cumbersome nature of the devices used make it difficult to generalise these results, and more comparative data are needed.

21.5.3 Positive Pressure Ventilation

Various modes of positive pressure ventilation have been proposed, including assist-control ventilation, pressure-support ventilation and assist-pressure controlled ventilation. All modes have their advantages and their limitations, and important clinical results have been obtained with almost all. Volume-targeted modes are more sensitive to leaks, and tidal volumes exceeding usual settings have been recommended. Because the peak mask pressure is not limited, a certain number of side effects may be favoured by the use of this modality such as high peak pressures inducing poor tolerance, leaks, and gastric insufflation (Meduri et al. 1996; Soo Hoo et al. 1994; Vitacca et al. 1993). Pressure-limited modes may help in improving tolerance. A randomised clinical trial comparing assist-control and PSV has shown that fewer side effects are observed with the latter (Vitacca et al. 1993). During PSV, the cycling from inspiration to expiration may not be operative in case of leaks because neither the flow descent nor the increase in pressure is detected (Calderini et al. 1999). An adjustable flow threshold may be used to solve this problem, as well as an inspiratory time limit, such as with assist-pressure controlled ventilation. Girault et al. performed an interesting comparison of assist-control and pressure-support ventilation in a group of stable patients with COPD (Girault et al. 1997). The two modes markedly reduced the work of breathing, although the reduction was greater with assist-control (it is worth mentioning that the two modalities were not matched in terms of mean airway pressure delivered by the ventilator). The comfort scale, however, was better for pressure-support ventilation. A successful experience has also recently been reported using proportional-assist ventilation in non-COPD patients with various forms of acute respiratory failure (Patrick et al. 1996).

The importance of the mode may differ in case of hypoxaemic or in case of hypercapnic ventilatory failure. Mancebo et al. have simulated conditions of high ventilatory demand through CO_2 inhalation, as present in hypoxaemic respiratory failure, and observed that ventilatory support delivered with intermittent positive pressure breathing (IPPB) induced extra work of breathing, which made the amount of total effort during assisted ventilation markedly superior to the situation of unassisted breathing (Mancebo et al. 1995). This suggests that the ventilatory equipment used is probably critical in situations of high ventilatory demand and probably explains some failures of the technique in hypoxaemic respiratory failure.

Thus, although different modes of ventilation can be used with success, their effects are probably not equivalent in different conditions of respiratory failure. Pressure-targeted modes are by far the most frequently used, and among them is the combination of pressure support and PEEP. This combination has indeed been shown by different authors to be the most effective in reducing patients' respiratory effort in case of COPD (Appendini et al. 1994; Nava et al. 1993).

21.6 Clinical Results

Four large prospective randomised studies (Bott et al. 1993; Brochard et al. 1995; Kramer et al. 1995; Plant et al. 2000) of patients with chronic obstructive pulmonary disease demonstrated that important benefits could be obtained, as already suggested by a number of previous series with historical or matched control groups (Brochard et al. 1990; Fernandez et al. 1993; Vitacca et al. 1993). In a study by Bott et al., 60 patients with acute exacerbation of chronic respiratory failure were randomised to noninvasive nasal positive pressure ventilation or to standard medical treatment (Bott et al. 1993). Improvement in arterial pH was significantly greater compared with the standard group, and a reduction in breathlessness was observed in the NIV group. A benefit in terms of mortality also existed for the patients in the NIV group who tolerated the technique (after excluding four patients who did not tolerate NIV). In a study by Kramer et al., a major reduction in the need for ETI was observed in the treated group, essentially explained by the subgroup of patients with COPD (Kramer et al. 1995).

In a study by Brochard and co-workers, 85 COPD patients were randomised to treatment with or without face-mask pressure-support ventilation (Brochard et al. 1995). The disease in the two groups was of comparable severity (based on the number of patients with frank respiratory acidosis, hypoxaemia, encephalopathy). The ETI rate reached 74% of the patients in the control group and only 26% in the new-treatment group. This reduction was associated with fewer complications during the ICU stay, reduced length of hospital stay and, more importantly, a significant reduction in mortality (from 29% to 9%). The hospital mortality among patients requiring ETI remained similar in both groups (close to 30%), suggesting that the overall benefit observed regarding mortality under NIV was explained essentially by a reduction in the need for ETI in this group.

Plant et al. recently completed an important study of more than 230 patients with COPD treated in respiratory wards with either NIV or a standard medical treatment (Plant et al. 2000). A significantly smaller number of patients met pre-defined criteria for intubation in the NIV group, and the in-hospital mortality was significantly reduced. Importantly, the authors of the study spent a median of 7.5 h per centre in the 3 months preceding the study and an additional 0.9 h per centre once the study had begun, on training the personnel and teaching about NIV. This emphasises the importance of education for the success of the technique, and under-education may explain poorer results in other studies (Wood et al. 1998).

Until recently, the most striking data showing beneficial effects of NIV concerned patients with acute respiratory acidosis in whom hypoxaemia was not the major reason for respiratory failure. Antonelli and colleagues recently published the first relatively large randomised controlled study demonstrating important benefits in a group of non-COPD patients (Antonelli et al. 1998). In a group of 64 patients with hypoxaemic respiratory failure and a gradual deterioration in clinical conditions, patients were randomised at the time they reached pre-defined criteria for intubation. One group received ETI and mechanical ventilation, and the other was treated with NIV through a face mask using pressure support and PEEP. The initial improvement in oxygenation was similar with the two modes of support. Ten of 32 patients in the NIV group eventually required ETI, but several benefits were also observed in this group. Patients surviving the ICU had a shorter duration of ventilation and length of stay in the ICU and suffered from fewer complications, and the group showed a trend towards a lower mortality despite similar severity (28% vs 47%). A post-hoc analysis of the data suggested that the subgroup of patients with the lowest degree of severity on admission was the one most likely to benefit from NIV. The data from this study emphasise the potential of this technique to reduce iatrogenic complications. One concern in this study, however, is the very high mortality observed among the NIV patients eventually requiring ETI. In another series of solid-organ-transplant patients, the same group found again beneficial results in using NIV as a preventive measure during episodes of acute hypoxaemic respiratory failure (Antonelli et al. 2000). Both length of stay and ICU mortality, but not hospital mortality, were significantly reduced by using NIV. In a multicentre randomised trial, Confalonieri et al. found that NIV was also beneficial in community-acquired pneumonia with criteria for severity. Once again, however, these important results (mortality) were explained only by the subgroup of patients with COPD (Confalonieri et al. 1999).

Recently, Martin et al. (Martin et al. 2000), have compared in a randomised controlled trial the effects of NIV ($n=32$) with those of standard treatment ($n=29$) in patients with ARF (grouped into COPD or non-COPD-related pulmonary process). The rate of ETI was significantly lower in the NIV group than in controls (6.38 intubations vs 21.25 intubations per 100 ICU days, respectively, $p=0.002$). Patients with hypoxaemic ARF in the NIV group had a lower ETI rate than the control group (7.46 intubations vs 22.64 intubations per 100 ICU days, respectively, $p= 0.02$). A trend was observed to a decreased ETI rate in hypercapnic ARF patients treated with NIV, but the difference was not significant, probably because the sample population in this patient subgroup was too small. Mortality in the ICU was similar in the NIV and standard treatment groups.

Because not all patients with COPD can be treated with NIV, some will ultimately require ETI and conventional mechanical ventilation. Nava and colleagues showed that switching to NIV after 48 h of mechanical ventilation definitively shortened the duration of invasive mechanical ventilation (Nava et al. 1998). This approach increased the weaning success rate and reduced the time in the ICU, with a better survival at day 60 (92% vs 72%) compared with a standard approach. Girault et al. repeated the study and found again a reduction in the duration of ETI (Girault et al. 1999). They found, however, that the total duration of ventilation (including mask ventilation) was increased by this approach. Further studies are therefore needed concerning this indication.

21.7 Patients with Contraindications to Endotracheal Intubation and Those Who Failed an Extubation Attempt

In cases of end-stage pulmonary disease (e.g., severe chronic obstructive lung disease, pulmonary fibrosis, lung cancer), lung function will eventually deteriorate to a point where invasive mechanical ventilatory support may only prolong the unavoidable process of dying. More often, however, respiratory failure is due to a reversible condition (e.g., congestive heart failure, bronchospasm, and pneumonia) that can be corrected if the patient is supported with NIV during treatment of an acute event.

Several reports have described the application of NPPV for patients with ARF who are poor candidates for ETI for a variety of reasons: advanced age or poor physiologic reserve, patients with advanced disease and those with "do not resuscitate" directives (Benhamou et al. 1992; Meduri et al. 1994). The overall success rate in these reports is around 60%–70%. Successfully treated patients rapidly improved with regard to gas exchange. Even when respiratory failure does not resolve, NIV can be effective in providing symptomatic relief of dyspnoea. Although indiscriminate use of NIV in patients with advanced disease is not justifiable, individual needs should be taken into careful consideration by the responsible physician.

Lastly, several reports and a case-control study suggested that NIV could be useful to avoid reintubation in patients developing respiratory distress after extubation (Hilbert et al. 1998). Again, prospective studies are needed to better delineate the role of NIV in this indication.

21.8 Impact of NIV on Nosocomial Infection

The occurrence of nosocomial infections is a major source of morbidity and mortality in critically ill patients. Among the various risk factors for acquiring an infection in the ICU, the use of invasive devices such as intravenous catheters, urinary catheters, and endotracheal tubes is the leading factor. Whereas many of these devices cannot be avoided in the routine care of the patients, NIV may be a way to deliver ventilation through a face mask and avoid one of the major risk factors for pneumonia. This approach may reduce the risk of nosocomial pneumonia because it does not bypass the natural barriers provided by the upper airways, and it reduces the duration of mechanical assistance, the need for sedation, and the length of stay in the ICU. In addition, the global invasiveness of care is usually reduced in patients treated with NIV.

The beneficial impact of this technique on nosocomial infections has been suggested by several prospective randomised trials. In the randomised controlled trial of patients with COPD carried out by Brochard et al., NIV reduced the total number of complications associated with mechanical ventilation, and the rate of nosocomial pneumonia was reduced from 17% to 5% (Brochard et al. 1995). Using NIV as a means of shortening the duration of invasive mechanical ventilation, Nava et al. found that no patient developed nosocomial pneumonia, versus 28% in the group weaned invasively (Nava et al. 1998). Antonelli et al. showed that nosocomial sinusitis and pneumonia were significantly reduced by the use of NIV (Antonelli et al. 1998). Other large series also found a decreased incidence of infections with NIV, by means of multivariate analysis including all patients supported by either invasive or noninvasive techniques of ventilatory support (Nourdine et al. 1999). To address the question of the impact of NIV applied in routine practice, Girou et al. performed a matched case-control study (Girou et al. 2000). Indeed, over the past few years there has been a progressive increase in the frequency of use of NIV. Therefore, during this period the number of patients eligible for NIV who were effectively ventilated noninvasively also increased significantly. A total of 56 patients treated with NIV were compared with 56 mechanically ventilated patients matched on diagnosis and severity. The incidences of nosocomial infections and of nosocomial pneumonia were significantly lower among the NIV patients (18% vs 68% and 7% vs 23%, $p<0.03$). Similarly, the daily risk of acquiring an infection, the proportion of patients receiving antibiotics, the duration of ventilation and of ICU stay, and the crude mortality (4% vs 25%, $p=0.002$) were all lower among NIV patients. A multivariate analysis identified NIV as an independent factor linked with a reduced probability of nosocomial pneumonia and death in COPD patients.

21.9 Current Use of Noninvasive Ventilation

Together with the French Society of Intensive Care Medicine (SRLF), we undertook a prospective survey in 42 French ICUs (Carlucci et al. 2001). All the patients who required ventilatory support were included: 581 had ETI and conventional mechanical ventilation (i.e. ETI group) and 108 had NIV: the latter represented 16% of all patients and 35% of the patients admitted without ETI in the ICUs and needing ventilatory support. NIV was never used in patients with coma; it was used in fewer than 20% of all hypoxaemic ARF patients, and in half of the patients with hypercapnic respiratory failure. In 40% of cases, NIV was followed by ETI. There was a lower incidence of nosocomial pneumonia in the NIV group (8%) vs the ETI group (20%), $p<0.01$. A logistic regression analysis showed that the need for ETI (initial and/or secondary) was the major risk factor for nosocomial pneumonia. The mortality was also significantly lower in the NIV vs the ETI group ($p=0.002$). Multiple regression analysis found SAPS II, MacCabe score, and hypoxaemic ARF to be the risk factors explaining mortality. The success of NIV was an independent protective factor ($p=0.002$). In the NIV group, SAPS II and a poor clinical tolerance (assessed by a semi-quantitative score) were factors predictive of the need for secondary ETI. In conclusion, NIV was used in 35% of the nonintubated patients admitted to the ICUs when ventilatory support was required, but it was followed by ETI in 40% of cases. When successful, however, NIV was associated with a lower risk of pneumonia and death. Technical improvements and better management to increase tolerance seem necessary for a higher success rate.

21.10 Conclusion

NIV can be extremely effective in reversing severe physiological abnormalities observed in frank hypercapnic ventilatory failure, such as those observed in acute-on-chronic respiratory failure. Its use may reduce the need for ETI and improve the outcome of such patients. It may also be useful in selected group of patients with hypoxaemic respiratory failure, although selection of patients and administration of the ventilatory support may prove to be more difficult in this group. Lastly, motivation of the staff and education of the personnel are essential for the success of the technique.

Acknowledgements. The authors thank Florence Picot for typing the manuscript.

21.11 References

Antonelli M, Conti G, Rocco M, Bufi M, De Blasi RA, Vivino G, Gasparetto A, Meduri GU (1998) A comparison of noninvasive positive-pressure ventilation and conventional mechanical ventilation in patients with acute respiratory failure. N Engl J Med 339:429–435

Antonelli M, Conti G, Bufi M, Costa M, Lappa A, Rocco M, Gasparetto A, Meduri G (2000) Noninvasive ventilation for treatment of acute respiratory failure in patients undergoing solid organ transplantation: a randomized trial. JAMA 283:235–241

Appendini L, Patessio A, Zanaboni S, Carone M, Gukov B, Donner CF, Rossi A (1994) Physiologic effects of positive end-expiratory pressure and mask pressure support during exacerbations of chronic obstructive pulmonary disease. Am J Respir Crit Care Med 149:1069–1076

Aslanian P, El Atrous S, Isabey D, Valente E, Corsi D, Harf A, Lemaire F, Brochard L (1998) Effects of flow triggering on breathing effort during partial ventilatory support. Am J Respir Crit Care Med 157:135–143

Benhamou D, Girault C, Faure C, Portier F, Muir JF (1992) Nasal mask ventilation in acute respiratory failure. Experience in elderly patients. Chest 102:912–917

Bersten AD, Holt AW, Vedig AE, Skowronski GA, Baggely CJ (1991) Treatment of severe cardiogenic pulmonary edema with continuous positive airway pressure delivered by face mask. N Engl J Med 325:1825–1830

Bott J, Carroll MP, Conway JH, Klilty SEJ, Ward EM, Brown AM, Paul EA, Elliott MW, Godfrey RC, Wedzicha JA, et al (1993) Randomised controlled trial of nasal ventilation in acute ventilatory failure due to chronic obstructive airways disease. Lancet 341:1555–1557

Brochard L, Isabey D, Piquet J, Amaro P, Mancebo J, Messadi AA, Brun-Buisson C, Rauss A, Lemaire F, Harf A (1990) Reversal of acute exacerbations of chronic obstructive lung disease by inspiratory assistance with a face mask. N Engl J Med 323:1523–1530

Brochard L, Mancebo J, Wysocki M, Lofaso F, Conti G, Rauss A, Simonneau G, Benito S, Gasparetto A, Lemaire F, et al (1995) Noninvasive ventilation for acute exacerbations of chronic obstructive pulmonary disease. N Engl J Med 333:817–822

Buda AJ, Pinsky MR, Ingels NB, Daughters GT, Stinson EB, Alderman EL (1979) Effect of intrathoracic pressure on left ventricular performance. N Engl J Med 301:453–59

Bunburaphong T, Imanaka H, Nishimura M, Hess D, Kacmarek RM (1997) Performance characteristic of bilevel pressure ventilators: a lung model study. Chest 111:1050–1060

Calderini E, Confalonieri M, Puccio PG, Francavilla N, Stella L, Gregoretti C (1999) Patient-ventilator asynchrony during noninvasive ventilation: the role of expiratory trigger. Intensive Care Med 25:662–667

Carlucci A, Richard JC, Wysocki M, Lepage E, Brochard L, and the SRLF collaborative group on mechanical ventilation (2001) Noninvasive versus conventional mechanical ventilation. An epidemiological survey. Am J Respir Crit Care Med 163:874–880

Carrey Z, Gottfried SB, Levy RD (1990) Ventilatory muscle support in respiratory failure with nasal positive pressure ventilation. Chest 97:150–158

Confalonieri M, Potena A, Carbone G, Della Porta R, Tolley E, Meduri G (1999) Acute respiratory failure in patients with severe community-acquired pneumonia. A prospective randomized evaluation of noninvasive ventilation. Am J Respir Crit Care Med 160:1585–1591

Corrado A, Bruscoli G, Messori A, et al (1992) Iron lung treatment of subjects with COPD in acute respiratory failure. Evaluation of short- and long-term prognosis. Chest 101:692–696

Corrado A, Gorini M, Villella G, De Paola E (1996) Negative pressure ventilation in the treatment of acute respiratory failure: an old noninvasive technique reconsidered. Eur Respir J 9:1531–1544

Corrado A, Gorini M, Ginanni R, Pelagatti C, Villella G, Buoncristiano U, Guidi F, Pagni E, Peris A, De Paola E (1998) Negative pressure ventilation versus conventional mechanical ventilation in the treatment of acute respiratory failure in COPD patients. Eur Respir J 12:519–525

Delclaux C, L'Her E, Alberti C, Mancebo J, Abroug F, Conti G, Guérin C, Schortgen F, Lefort Y, Antonelli M, et al (2000) Treatment of acute hypoxemic nonhypercapnic respiratory insufficiency with continuous positive airway pressure delivered by a face mask. A randomized controlled trial. JAMA 284:2352–2360

Diaz O, Iglesias R, Ferrer M, Zavala E, Santos C, Wagner PD, Roca J, Rodriguez-Roisin R (1997) Effects of noninvasive ventilation on pulmonary gas exchange and hemodynamics during acute hypercapnic exacerbations of chronic obstructive pulmonary disease. Am J Respir Crit Care Med 156:1840–1845

Ferguson GT, Gilmartin M (1995) CO_2 rebreathing during BiPAP ventilatory assistance. Am J Respir Crit Care Med 151:1126–1135

Fernandez R, Blanch L, Valles J, Baigorri F, Artigas A (1993) Pressure support ventilation via face mask in acute respiratory failure in hypercapnic COPD patients. Intensive Care Med 19:456–461

Girault C, Richard JC, Chevron V, Tamion F, Pasquis P, Leroy J, Bonmarchand G (1997) Comparative physiologic effects of noninvasive assist-control and pressure support ventilation in acute hypercapnic respiratory failure. Chest 111:1639–1648

Girault C, Daudenthun I, Chevron V, Tamion F, Leroy J, Bonmarchand G (1999) Noninvasive ventilation as a systematic extubation and weaning technique in acute on chronic respiratory failure. A prospective, randomized controlled study. Am J Respir Crit Care Med 160:86–92

Girou E, Schortgen F, Delclaux C, Brun-Buisson C, Blot F, Lefort Y, Lemaire F, Brochard L (2000) Association of noninvasive ventilation with nosocomial infections and survival in critically ill patients. JAMA 284:2361–2367

Goldberg P, Reissmann H, Maltais F, Ranieri M, Gottfried SB (1995) Efficacy of noninvasive CPAP in COPD with acute respiratory failure. Eur Respir J 8:1894–1900

Hilbert G, Gruson D, Portel L, Gbikpi-Benissan G, Cardinaud JP (1998) Noninvasive pressure support ventilation in COPD patients with postextubation hypercapnic respiratory insufficiency. Eur Respir J 11:1349–1353

Hoffmann B, Welte T (1999) The use of noninvasive pressure support ventilation for severe respiratory insufficiency due to pulmonary oedema. Intensive Care Med 25:15–20

Jaber S, Fodil R, Carlucci A, Boussarsar M, Pigeot J, Lemaire F, Harf A, Lofaso F, Isabey D, Brochard L (2000) Noninvasive ventilation with helium-oxygen in acute exacerbations of chronic obstructive pulmonary disease. Am J Respir Crit Care Med 161:1191–1200

Jolliet P, Tassaux D, Thouret JM, Chevrolet JC (1999) Beneficial effects of helium:oxygen versus air:oxygen noninvasive pressure support in patients with decompensated chronic obstructive pulmonary disease. Crit Care Med 27:2422–2429

Kramer N, Meyer TJ, Meharg J, Cece RD, Hill NS (1995) Randomized, prospective trial of noninvasive positive pressure ventilation in acute respiratory failure. Am J Respir Crit Care Med 151:1799–1806

Lenique F, Habis M, Lofaso F, Dubois-Randé JL, Harf A, Brochard L (1997) Ventilatory and hemodynamic effects of continuous positive airway pressure in left heart failure. Am J Respir Crit Care Med 155:500–505

L'Her E, Moriconi M, Texier F, Bouquin V, Kaba L, Renault A, Garo B, Boles JM (1998) Non-invasive continuous positive airway pressure in acute hypoxaemic respiratory failure – experience of an emergency department. Eur J Emerg Med 5:313–318

Lin M, Yang YF, Chiang HT, Chang MS, Chiang BN, Cheitlin MD (1995) Reappraisal of continuous positive airway pressure therapy in acute cardiogenic pulmonary edema. Short-term results and long-term follow-up. Chest 107:1379–1386

Lofaso F, Brochard L, Hang T, Touchard D, Harf A, Isabey D (1995) Evaluation of carbon dioxide rebreathing during pressure support with BiPAP devices. Chest 108:772–778

Lofaso F, Brochard L, Hang T, Lorino H, Harf A, Isabey D (1996) Home vs intensive-care pressure support devices : experimental and clinical comparison. Am J Respir Crit Care Med 153:1591–9

Lofaso F, Aslanian P, Richard JC, Isabey D, Hang T, Corriger E, Harf A, Brochard L (1998) Expiratory valves used for home devices: experimental and clinical comparison. Eur Respir J 11:1382–1388

Mancebo J, Isabey D, Lorino H, Lofaso F, Lemaire F, Brochard L (1995) Comparative effects of pressure support ventilation and intermittent positive pressure breathing (IPPB) in non-intubated healthy subjects. Eur Respir J 8:1901–1909

Martin TJ, Hovis JD, Costantino JP, Bierman MI, Donahoe MP, Rogers RM, Kreit JW, Sciurba FC, Stiller RA, Sanders MH (2000) A randomized, prospective evaluation of noninvasive ventilation for acute respiratory failure. Am J Respir Crit Care Med 161:807–813

Masip J, Betbesé A, Paez J, Vecilla F, R C, Padro J, Paz M, de Otero J, Ballus J (2000) Non-invasive pressure support ventilation versus conventional oxygen therapy in acute cardiogenic pulmonary oedema: a randomised trial. Lancet 356:2126–2132

Meduri GU, Fox RC, Abou-Shala N, Leeper KV, Wunderink RG (1994) Noninvasive mechanical ventilation via face mask in patients with acute respiratory failure who refused endotracheal intubation. Crit Care Med 22:1584–1590

Meduri GU, Turner RE, Abou-Shala N, Wunderink R, Tolley E (1996) Noninvasive positive pressure ventilation via face mask. First-line intervention in patients with acute hypercapnic and hypoxemic respiratory failure. Chest 109:179–193

Mehta S, Gregory DJ, Woolard RH, Hipona RA, Connolly EM, Cimini DM, Drinkwine JH, Hill NS (1997) Randomized, prospective trial of bilevel versus continuous positive airway pressure in acute pulmonary edema. Crit Care Med 25:620–628

Miro AM, Shivaram U, Hertig I (1993) Continuous positive airway pressure in COPD patients in acute respiratory failure. Chest 103:266–268

Nava S, Ambrosino N, Rubini F, Fracchia C, Rampulla C, Torri G, Calderini E (1993) Effect of nasal pressure support ventilation and external PEEP on diaphragmatic activity in patients with severe stable COPD. Chest 103:143–150

Nava S, Bruschi C, Rubini F, Palo A, Iotti G, Braschi A (1995) Respiratory response and inspiratory effort during pressure support ventilation in COPD patients. Intensive Care Med 21: 871–879

Nava S, Ambrosino N, Bruschi C, Confalonieri M, Rampulla C (1997a) Physiological effects of flow and pressure triggering during non-invasive mechanical ventilation in patients with chronic obstructive pulmonary disease. Thorax 52:249–254

Nava S, Evangelisti I, Rampulla C, Compagnoni ML, Fracchia C, Rubini F (1997b) Human and financial costs of noninvasive mechanical ventilation in patients affected by COPD and acute respiratory failure. Chest 111:1631–1638

Nava S, Ambrosino N, Clini E, Prato M, Orlando G, Vitacca M, Brigada P, Fracchia C, Rubini F (1998) Noninvasive mechanical ventilation in the weaning of patients with respiratory failure due to chronic obstructive pulmonary disease. A randomized, controlled trial. Ann Intern Med 128:721–728

Navalesi P, Fanfulla F, Frigerio P, Gregoretti C, Nava S (2000) Physiologic evaluation of noninvasive mechanical ventilation delivered with three types of masks in patients with chronic hypercapnic respiratory failure. Crit Care Med 28:1785–1790

Nourdine K, Combes P, Carton M, Beuret P, Cannamela A, Ducreux J (1999) Does noninvasive ventilation reduce the ICU nosocomial infection risk? A prospective clinical survey. Intensive Care Med 25:567–573

Patrick W, Webster K, Ludwig L, Roberts D, Wiebe P, Younes M (1996) Noninvasive positive-pressure ventilation in acute respiratory distress without prior chronic respiratory failure. Am J Respir Crit Care Med 153:1005–1011

Petrof BJ, Legaré M, Goldberg P, Milic-Emili J, Gottfried SB (1990) Continuous positive airway pressure reduces work of breathing and dyspnea during weaning from mechanical ventilation in severe chronic obstructive pulmonary disease (COPD). Am Rev Resp Dis 141: 281–289

Plant P, Owen J, Elliott M (2000) Early use of non-invasive ventilation for acute exacerbations of chronic obstructive pulmonary disease on general respiratory wards: a multicentre randomised controlled trial. Lancet 355:1931–1935

Räsänen J, Heikkilä J, Downs J, Nikki P, Vaisänen IT, Viitanen A (1985) Continuous positive airway pressure by face mask in acute cardiogenic pulmonary edema. Am J Cardiol 55:296–300

Richards G, Cistulli P, Ungar R, Berthon-Jones M, Sullivan C (1996) Mouth leak with nasal continuous positive airway pressure increases nasal airway resistance. Am J Respir Crit Care Med 154:182–186

Rusterholtz T, Kempf J, Berton C, Gayol S, Tournoud C, Zaehringer M, Jaeger A, Sauder P (1999) Noninvasive pressure support ventilation (NIPSV) with face mask in patients with acute cardiogenic pulmonary edema. Intensive Care Med :21–28

Smith TC, Marini JJ (1988) Impact of PEEP on lung mechanics and work of breathing in severe airflow obstruction. J Appl Physiol 65:1488–1499

Soo Hoo GW, Santiago S, Williams AJ (1994) Nasal mechanical ventilation for hypercapnic respiratory failure in chronic obstructive pulmonary disease: determinants of success and failure. Crit Care Med 22:1253–1261

Thorens JB, Ritz M, Reynard C, Righetti A, Vallotton M, Favre H, Kyle U, Jolliet P, Chevrolet JC (1997) Haemodynamic and endocrinological effects of noninvasive mechanical ventilation in respiratory failure. Eur Respir J 10:2553–2559

Vitacca M, Rubini F, Foglio K, Scalvani S, Nava S, Ambrosino N (1993) Noninvasive modalities of positive pressure ventilation improve the outcome of acute exacerbations in COLD patients. Intensive Care Med 19:450–455

Warren PM, Flenley DC, Millar JC, Avery A (1980) Respiratory failure revisited: acute exacerbations of chronic bronchitis between 1961–1968 and 1970–1976. Lancet 1:467–471

Wood KA, Lewis L, Von Harz B, Kollef MH (1998) The use of noninvasive positive pressure ventilation in the emergency department: results of a randomized clinical trial. Chest 113:1339–1346

22 Unplanned Extubation

A.J. Betbesé and J. Mancebo

22.1 Introduction

Unplanned extubation is defined as the expulsion of the endotracheal tube. It may be deliberate, e.g., as a result of patient agitation or lack of cooperation, or accidental, e.g., due to rupture of the endotracheal cuff, nursing procedures such as change of position or washing, X-ray procedures, coughing, or other unintentional events.

Endotracheal intubation has been routine practice for intensivists since the introduction of mechanical ventilation. However, although endotracheal intubation and mechanical ventilation are lifesaving techniques, they may potentially increase the risk of complications [1–4]. One of the most frequent of these, related to the tube itself, is endotracheal unplanned extubation (EUE), estimated to occur in 8.5%–13% of intubated mechanically ventilated patients [1, 5–7]. Moreover, EUE is a potentially serious complication, as some patients may need reintubation while in a very poor clinical condition, which may account for an increase in morbidity and even mortality [6–14]. Factors contributing to unplanned extubation are not well understood. In this review of the literature we discuss incidence, factors predisposing to unplanned extubation, and prognostic factors in the reintubation of self-extubated patients. Table 22.1 shows the most recent and complete studies on unplanned extubations.

22.2 Studies of Unplanned Extubation

In a multicentric study performed in multidisciplinary and medical intensive care units over a 2-month period, Boulain et al. [8] recorded 57 episodes of self-extubation in 46 patients from a total of 426 mechanically ventilated patients, representing an incidence of 10.8% unplanned extubations; 61% of these patients required reintubation. The percentage of reintubations following EUE was higher than the reintubation rate for non-self-extubated patients (10%), but a significant difference was found when comparing the reintubation rate between patients with chronic respiratory failure (88%) and patients without chronic respiratory failure (43%). Chronic respiratory failure, endotracheal tube fixation with only thin adhesive tape, orotracheal intubation, and the lack of intravenous sedation were identified as factors contributing to unplanned extubation. Two patients

Table 22.1. Description of the most important items in unplanned extubation studies

Reference	Setting	Study type, length (months)	n	(%)	Incidence (100p-vd)	Reintubation (%)	Factors for EUE	Factors for reintubation	DSE (%)	ASE (%)	Complications	Deaths
[5]	Medical-surgical	Prospective	29	13	–	–	–	–	–	–	–	–
[8]	Eleven hospitals, medical-surgical	Prospective, 2	57	10.8	1.4	61	CRF; lack strong fixation ETT; orotracheal intubation	CRF	72	28	Pneumonia; laryngeal edema; cardiac arrest	Yes
[11]	Multidisciplinary	Retrospective	81	–	–	48	–	>6 assisted breaths/min; pH>7.45; PaO$_2$/FiO$_2$ <250; highest heart rate>120; mental status other than alert; 3 or more factors	–	–	Aspiration; tachycardia; bradycardia; bronchospasm; difficult orotracheal intubation	No
[1]	Multidisciplinary	Prospective, 5	30	8.5	–	47	–	–	–	–	Pneumonia	–
[7]	Multidisciplinary	Prospective, 12	12	11	2.6	31	Age (older); sex (male)	–	77	23	Tachycardia; hypotension	No
[9]	Medical	Retrospective, 24	23	7	–	78	–	Pulmonary disease; FiO$_2$>0.4; VE>7 l/min	91.3	8.7	–	–
[19]	Medical-surgical	Prospective, 18	102	14	–	88	–	–	39	61	–	–

Table 22.1. *Continued.*

Reference	Setting	Study type, length (months)	n	(%)	Incidence (100p-vd)	Reintubation (%)	Factors for EUE	Factors for reintubation	DSE (%)	ASE (%)	Complications	Deaths
[24]	Medical-surgical	Case-control, prospective, 12	50; 100 controls	–	–	74	Smoker; nosocomial infection; medical patient; ICU length; hospital length; agitation	–	–	–	Laryngeal or vocal trauma; ventricular tachycardia; aspiration	No
[25]	Medical	Case-control, prospective, 15	66	15.9	–	34.8	Orotracheal intubation; Ramsay≥2	Glasgow <11; PaO$_2$/FiO$_2$<200; accidental EUE	87.1	13.9	Stridor; Arrhythmias	Yes
[10]	Multidisciplinary	Prospective, 8	76	9.1	–	–	–	–	–	–	–	–
[22]	–	Retrospective, 36	153	9.3	–	49	–	–	68	28	–	–
[23]	Multidisciplinary	Prospective, 4	13	3	–	46	–	VE>14 l/min; Days of orotracheal intubation	92.3	7.7	–	No
[6]	Medical	Prospective, 8	27	12	–	74	CRF	–	77.8	22.2	Pulmonary edema; Cardiac arrest; Laryngeal bleeding	Yes
[28]	Multidisciplinary	Prospective, 32	59	7.3	–	45.8	–	Weaning; DMV	77.9	22.1	–	No

(%) percentage of unplanned extubation episodes; *n*, Number of episodes of endotracheal self-extubation; *100 p-vd*, incidence of unplanned extubation in 100 patient-ventilator days; *EUE*, endotracheal unplanned extubation; *DSE*, deliberate self-extubation; *ASE*, accidental self-extubation; *CRF*, chronic respiratory failure; *ETT*, endotracheal tube; *VE*, minute ventilation; *DMV*, days of mechanical ventilation.

self-extubated four times, which suggests that patients who do so once are at risk of self-extubating again. Several authors recommend the routine use of hand and/or thorax restraints in the case of patients likely to self-extubate. Although nosocomial pneumonia is one of the most common complications of reintubation following self-extubation, in this study no statistical differences were observed in the incidence of this event between patients with EUE (8.7%) and non-EUE (5.8%). The mortality was not affected by self-extubation.

Levy et al. [15] compared four different methods of securing the endotracheal tube, evaluating tube migration, patient comfort, oral hygiene, and skin integrity, as well as nurses' or respiratory therapists' maintenance time. This study concluded that adhesive tape and twill tape were more effective than bite blockers. Tominaga et al. [16] described a decrease in accidental unplanned extubation with the use of water-resistant tape to secure endotracheal tubes and routine use of hand restraints. In this case, hospital policy limited the use of hand restraints for ethical reasons. Accidental self-extubation increased from 2% (use of waterproof tape, hand restraints, and adequate sedation) to 6% after hand restraints were restricted owing to ethical problems. Hand restraints presented an ethical problem in some intensive care units. In 1992, the Food and Drug Administration published an article alerting health professionals to concerns raised by increased reports of injuries and deaths associated with the incorrect use of protective restraint devices [17].

Listello et al. [11] retrospectively recorded 81 incidents of EUE; reintubation was required in 48% of these cases, most (85%) in the first hour. They found that the majority of EUEs occurred at night. Five patients self-extubated twice and two patients three times, similar to data observed in Boulain's study [8]. These authors describe a model that correctly predicted reintubation in 92% of cases when the presence of four or more of the following seven predictive factors was verified:

1. Assist-controlled ventilation or synchronous intermittent mandatory ventilation at a rate over 6/min
2. pH before EUE 7.45 or greater
3. PaO_2/FiO_2 below 250 mm Hg
4. Highest heart rate 24 h before EUE above 120 beats/min
5. Presence of three or more coexisting medical disorders
6. Mental status other than alert
7. Indication for intubation other than preoperative

The presence of three of these factors correctly predicted reintubation in 83%. Following this retrospective period, the model was validated in the new cases of EUE with a correct prediction of 75%.

Quality-control programs seem to be extremely effective in decreasing the rate of EUE. One month after prospectively recording EUE, Maguire et al. [18] designed a corrective action plan to teach nurses and house staff about the problem of EUE, with daily assessment on rounds of patient risk (anxiety, history of previous EUE, and routine care intervention) of EUE and careful documentation of the EUE episodes. Follow-up revealed a significant reduction in the EUE rate, but not total elimination. Similarly, Carrión et al. [19] designed a prospective, observational and interventional study in three consecutive 6-month periods. Following the first and second periods, information about unplanned removal of tubes and lines and instructions for greater vigilance were given, the ETT position at teeth was marked, and specific measures such as limiting upper extremity access to 20 cm from tubes or lines were introduced. This educational program significantly reduced the deliberate EUE rate. Some articles demonstrate that the duration of weaning and mechanical ventilatory support was reduced when a protocol for weaning from mechanical ventilation was applied [20, 21]. Chiang et al. [10] concluded that a continuous quality-improvement program was effective in reducing the overall incidence of unplanned endotracheal extubation. The major components of the program were the organization of a multidisciplinary task force (including intensivists, respiratory therapists, and nursing staff), collection of all pertinent data regarding all episodes of unplanned extubation, standardization of procedures such as hand restraints or securing of the endotracheal tube, avoidance of delayed extubation using weaning protocols, and development of guidelines for the use of sedatives and actions to solve identified problems. In their 3-year study, Soni et al. [22] concluded that the incidence of unplanned extubations can be decreased significantly by means of teaching and frequent in-service training of staff, although the problem cannot be eliminated completely. Tindol et al. [23] documented a low incidence of EUE and attributed this to staff vigilance and nasal intubation. Other studies, however, found orotracheal intubation to be a risk factor in a greater number of unplanned extubations [8].

Other studies have tried to find prognostic factors associated with unplanned extubation using case-control subjects. In one such study performed by Atkins et al. [24], self-extubated patients were compared with two control subjects, based on gender, age, primary discharge diagnosis, and time of hospitalization. The comparison showed that those who self-extubated were smokers and more likely to be medical rather than surgical patients. Other factors associated with self-extubation were an abnormal blood urea nitrogen (below 10 or above 50 mg/dl), abnormal $PaCO_2$ (below 20 or above 50 mmHg), agitation, and physical restraint (in this case, the physical restraints were probably applied because of agitation). Patients who suffered an unplanned extubation needed more frequent reintubation, and the length of stay in the ICU and in hospital was longer. The reintubation rate was 74% in the self-extubated group, while none of the controls needed reintubation after elective extubation; this seems to indicate that this control group was probably slowly weaned. No differences in mortality were found.

Chevron et al. [25] designed a prospective case-control study. In the first phase, lasting 10 months, 40 EUEs occurred (incidence 14%) and these patients were compared with 74 ventilated controls. Patients with EUE presented a Ramsay score of 1 in 60% of cases while the Ramsay score in control subjects was ≥2 in 81% of cases; physical restraints were used in 74% of EUE patients but in only 55% of controls; and the route of intubation was oral in 33% of EUE patients but in only 15% of controls. Surprisingly, in contrast with the previous report by Atkins et al., the control group had a longer duration of mechanical ventilation and more days of hospitalization. The data obtained by Chevron et al. might also indicate that intubation and mechanical ventilation were unduly prolonged in the control group. These last results show that it is indeed difficult to define factors associated with EUE, probably because EUE depends on the type of patient (medical or surgical), the patient:nurse ratio, the guidelines used to administer sedatives, the protocol employed to wean patients from mechanical ventilation, and the use of restraints, among other factors.

Although it is reasonable to assume that the nursing workload could play an important role in predicting EUE, in this study by Chevron et al., statistical differences between EUE and controls were not established. The second phase of the study compared those patients with EUE requiring reintubation with those who did not. Mortality was 39% in reintubated patients, compared with 2.6% of patients who were not reintubated. Glasgow Coma Score below 11, PaO_2/FiO_2 under 200 mmHg, and accidental extubation were the factors that logistic regression analysis defined as independent predictors of reintubation.

Reintubation after EUE should not be considered mandatory in every patient who presents with an EUE, and noninvasive mechanical ventilation could avoid some reintubations, probably in patients with chronic obstructive pulmonary disease [26]. On the other hand FiO_2 ≤0.4 seems to predict a lack of need for reintubation of EUE patients [9].

Recently, Epstein et al. [27] performed a case-control study involving 75 patients with unplanned extubation and 150 patients as controls matched for APACHE II score, presence of co-morbid conditions, age, indication for mechanical ventilation, and gender. They conclude that unplanned extubation is not associated with increased mortality when compared with matched controls, although they observed an increase in days of mechanical ventilation, ICU, and hospital stay, and in need for chronic care in the unplanned extubation group. When mortality was compared between the group that needed reintubation and the group that did not, they observed an increase in mortality in the reintubated unplanned extubation group. They also observed statistical differences regarding the need for reintubation on comparing patients in weaning trials (44%) and those with full ventilatory support (76%). These data are similar to ours.

We designed a prospective study [28] of unplanned extubation over a 32-month period. Fifty-nine episodes of EUE were observed in 55 of 750 patients (frequency 7.3%) who required mechanical intubation for more than 48 h from a total of 1085 patients admitted to our ICU. EUEs were deliberate in 77.9% and accidental in 22.1%. Twenty-seven episodes (45.8%) occurred in patients on full mechanical ventilatory support and 32 (54.2%) during the period of weaning from mechanical ventilation. This parameter had not been studied previously, and we observed that it played an important role in determining the subsequent need for reintubation.

The results of our study indicate that the need for reintubation after an episode of EUE depends mainly on whether or not the patient is in the weaning phase of mechanical ventilation. Patients presenting EUE during weaning required significantly fewer reintubations than those who were not in weaning (odds ratio 6.6). Only 15.6% of EUE patients who were being weaned from mechanical ventilation (5/32) needed reintubation; reintubation was mandatory in 81.5% of EUE patients (22/27) receiving full mechanical ventilatory support ($p<0.001$). In view of these results, it is conceivable that the process of weaning may be longer than necessary in some patients. Indeed, at least 15% of patients being weaned from mechanical ventilation could have been extubated earlier in our study, as they did not require reintubation.

Although it has been shown that protocol-directed weaning strategies may significantly shorten the duration of mechanical ventilation, our data suggest that, at least in our institution, such strategies could be further improved, especially those concerning CPAP or a T-piece trial. Only 8.3% of patients who were being weaned with these techniques needed reintubation, whereas 37.5% of patients under weaning with pressure support were reintubated. This difference is not statistically significant, but it suggests that the duration of spontaneous breathing with a T-piece or CPAP could be shortened. Our results also indicate that a conservative attitude is advisable with respect to EUE. Reintubation was required in 27 episodes (45.8%) of EUE. The need for reintubation after EUE was 36.9% in deliberate self-extubation patients and 76.9% in accidental self-extubation patients ($p=0.01$). A multiple logistic regression analysis was performed to determine the variables independently associated with the need for reintubation: Days of mechanical ventilation were significantly associated with the need for reintubation, and weaning was associated with no need for reintubation. The model correctly classified the need for reintubation in 84.7% of cases (50/59). These data suggest that some patients are under mechanical ventilation longer than necessary.

The rather high level of accidental EUE (22.1%) found in our study decreased significantly after these results were published and new strategies were applied to solve the problem. In the past 12 months only two accidental EUEs from a total of 20 episodes of EUE (10%) have been reported. This decreased incidence of EUE confirms the assumption that quality-control programs reduce complications of mechanical ventilation. Reintubation was needed following these two accidental EUEs, and these patients were under full mechanical ventilatory support. Reintubation was needed in 9/18 (50%) of deliberate EUEs. Only one of these nine reintubated patients who deliberately extubated was in weaning from mechanical ventilation. Although the incidence of reintubation in this group seems low, the use of noninvasive mechanical ventilation avoided reintubation in three of the nine non-reintubated patients.

22.3 Conclusion

In order to decrease the number of unplanned extubations greater vigilance is recommended during daily procedures such as positional changes, washing, and X-rays. Marking the position of tubing at the teeth, use of sedation scales, careful endotracheal tube fixation, clinical assessment of weaning from mechanical ventilation at least once per day, by means of an institutional protocol, more surveillance of the high-risk self-extubation patients (such as agitated patients, patients with a prior unplanned extubation, history of alcoholism, or chronic obstructive pulmonary disease), and use of hand restraints when appropriate could also reduce accidental unplanned extubations. Finally, in our opinion, it seems that the incidence of unplanned extubation can also be used as an indicator of quality nursing and medical care in most intensive care units: a high incidence of EUE and a low incidence of reintubation of these patients seems to indicate that patients are slowly weaned from mechanical ventilatory support. On the other hand, a high incidence of accidental EUE seems to indicate that improvements are needed in clinical care.

Acknowledgements. We acknowledge Ms. Carolyn Newey for her translation of the manuscript.

22.4 References

1. Zwillich CW, et al (1974) Complications of assisted ventilation: a prospective study of 354 consecutive episodes. Am J Med 57:161–170
2. Craven DE, et al (1986) Risk factors for pneumonia and fatality in patients receiving continuous mechanical ventilation. Am Rev Respir Dis 133:792–796
3. Torres A, et al (1990) Incidence, risk, and prognosis factors of nosocomial pneumonia in mechanically ventilated patients. Am Rev Respir Dis 142:523–528
4. Levine SA, Niederman MS (1991) The impact of tracheal intubation on host defenses and risks for nosocomial pneumonia. Clin Chest Med 12:523–543
5. Stauffer JL, et al (1981) Complications and consequences of endotracheal intubation and tracheotomy: a prospective study of 150 critically ill adult patients. Am J Med 70:65–76
6. Vassal T, et al (1993) Prospective evaluation of self-extubations in a medical intensive care unit. Intensive Care Med 19:340–342
7. Coppolo DP, May JJ (1990) Self-extubations: a 12-month experience. Chest 98:165–169
8. Boulain T and the Association des Réanimateurs de Centre-Ouest (1998) Unplanned extubations in the adult intensive care unit. Am J Respir Crit Care Med 157:1131–1137
9. Whelan Jet, al (1994) Unplanned extubation. Predictors of successful termination of mechanical ventilatory support. Chest 105:1808–1812
10. Chiang AA, et al (1996) Effectiveness of a continuous quality improvement program aiming to reduce unplanned extubation: a prospective study. Intensive Care Med 22:1269–1271
11. Listello D, Sessler CN (1994) Unplanned extubation. Clinical predictors for reintubation. Chest 105:1496–1503
12. Little LA, et al (1990) Factors affecting accidental extubations in neonatal and pediatric intensive care patients. Crit Care Med 18:163–165
13. Christie JM, et al (1996) Unplanned endotracheal extubation in the intensive care unit. J Clin Anesth 8:289–293
14. Scott PH, et al (1985) Predictability and consequences of spontaneous extubation in a pediatric ICU. Crit Care Med 13:228–232
15. Levy H, Griego L (1993) A comparative study of oral endotracheal tube securing methods. Chest 104:1537–1540
16. Tominaga GT, et al (1995) Decreasing unplanned extubations in the surgical intensive care unit. Am J Surg 170:586–590
17. Nightingale SL (1992) Warning about use of protective restraint devices. JAMA 267:1442
18. Maguire GP, et al (1994) Unplanned extubation in the intensive care unit: a quality-of-care concern. Crit Care Nurs Q 17:40–47
19. Carrión MI, et al (2000) Accidental removal of endotracheal and nasogastric tubes and intravascular catheters. Crit Care Med 28:63–66
20. Ely EW, et al (1996) Effect on the duration of mechanical ventilation of identifying patients capable of breathing spontaneously. N Engl J Med 335:1864–1869
21. Kollef MH, et al (1997) A randomized, controlled trial of protocol-directed versus physician-directed weaning from mechanical ventilation. Crit Care Med 25:567–574

22. Soni A, et al (1997) Unplanned extubations: a prospective 3-year study. Chest 112:127S
23. Tindol GA, et al (1994) Unplanned extubations. Chest 105:1804–1807
24. Atkins PM, et al (1997) Characteristics and outcomes of patients who self-extubate from ventilatory support. Chest 112:1317–1323
25. Chevron V, et al (1998) Unplanned extubation: risk factors of development and predictive criteria for reintubation. Crit Care Med 26:1049–1053
26. Wysocki M, et al (1993) Noninvasive pressure support ventilation in patients with acute respiratory failure. Chest 103:907–913
27. Epstein SK, et al (2000) Effect of unplanned extubation on outcome of mechanical ventilation. Am J Respir Crit Care Med 161:1912–1916
28. Betbesé AJ, et al (1998) A prospective study of unplanned extubation in intensive care unit patients. Crit Care Med 26:1180–1186

23 Extubation Failure: Can It Be Prevented or Predicted?

S.K. Epstein

23.1 Introduction

For the past 30 years extensive research has focused on determining readiness for weaning from mechanical ventilation (liberation) and on the mode of ventilator support that best accelerates the process of progressive withdrawal for those who prove difficult to liberate (Brochard et al. 1994; Ely et al. 1996; Esteban et al. 1995, 1997; Kollef et al. 1997). Once a patient no longer requires ventilatory support, the clinician must address a separate and distinct question. Can the patient tolerate extubation or the removal of the translaryngeal endotracheal tube? Over the past decade, the process and outcome of extubation have received increasing attention. One limiting factor is that many investigators have combined liberation and extubation failure into a single entity. In contrast, recent work clearly indicates that these are distinct processes with discrete pathophysiological causes and unique outcomes.

23.2 Frequency and Risk Factors for Extubation Failure

Extubation failure is usually represented as the number of patients requiring reinstitution of ventilatory support within 24–72 h of planned extubation divided by the total number of patients extubated. Planned extubation implies that removal of the translaryngeal endotracheal tube has occurred after the patient has satisfied specific criteria both prior to and during a spontaneous breathing trial (Brochard et al. 1994; Esteban et al. 1995, 1997, 1999a; Vallverdu et al. 1998). In contrast, few studies have utilized strict objective criteria to determine tolerance for extubation and the need for reintubation. There is also little agreement on what constitutes an acceptable extubation failure rate. Centers reporting very low rates may be needlessly keeping patients on prolonged mechanical ventilation. In contrast, high failure rates may indicate insufficient assessment prior to extubation.

Numerous factors may affect the frequency of extubation failure:

- Type of patient (e.g., medical)[a]
- Older age[a]
- Male gender[b]
- Initial severity of illness

- Indication for mechanical ventilation (e.g., etiology of acute respiratory failure)
- Use of continuous intravenous sedation[a]
- Need for transport out of the ICU[b]
- Increased duration of mechanical ventilation prior to extubation[a]
- Severity of illness at weaning onset[a]
- Duration or number of individual spontaneous breathing trials prior to extubation
- Mode of ventilator support prior to extubation
- Protocol-directed weaning

    [a] Probably related to increased frequency of extubation failure
    [b] Possibly related to increased frequency of extubation failure

The risk of extubation failure ranges from 1% to 20%, being lowest for postoperative cardiac surgical, general surgical, and trauma populations and highest for patients in medical or multidisciplinary ICUs (Daley et al. 1996; Demling et al. 1988; Ely et al. 1996; Epstein et al. 1997; Esteban et al. 1997, 1999a; Leith and Bradley 1976; Tahvanainen et al. 1983). Patients requiring reintubation tend to be older than those successfully extubated, with risk highest for patients more than 70 years old (Capdevila et al. 1995; Del Rosario et al. 1997; Engoren et al. 1999; Epstein et al. 1997; Esteban et al. 1997; Rady and Ryan 1999). Some studies have noted the highest extubation failure rates for neurological patients (Vallverdu et al. 1998), cardiac patients (Del Rosario et al. 1997; Epstein et al. 1997), or patients with COPD (Esteban et al. 1997), while other investigators have found no difference based on the etiology of acute respiratory failure.

The duration of mechanical ventilation may influence extubation failure rate because of the time-dependent effects on airway complications and ventilator-associated pneumonia. At least three studies noted a longer duration of ventilation prior to extubation in patients who failed (Del Rosario et al. 1997; Lee et al. 1994; Rady and Ryan 1999) while others have noted no difference (Capdevila et al. 1995; Epstein et al. 1997; Esteban et al. 1997; Tahvanainen et al. 1983). To date, no study has shown that a shorter duration of ventilation prior to extubation predisposes to extubation failure.

The ideal duration of an individual weaning or spontaneous breathing trial (SBT) remains a subject of controversy, with most investigators employing trials lasting 30–120 min. Too brief a trial may result in premature extubation and culminate in extubation failure. In contrast, when the work imposed by the endotracheal tube or ventilatory circuit is excessive an overly long trial could result in "iatrogenic" weaning failure. In general, extubation failure rates appear similar when studies using different trial durations are compared. In the only direct comparison, Esteban et al. randomized 526 medical and surgical patients to an initial T-piece trial of either 30 or 120 min duration and found similar 48-h reintubation rates (30 min, 13.5% vs. 120 min, 13.4%) (Esteban et al. 1999a). Another consideration is the mode of ventilation used to prior to extubation, which may influence extubation failure frequency because modes providing partial support may over-assist the patient still experiencing an imbalance between respiratory load and demand. In general, the frequency of extubation failure appears similar for unassisted and partial support modes (Brochard et al. 1994; Esteban et al. 1995; Jones et al. 1991). In a direct comparison, Esteban and colleagues found nearly identical rates of extubation failure comparing an initial 2-h T-piece trial with a 2-h trial of PSV 7 cmH$_2$O (18.5% vs 18.8%) (Esteban et al. 1997). Though further investigation is needed, these studies do not indicate that pre-extubation mode of ventilation or duration of the trial affect extubation outcome.

Protocol-directed weaning has been shown to reduce both the duration of mechanical ventilation and the duration of weaning (Ely et al. 1996; Kollef et al. 1997; Saura et al. 1996). Although Ely and colleagues noted a trend toward a lower extubation failure rate (3% vs 8%, p=0.08) comparing protocol-directed with traditional physician-directed weaning (Ely et al. 1996), three other studies were unable to confirm this observation (Horst et al. 1998; Kollef et al. 1997; Saura et al. 1996).

23.3 Etiology of Extubation Failure

Although weaning failure may result from hypoxemia or encephalopathy, the principal mechanism appears to be an imbalance between respiratory load and respiratory muscle capacity (Jubran and Tobin 1997; Vassilakopoulos et al. 1998). In addition, the change to negative pressure breathing through a T-piece can result in cardiac failure by increasing left ventricular preload and afterload (Lemaire et al. 1988). When patients are weaned with positive pressure, the change to negative intrathoracic pressure may occur only *after* extubation. This may explain why up to one third of patients fail extubation because of cardiac failure, with the incidence lowest for T-piece (Capdevila et al. 1995; Esteban et al. 1999a; Vallverdu et al. 1998) and highest for partial support modes (Epstein 1995; Epstein and Ciubotaru 1998; Tahvanainen et al. 1983). In addition to these factors, extubation failure may also result from upper airway obstruction or an inability to manage secretions, factors that become manifest only after removal of the translaryngeal endotracheal tube. Intubation can result in laryngotracheal injury, which tends to occur more frequently with increasing duration of intubation and with female gender (Epstein 2000). Similarly, laryngeal dysfunction can lead to aspiration and, together with expiratory muscle weakness and consequent ineffective cough, result in inadequate clearing of secretions from the tracheobronchial tree (Epstein 2000).

The purpose of an SBT is to ensure the absence of an imbalance between load and capacity, indicating adequate recovery and low risk for "premature extubation". Although no differences were noted when 30 and 120 min T-piece trials were compared, it may be that these durations are inadequate to fully assess the interaction between load and capacity. Alternatively, SBTs may precipitate respiratory muscle fatigue that becomes clinically detectable only after extubation. (Murciano et al. 1988)

23.4 Outcome for Extubation Failure

Recent investigations indicate that failed extubation is associated with increased hospital mortality. Mortality appears to depend upon the patient population, with rates of 10% or lower seen in trauma units and substantially higher rates (10%–43%) in general surgical, cardiothoracic surgical, or medical ICUs (Daley et al. 1996; Demling et al. 1988; Engoren et al. 1999; Epstein et al. 1997; Epstein 2000; Esteban et al. 1997, 1999a; Lee et al. 1994; Rady and Ryan 1999; Vallverdu et al. 1998). Extubation failure also results in a marked increase in the duration of mechanical ventilation, ICU and hospital stay, and need for tracheostomy (Daley et al. 1996; Epstein and Ciubotaru 1998; Esteban et al. 1997, 1999a). The etiology of extubation failure also influences outcome, with mortality lowest for airway problems (upper airway obstruction, aspiration, excess pulmonary secretions) and highest when reintubation is required for other causes (Daley et al. 1996; Epstein and Ciubotaru 1998; Esteban et al. 1997, 1999a).

Several hypotheses have been generated to explain the high mortality seen with extubation failure: sicker patient population (increased severity of illness, more chronic disease); direct complications of reintubation; adverse effect of prolonged mechanical ventilation: clinical deterioration between extubation and reintubation. Greater severity of illness or chronic disease does not provide a sufficient explanation, because two studies – adequately controlled for these factors and using multivariate techniques – found extubation failure to be a strong independent predictor of hospital death (Epstein et al. 1997; Esteban et al. 1997). Reintubation itself may potentially contribute to excess hospital mortality by increasing the risk of nosocomial pneumonia (Torres et al. 1995). More recently, three separate investigations were unable to demonstrate an increased mortality attributable to complications resulting from reintubation after extubation failure (Epstein and Ciubotaru 1998; Esteban et al. 1997, 1999a). Therefore, although complications of reintubation are numerous, this does not appear to translate into excess mortality. Other complications of mechanical ventilation increase with time spent on the ventilator (Fagon et al. 1993). Because extubation failure substantially lengthens the duration of mechanical ventilation (Epstein et al. 1997), excess mortality could result from increasing exposure to potentially life-threatening complications. Unfortunately, insufficient research exists to fully evaluate this hypothesis.

Delay in reintubation may be a crucial component, because clinical deterioration can occur before adequate ventilatory support is reestablished. For example, a reduced incidence of pneumonia was found in patients who were reintubated immediately compared with those with delayed reintubation (Torres et al. 1995). In addition, the data from two previously published studies indicated that mortality was higher when reintubation occurred more than 12 h after extubation (Demling et al. 1988; Tahvanainen et al. 1983). This was confirmed by a large international observational study that revealed lower mortality when reintubation occurred within 12 h of extubation (Esteban et al. 1999b). In a study of 74 medical patients reintubated within 72 h of extubation, mortality was lowest for those reintubated within 12 h and increased steadily with duration of time to reestablishment of ventilator support (Epstein and Ciubotaru 1998). After controlling for severity of illness, presence of significant co-morbid conditions, organ failure, and cause of reintubation, time to reintubation was found to be an independent predictor of outcome.

23.5 Prediction of Extubation Failure

The frequency of reintubation and the adverse impact on survival indicate that accurate prediction of extubation outcome is important. Precise forecasting of extubation outcome could also improve ICU bed management. For example, patients highly likely to be successfully extubated may be appropriate for early transfer from the ICU, once extubated. Conversely, those at higher, but not prohibitive, risk for extubation failure require a longer period of ICU observation to facilitate rapid identification of clinical worsening and timely reinstitution of ventilatory support.

Currently, most clinicians assess patient readiness for both liberation from ventilator support and extubation by conducting a trial of spontaneous breathing. The SBT is carried out only after the patient has demonstrated clinical recovery and hemodynamic stability and has satisfied one or more of the classical weaning parameters. Patients tolerating an SBT are then extubated as long as they are judged sufficiently able to protect their airway and manage respiratory secretions. The best manner for conducting a SBT has been under active investigation for some time. Theoretically, there are reasons to suspect that unassisted breathing (T-piece) or partially assisted breathing with low levels of (PSV) or CPAP may be advantageous. Some investigators have demonstrated that the endotracheal tube can impose an additional work load. This may worsen for a tube maintained for a prolonged period of time due to kinking of the tube or inspissation of secretions which narrow the lumen and increase resistance (Wright et al. 1989). One would therefore anticipate that low levels of inspiratory PSV to overcome this imposed work would best reflect the load the patient will face after extubation. In fact, Brochard et al. demonstrated that the amount of PSV needed to overcome this imposed load ranged broadly from 3 to 14 cmH_2O. In contrast, recent studies suggest that post-extubation work equals (Straus et al. 1998) or exceeds (Nathan et al. 1993) that seen with the endotracheal tube in place. This suggests that unassisted breathing would best approximate post-extubation work. Under these circumstances, applying PSV would then lead to an underestimation of post-extubation work and an increased likelihood of extubation failure. In fact, Esteban and co-workers (Esteban et al. 1997) found no difference in extubation failure rate comparing 2-h trials of either T-piece or PSV at 7 cmH_2O, though the trial failure rate was higher for the former. Similarly, these investigators found no difference in extubation failure rate for patients undergoing a 30-min compared with those undergoing a 120-min T-piece trial. This latter observation raises the question of whether a trial of spontaneous breathing is necessary prior to extubation. To address this question, Zeggwagh et al. proceeded directly to extubation after medical ICU patients had demonstrated clinical improvement or recovery, adequate mental status, temperature <38°C, respiratory rate <35 breaths/min, SaO_2 >90% on FiO_2 ≤0.40, Hb >10, and hemodynamic stability. Of the 119 episodes of extubation, 44 (37%) resulted in reintubation, a rate 2–3 times that noted for patients extubated only after passing an SBT (Zeggwagh et al. 1999). Conversely, in a pathophysiologic study, Vassilakopoulos and colleagues noted that no patient tolerating a 6-h T-piece trial required reintubation (Vassilakopoulos et al. 1998). These studies reinforce the importance of the SBT and raise the possibility that trials longer than 2 h may be useful in some patient populations.

A major question is whether physiologic measurements can be used to further improve extubation prediction and, beyond that, outcome. Many predictors, e.g., negative inspiratory force (NIF), maximal inspiratory pressure (MIP), frequency-tidal volume ratio (f/V_T), were initially conceived based on their capacity to reflect the pathophysiology of weaning failure, an imbalance between respiratory capacity and load. Although capacity-load imbalance can lead to extubation failure, evidence suggests that there are frequently other causes. This difference in pathophysiology provides some explanation for the observation that, in general, most "weaning predictors" are less accurate in predicting extubation outcome than weaning outcome. In addition, successful completion of an SBT itself is associated with a high probability of extubation success (0.80–0.95). To further improve on this probability, an extubation predictor will have to be highly accurate (e.g., high sensitivity and specificity). Another confounding factor is that many investigators have lumped together weaning and extubation failure, making it difficult to separate out prediction of extubation outcome.

The accuracy of traditional weaning predictors (e.g. MIP, vital capacity, minute ventilation, maximal voluntary ventilation, PaO_2/FiO_2), measured just prior to an SBT, is lower when applied to extubation prediction. Although positive test results are strongly associated with extubation success (e.g., positive predictive values, 0.74–0.93), this offers only marginal improvement from prediction based solely on successful completion of an SBT. In contrast, more than 50% of patients having a test result that predicts failure are still successfully extubated after passing an SBT (e.g., negative predictive value is poor).

Breathing pattern (f/V_T), assessed immediately upon disconnection from the ventilator, accurately predicts weaning outcome (Yang and Tobin 1991). Fewer studies have exclusively examined the accuracy of f/V_T in predicting extubation outcome, and these suggest that breathing pattern may have limited utility in predicting extubation outcome. Some studies (Capdevila et al. 1995; Del Rosario et al. 1997; Farias et al. 1998; Murciano et al. 1988), but not others (Epstein et al. 1997; Esteban et al. 1997; Krieger et al. 1989), have noted higher mean f/V_T values for patients with failure than for those with extubation success. Positive predictive values are similar to those for weaning outcome when a threshold of 100 breaths/min/l is used (Epstein 1995). Nevertheless, approximately 20% of patients predicted to succeed still fail (the f/V_T is a false positive), perhaps reflecting the distinct pathophysiologic causes of extubation failure, including upper airway obstruction, excess pulmonary secretions, or the development of a new process (Epstein 1995). Another explanation is that the best threshold value may be lower for certain patient populations. For example, patients with COPD may make "undetected" respiratory efforts that are uncovered only when an esophageal balloon is in place and demonstrates a negative intrathoracic pressure swing (Purro et al. 2000). Although using a lower threshold value may decrease the number of false-positive predictions, it may also result in a higher number of false negatives (e.g., patients predicted to fail who actually can be successfully extubated). The negative predictive value of the f/V_T is substantially lower for extubation than for weaning outcome (Epstein 1995; Epstein and Ciubotaru 1996; Lee et al. 1994). The probability of extubation failure is increased when rapid shallow breathing is present, but the majority of patients can *still* be successfully extubated. It is unclear whether assessment of the f/V_T (or other parameters) at the completion of the SBT, just prior to extubation, will improve predictive accuracy.

Patients incapable of protecting the airway and expelling secretions with an effective cough are at increased risk for extubation failure. Traditional assessment has consisted of ensuring an adequate gag reflex, demonstrating a cough reflex when stimulated with a suction catheter, and by determining the absence of "excess" secretions, but these criteria have not been standardized. A "sawtooth" pattern on the flow-volume curve indicates the presence of excess airway secretions but does not provide quantitative information (Jubran and Tobin 1994). Although the criteria are not specifically delineated, investigators have tried assessing "effective cough" as a predictor of extubation outcome (Capdevila et al. 1995). In a preliminary report using qualitative assessments made by a single observer, it was noted that patients with moderate or large amounts of secretions were more than seven times as likely to develop extubation failure as those with small amounts of secretions (Khamiees et al. 2000). Patients with weak coughs were more than five times as likely to fail extubation. Five of six patients with both weak coughs and moderate or large amounts of secretions required reintubation within 72 h. Coplin et al. used a six-part semi-quantitative Airway Care Score (ACS: spontaneous cough, gag, sputum quantity, sputum viscosity, suctioning frequency, sputum character) to assess extubation outcome in brain-injured patients (Coplin et al. 2000). Measurements of the ACS made on the day of extubation were not predictive of extubation outcome. In contrast, two individual components (spontaneous cough and suctioning frequency), measured at the time that ventilatory support was no longer required, were predictive of eventual extubation success. Quantitative measurements may prove more useful in predicting extubation outcome. For example, one study found that unassisted or assisted (after abdominal thrust timed to glottic opening) peak cough flows could predict extubation/decannulation outcome in patients with primarily neuromuscular disease (Bach and Saporto 1996). Vallverdu et al. used a unidirectional valve and a 25–30 s expiratory port occlusion (permitting inspiration but not expiration) to measure maximal expiratory pressure (MEP) (Vallverdu et al. 1998). In acute respiratory failure patients and neurological patients, but not in those with COPD, the MEP was lower for those who failed weaning. A lower MEP, which may indicate increased risk for ineffective cough, independently predicted failure among neurological patients, most of whom were extubation failures.

It is difficult to fully evaluate upper airway patency in the presence of an endotracheal tube capable of stenting open the airway. Fisher and Raper reported the association of increased risk for post-extubation stridor and the absence of an audible air-leak after deflation of the endotracheal tube balloon (qualitative cuff-leak test) (Fisher and Raper 1992). Marik applied the qualitative cuff leak test to 100 noncardiothoracic patients intubated for greater than 24 h (Marik 1996). Of the 94 patients with a leak none developed stridor, while stridor occurred in two of six without a leak. To provide a more objective measurement, Miller and Cole studied the utility of a quantitative cuff-leak test, determined within 24 h of extubation, in 100 episodes of mechanical ventilation in 88 medical intensive care unit patients (Miller and Cole 1996). The cuff-leak volume was measured as the average difference between inspiratory and expiratory volume (after balloon deflation), recorded for six consecutive breaths during assist-control ventilation. With post-hoc analysis, a threshold cuff-leak volume of 110 ml was found to be predictive of post-extubation upper airway obstruction. When the volume was greater than 110 ml, 98% of patients did not have stridor, while 80% of patients developed stridor when the volume was less than 110 ml. More recently, Engoren evaluated the quantitative cuff-leak test determined just prior to extubation in 524 postoperative cardiothoracic surgical patients (Engoren 1999). While three patients with leak volumes >110 ml developed stridor, upper airway obstruction did not occur in the 20 patients with a positive cuff-leak test (leak <110 ml). The impact of the test may also be limited because reintubation is often not required to treat post-extubation stridor, and the mortality of those needing reinsertion of the endotracheal tube is similar to that of successfully extubated patients. Therefore, prior to broad application, further study of the quantitative cuff-leak test is warranted.

Measurements of work of breathing have been used to assess weaning outcome, but relatively few studies have examined their value in predicting extubation outcome. For example, two studies found that approximately 90% of trauma patients with tachypnea during a room-air CPAP trial were successfully extubated if either the total WOB was ≤ 1.1 J/l or physiologic WOB (total WOB minus imposed WOB) was ≤ 0.8 J/l (DeHaven et al. 1996; Kirton et al. 1995). These investigations did not examine the accuracy of an elevated physiologic work of breathing in predicting extubation outcome. Using esophageal manometry, Levy and co-workers observed that nine of ten patients were successfully extubated despite a markedly elevated WOB measured during PSV (Levy et al. 1995). At the present time, it is uncertain whether WOB measurements will identify patients who pass a weaning trial but fail extubation.

Airway occlusion pressure measured at 100 ms (P_{100} or $P_{0.1}$) reflects respiratory drive, demand on the respiratory system, and has recently been used to predict extubation outcome. This approach is increasingly attractive because some modern ventilators, taking advantage of the time delay required to open the demand value, are capable of providing on-line assessment of airway occlusion pressure. In a small study of patients with COPD, the $P_{0.1}$ fell significantly from 7.4 to 3.9 cmH_2O in those successfully extubated, while there was no improvement in extubation failure patients (Murciano et al. 1988). In a physiologic study, Del Rosario et al. observed a higher $P_{0.1}$ and $P_{0.1}$ corrected for maximal inspiratory pressure ($P_{0.1}$/PImax) among patients with extubation failure (Del Rosario et al. 1997). Capdevila and co-workers found higher $P_{0.1}$ and $P_{0.1}$/MIP values, measured after 20 min of spontaneous breathing, among patients who subsequently required reintubation (Capdevila et al. 1995). Using post-hoc threshold values of 0.5 cmH_2O and 0.09, these authors noted positive predictive values of 0.96 and 1.00 and negative predictive values of 0.65 and 0.92, respectively. Although these data are encouraging, prospective studies using predefined thresholds are not yet available. Airway occlusion measurements made prior to extubation may not identify patients at risk for extubation failure from causes that become evident only after extubation. Hilbert and co-workers, studying COPD patients, measured the $P_{0.1}$ prior to and 90 min *after* extubation while patients breathed on pressure support via a full face mask (Hilbert et al. 1998b). Only the $P_{0.1}$ measured after extubation accurately identified patients destined to develop respiratory distress after extubation.

Careful observation is used to assess tolerance for an SBT, but it is possible that trends in these parameters during the trial may better predict extubation outcome. To address this issue, Esteban and co-workers investigated changes in four parameters (respiratory frequency, heart rate, systolic arterial pressure, and oxygen saturation) recorded every 15 min during either a T-piece or a PSV trial (Esteban et al. 1997, 1999a). With the incremental area under the curve used as a summary statistic, changes in these variables did not distinguish patients who eventually required reintubation from those successfully extubated. Although Murciano et al. also noted no change in routinely measured parameters, they did not find electromyographic evidence suggestive of diaphragmatic fatigue among patients who failed extubation (Murciano et al. 1988). The implication is that current methods for assessing load-capacity imbalance during an SBT, using vital signs and gas exchange, may not be sufficiently sensitive to detect impending respiratory muscle fatigue.

Several other approaches to prediction of extubation outcome have been studied. In a large retrospective study, numerous operative factors appeared to predict extubation failure after cardiac surgery (Rady and Ryan 1999). In a retrospective analysis, a multivariate model that included operating-room time, respiratory rate, vital capacity, and presence of COPD accurately predicted the need for reintubation in cardiac surgical patients (Engoren et al. 1999). In an older study, reintubated patients were noted to have lower urine volume and lower respiratory quotients and were more likely to have positive blood cultures 3 days prior to extubation (Tahvanainen et al. 1983). Capdevila et al. found that failed extubation occurred in approximately 50% of patients with either a new infiltrate or pleural effusion on chest radiograph (Capdevila et al. 1995).

In summary, although many parameters have been assessed, accuracy for predicting extubation outcome is suboptimal. Several parameters appear promising, such as assessment of respiratory secretions and the $P_{0.1}$/MIP, but further confirmation of accuracy is required before general application can be recommended. At the present time, successful completion of a spontaneous breathing trial appears to be the best predictor of favorable extubation outcome.

23.6 Prevention of Extubation Failure

Ideally, precise classification of patients at risk for extubation failure would allow for postponement of tube removal until the relevant pathophysiologic process had been corrected. As noted above, currently available predictive instruments are not sufficiently accurate, and up to 20% of patients will require reintubation after extubation. When signs of extubation failure occur, therapeutic measures aimed at the specific etiology for failure should be instituted immediately and their efficacy rapidly assessed. It is our experience that physicians are often hesitant to reintubate because extubation failure may imply that an error in decision-making (e.g., premature extubation) has occurred. To avoid confirmation that an error in judgement has occurred, physicians may unintentionally delay reintubation waiting for medical therapy to be effective. Such delays in reestablishing ventilatory support may result in poorer outcomes.

Understandably, many physicians may hesitate to reintubate patients when only early signs of distress are present, because of the invasive nature of the procedure. In contrast, a number of studies have examined the role of noninvasive ventilation (NIV) in preventing or treating extubation failure (Table 23.1). Investigations have consisted of uncontrolled, case-controlled, and randomized controlled design where extubation failure was studied exclusively or as a subgroup of a larger patient population. Both uncontrolled and controlled studies with subgroup analysis suggest that when NIV is used reintubation is required in 0%–42% of patients with

Table 23.1. Studies of NIV to prevent or treat extubation failure

Reference	No. of patients with NIV (controls)	Study design	Type of NPV	Reintubation, n (%)
Meduri et al. 1991	7	Uncontrolled subgroup	NIPSV	14
Pennock et al. 1991	23	Uncontrolled, postoperative	Bi-level positive pressure	26
Wysocki et al. 1993	6	Uncontrolled subgroup	NIPSV	17
Chiang and Lee (1995)	19	Uncontrolled	Bi-level Positive pressure nasal mask	42
Wysocki et al. 1995	4 (4)	RCT subgroup	NIPSV	0 (NR)
Meduri et al. (1996)	39	Uncontrolled subgroup	NIPSV	35
Leitch et al. 1996	34	Uncontrolled subgroup	CPAP	6
Alsous et al. 1999	10	Uncontrolled subgroup	Bi-level positive pressure	20
Hilbert et al. (1998a)	30 (30)	Case-control (historical)	NIPSV	20 (67)
Munshi et al. (1999)	72	Uncontrolled	NIPSV/CPAP	28
Jiang et al. (1999)	47 (46)	RCT[a] (including unplanned extubation)	Bi-level positive pressure face mask	28 (15)
Wu et al. (2000)	126 (124)	RCT[a]	Bi-level positive pressure face mask	17 (11)
Keenan et al. (2000)	36 (39)	RCT[b]	NR	72 (69)

[a]All extubated patients were studied.
[b]Only patients with signs of extubation failure were studied.
Abbreviations: *RCT*, randomized controlled trial; *NR*, not reported; *NIPSV*, noninvasive pressure-support ventilation delivered via a standard ICU ventilator.

signs of extubation failure. In one large observational study, NIV was effective in 26 of 39 patients (17 with COPD) with post-extubation hypercapnic respiratory failure, including three in whom upper airway obstruction was the principal etiology (Meduri et al. 1996). In that study, noninvasive pressure support was titrated to a respiratory rate of 25 breaths/min and a tidal volume of 7 ml/kg, with 86% of patients subsequently demonstrating correction or improvement in arterial blood gases. In a prospective, uncontrolled study of 19 patients (14 planned and five unplanned extubations) with post-extubation respiratory distress, use of nasal bi-level positive pressure ventilation prevented reintubation in 11 patients (Chiang and Lee 1995). Success was heralded by a significant reduction in respiratory rate within 1 h of instituting NIV, while failure was attributable to either mouth leaks or excess secretions. Munshi et al. used mask or nasal CPAP or bi-level positive pressure ventilation in 72 trauma patients with post-extubation hypoxemia and prevented reintubation in 52 patients (Munshi et al. 1999). Hilbert and colleagues performed a case-control study of noninvasive pressure support (NIPSV) in 30 COPD patients with hypercapnic respiratory failure within 72 h of extubation (Hilbert et al. 1998a). Compared with 30 historical matched controls managed by traditional means, fewer NIPSV patients required invasive ventilation (20% vs 67%) and the length of ICU stay was decreased (8 vs 14 days). Patients used NIPSV for at least 30 min out of every 4 h and averaged 5.2 days of use (6–7 h/day). Perhaps because of the small number of patients studied, the observed reduction in mortality did not achieve statistical significance. A recent preliminary report found no difference in reintubation rates or mortality for patients with post-extubation respiratory failure randomized to NIV compared with those receiving standard care (Keenan et al. 2000). The high reintubation rate in this well-done study suggests that "late" application of NIV may be ineffective and perhaps earlier intervention is warranted. In a randomized controlled study of *all* extubated patients (including unplanned extubations), no difference in likelihood of extubation failure was found when patients randomized to immediate post-extubation bi-level positive pressure ventilation (IPAP 12 cmH_2O and EPAP 5 cmH_2O) delivered by face mask were compared with those who received oxygen alone (Jiang et al. 1999). Similarly, a preliminary report of a randomized, controlled trial of 250 patients extubated only after tolerating 2 h of T-piece breathing also noted that routine application of bi-level positive pressure ventilation did not reduce the need for reintubation (Wu et al. 2000). Larger randomized, controlled trials examining the role of NIPPV in patients exhibiting early signs of extubation failure are not yet available.

23.7 Conclusion

Extubation failure occurs in up to 20% of patients, with the frequency dependent upon numerous factors including the patient population, age, duration of pre-extubation ventilation, and the use of continuous intravenous sedation. The causes of extubation failure are often distinct from those present in patients failing spontaneous breathing trials. Because the need for reintubation is associated with an increase in the duration of mechanical ventilation, ICU and hospital stay, and a substantial increase in hospital mortality, prediction of extubation outcome and prevention of extubation failure are critically important. Tests used to predict weaning outcome have proved much less precise in predicting extubation outcome. Mortality appears to increase with delayed reintubation, suggesting that clinical deterioration occurs during the period without ventilatory support. Therefore, rapid identification of patients at risk, followed by expeditious re-institution of ventilatory support, may improve the outcome for extubation failure.

23.8 References

Alsous F, Amoateng-Adjepong Y, Manthous CA (1999) Noninvasive ventilation: experience at a community teaching hospital. Intensive Care Med 25:458–463

Bach J, Saporto L (1996) Criteria for extubation and tracheostomy tube removal for patients with ventilatory failure. Chest 110:1566–1571

Brochard L, Rauss A, Benito S, et al (1994) Comparison of three methods of gradual withdrawal from ventilatory support during weaning from mechanical ventilation. Am J Respir Crit Care Med 150:896–903

Capdevila XJ, Perrigault PF, Perey PJ, et al (1995) Occlusion pressure and its ratio to maximum inspiratory pressure are useful predictors for successful extubation following T-piece weaning trial. Chest 108:482–489

Chiang A, Lee K (1995) Use of noninvasive ventilation via nasal mask in patients with respiratory distress after extubation. Chin Med J 56:94–101

Coplin WM, Pierson DJ, Cooley KD, et al (2000) Implications of extubation delay in brain-injured patients meeting standard weaning criteria. Am J Respir Crit Care Med 161:1530–1536

Daley B, Garcia-Perez F, Ross S (1996) Reintubation as an outcome predictor in trauma patients. Chest 110:1577–1580

DeHaven CB, Kirton OC, Morgan JP, et al (1996) Breathing measurement reduces false negative classification of tachypneic preextubation trial failures. Crit Care Med 24:976–980

Del Rosario N, Sassoon CS, Chetty KG, et al (1997) Breathing pattern during acute respiratory failure and recovery. Eur Respir J 10:2560–2565

Demling RH, Read T, Lind LJ, et al (1988) Incidence and morbidity of extubation failure in surgical intensive care patients. Crit Care Med 16:573–577

Ely EW, Baker AM, Dunagan DP, et al (1996) Effect on the duration of mechanical ventilation of identifying patients capable of breathing spontaneously. N Engl J Med 335:1864–1869

Engoren M (1999) Evaluation of the cuff-leak test in a cardiac surgery population. Chest 116:1029–1031

Engoren M, Buderer N, Zacharias A, et al (1999) Variables predicting reintubation after cardiac surgical procedures. Ann Thorac Surg 67:661–665

Epstein SK (1995) Etiology of extubation failure and the predictive value of the rapid shallow breathing index. Am J Respir Crit Care Med 152:545–549

Epstein SK (2000) Endotracheal extubation. Respir Care Clin N Am 6:321–360

Epstein SK, Ciubotaru RL (1996) Influence of gender and endotracheal tube size on preextubation breathing pattern. Am J Respir Crit Care Med 154:1647–1652

Epstein SK, Ciubotaru RL (1998) Independent effects of etiology of failure and time to reintubation on outcome for patients failing extubation. Am J Respir Crit Care Med 158:489–493

Epstein SK, Ciubotaru RL, Wong JB (1997) Effect of failed extubation on the outcome of mechanical ventilation. Chest 112:186–192

Esteban A, Frutos F, Tobin MJ, et al (1995) A comparison of four methods of weaning patients from mechanical ventilation. N Engl J Med 332:345–350

Esteban A, Alia I, Gordo F, et al (1997) Extubation outcome after spontaneous breathing trials with T-tube or pressure support ventilation. Am J Respir Crit Care Med 156:459–465

Esteban A, Alia I, Tobin M, et al (1999a) Effect of spontaneous breathing trial duration on outcome of attempts to discontinue mechanical ventilation. Am J Respir Crit Care Med 159:512–518

Esteban A, Anzueto A, Alia I, et al (1999b) Mortality of patients receiving mechanical ventilation. Am J Respir Crit Care Med 159:A47

Fagon JY, Chastre J, Hance AJ, et al (1993) Nosocomial pneumonia in ventilated patients: a cohort study evaluating attributable mortality and hospital stay. Am J Med 94:281–288

Farias JA, Alia I, Esteban A, et al (1998) Weaning from mechanical ventilation in pediatric intensive care patients. Intensive Care Med 24:1070–1075

Fisher MM, Raper RF (1992) The "cuff leak" test for extubation. Anaesthesia 47:10–12

Hilbert G, Gruson D, Portel L, et al (1998a) Noninvasive pressure support ventilation in COPD patients with postextubation hypercapnic respiratory insufficiency. Eur Respir J 11:1349–1353

Hilbert G, Gruson D, Portel L, et al (1998b) Airway occlusion pressure at 0.1 s ($P_{0.1}$) after extubation: an early indicator of postextubation hypercapnic respiratory insufficiency. Intensive Care Med 24:1277–1282

Horst HM, Mouro D, Hall-Jenssens RA, et al (1998) Decrease in ventilation time with a standardized weaning process. Arch Surg 133:483–488

Jiang J, Kao S, Wang S (1999) Effect of early application of biphasic positive airway pressure on the outcome of extubation in ventilatory weaning. Respirology 4:161–165

Jones D, Byrne P, Morgan C, et al (1991) Positive end-expiratory pressure vs T-piece extubation after mechanical ventilation. Chest 100:1655–1659

Jubran A, Tobin MJ (1994) Use of flow-volume curves in detecting secretions in ventilator-dependent patients. Am J Respir Crit Care Med 150:766–769

Jubran A, Tobin MJ (1997) Pathophysiologic basis of acute respiratory distress in patients who fail a trial of weaning from mechanical ventilation. Am J Respir Crit Care Med 155:906–915

Keenan SP, Powers C, Block G, et al (2000) Noninvasive ventilation (NPPV) for post-extubation respiratory distress: a randomized controlled trial. Am J Respir Crit Care Med 161:A263

Khamiees M, Raju P, Amoateng-Adjepong Y, et al (2000) Factors associated with extubation outcome. Am J Respir Crit Care Med 161:A792

Kirton OC, DeHaven CB, Morgan JP, et al (1995) Elevated imposed work of breathing masquerading as ventilator weaning intolerance. Chest 108:1021–1025

Kollef MH, Shapiro SD, Silver P, et al (1997) A randomized, controlled trial of protocol-directed versus physician-directed weaning from mechanical ventilation. Crit Care Med 25:567–574

Krieger BP, Ershowsky PF, Becker DA, et al (1989) Evaluation of conventional criteria for predicting successful weaning from mechanical ventilatory support in elderly patients. Crit Care Med 17:858–861

Lee KH, Hui KP, Chan TB, et al (1994) Rapid shallow breathing (frequency-tidal volume ratio) did not predict extubation outcome. Chest 105:540–543

Leitch EA, Moran JL, Grealy B (1996) Weaning and extubation in the intensive care unit. Clinical or index-driven approach. Intensive Care Med 22:752–759

Leith DE, Bradley M (1976) Ventilatory muscle strength and endurance training. J Appl Physiol 41:508–516

Lemaire F, Teboul J-L, Cinotti L, et al (1988) Acute left ventricular dysfunction during unsuccessful weaning from mechanical ventilation. Anesthesiology 69:171–179

Levy MM, Miyasaki A, Langston D (1995) Work of breathing as a weaning parameter in mechanically ventilated patients. Chest 108:1018–1020

Marik PE (1996) The cuff-leak test as a predictor of postextubation stridor: a prospective study. Respir Care 41:509–511

Meduri GU, Abou-Shala N, Fox RC, Jones CB, Leeper KV, Wunderik RG (1991) Noninvasive face mask mechanical ventilation in patients with acute hypercapnic respiratory failure. Chest 100:445–454

Meduri GU, Turner RE, Abou-Shala N, et al (1996) Noninvasive positive pressure ventilation via face mask: first-line intervention in patients with acute hypercapnic and hypoxemic respiratory failure. Chest 109:179–193

Miller R, Cole R (1996) Association between reduced cuff leak volume and postextubation stridor. Chest 110:1035–1040

Munshi IA, DeHaven B, Kirton O, et al (1999) Reengineering respiratory support following extubation: avoidance of critical care unit costs. Chest 116:1025–1028

Murciano D, Boczkowski J, Lecocguic Y, et al (1988) Tracheal occlusion pressure: a simple index to monitor respiratory muscle fatigue during acute respiratory failure in patients with chronic obstructive pulmonary disease. Ann Intern Med 108:800–805

Nathan SD, Ishaaya AM, Koerner SK, et al (1993) Prediction of minimal pressure support during weaning from mechanical ventilation. Chest 103:1215–1219

Pennock BE, Kaplan PD, Carlin BW, Sabangan JS, Magovern JA (1991) Pressure support ventilation with a simplified ventilatory support system administered with a nasal mask in patients with respiratory failure. Chest 100:1371–1376

Purro A, Appendini L, De Gaetano A, et al (2000) Physiologic determinants of ventilator dependence in long-term mechanically ventilated patients. Am J Respir Crit Care Med 161:1115–1123

Rady MY, Ryan T (1999) Perioperative predictors of extubation failure and the effect on clinical outcome after cardiac surgery. Crit Care Med 27:340–347

Saura P, Blanch L, Mestre J, et al (1996) Clinical consequences of the implementation of a weaning protocol. Intensive Care Med 22:1052–1056

Straus C, Louis B, Isabey D, et al (1998) Contribution of the endotracheal tube and the upper airway to breathing workload. Am J Respir Crit Care Med 157:23–30

Tahvanainen J, Salmenpera M, Nikki P (1983) Extubation criteria after weaning from intermittent mandatory ventilation and continuous positive airway pressure. Crit Care Med 11:702–707

Torres A, Gatell JM, Aznar E, et al (1995) Re-intubation increases the risk of nosocomial pneumonia in patients needing mechanical ventilation. Am J Respir Crit Care Med 152:137–141

Vallverdu I, Calaf N, Subirana M, et al (1998) Clinical characteristics, respiratory functional parameters, and outcome of two-hour T-piece trial in patients weaning from mechanical ventilation. Am J Respir Crit Care Med 158:1855–1862

Vassilakopoulos T, Zakynthinos S, Roussos C (1998) The tension-time index and the frequency/tidal volume ratio are the major pathophysiologic determinants of weaning failure and success. Am J Respir Crit Care Med 158:378–385

Wright PE, Marini JJ, Bernard GR (1989) In vitro versus in vivo comparison of endotracheal tube airflow resistance. Am Rev Respir Dis 140:10–16

Wu CP, Lin HI, Cheng CH, et al (2000) Noninvasive ventilation cannot decrease the extubation failure rate after 2-hour T-piece trial. Am J Respir Crit Care Med 161:A556

Wysocki M, Tric L, Wolff MA, Gertner J, Millet H, Herman B (1993) Noninvasive pressure support ventilation in patients with acute respiratory failure. Chest 103:907–913

Wysocki M, Tric L, Wolff MA, Millet H, Herman B (1995) Noninvasive pressure support ventilation in patients with acute respiratory failure. A randomized comparison with conventional therapy. Chest 107:761–768

Yang KL, Tobin MJ (1991) A prospective study of indexes predicting the outcome of trials of weaning from mechanical ventilation. N Engl J Med 324:1445–1450

Zeggwagh AA, Abouqal R, Madani N, et al (1999) Weaning from mechanical ventilation: a model for extubation. Intensive Care Med 25:1077–1083

24 Continuous Positive Airway Pressure in the Hypoxemic Patient

C. Delclaux, L. Brochard, and J. Mancebo

J. Mancebo was supported by FISss grants 91/174 and 93/711, and HF061 (Spain).

24.1 Introduction

Continuous positive airway pressure (CPAP) is a ventilatory technique by which the patient breathes spontaneously with a constant level of positive pressure during both inspiration and expiration. A tracing showing airway pressure, esophageal pressure, airflow, and tidal volume recorded in a patient breathing in CPAP mode is given in Fig. 24.1. Airway pressure (P_{aw}) is maintained almost constant throughout the breathing cycle. This is an important characteristic and, ideally, the P_{aw} gradient between inspiration and expiration should be identical to that observed during normal spontaneous breathing, the only difference being that breathing occurs above the atmospheric pressure at a level determined by the preset positive end-expiratory pressure (PEEP).

CPAP has been widely used to treat hypoxemic patients who are able to breathe spontaneously. The beneficial effects of CPAP in hypoxemic patients are presumably due to the increase in functional residual capacity induced by PEEP.

The effectiveness of CPAP in improving hypoxemia of patients suffering from cardiac edema was first described in 1935 [1, 2]; however, its widespread use began after 1971, when Gregory et al. [3] reported that this technique was of value in reversing the hypoxemia associated with idiopathic respiratory distress syndrome of the newborn. CPAP was used in intubated adult patients with acute respiratory failure by Civetta et al. [4] in 1972. Shortly thereafter, its use became generalized in both intubated patients and nonintubated patients ventilated via face masks. Despite a large number of physiological studies, only very few randomized controlled trials have allowed precise determination of the indications for CPAP.

24.2 Working Principles

There are two basic CPAP systems: those with continuous-flow circuits (which may be "homemade" systems), and those with demand valves (the vast majority

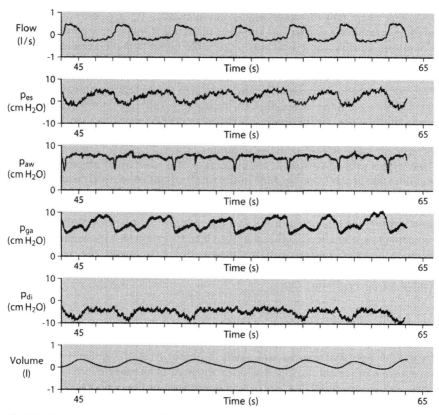

Fig. 24.1. From *top* to *bottom*: air flow (*flow*), esophageal pressure (P_{es}), airway pressure (P_{aw}), gastric pressure (P_{ga}), transdiaphragmatic pressure (P_{di}), and tidal volume (*volume*), obtained from a patient breathing in CPAP mode

of which are incorporated in intensive care mechanical ventilators). The two systems have different characteristics.

24.2.1 Continuous-Flow Circuits

Basically, continuous-flow circuits are built with an air-oxygen blender and a flowmeter, enabling delivery of an FiO_2 between 0.21 and 1 and a gas flow high enough to meet the patient's inspiratory demands. Inspired gases are heated and humidified adequately, usually by means of a cascade-type system. These systems should contain a manometer to control P_{aw}, positioned as close as possible to the patient's airway opening.

Various mechanisms are used to generate PEEP: underwater seal, threshold resistors, orificial resistances, etc. A common feature of these mechanisms is that many of them tend to increase PEEP when expiratory flow increases [5]. As valve resistance to air flow increases, higher fluctuations in P_{aw} are observed and the work of breathing is greater [6]. The ideal mechanism would be a pure nonresistive threshold valve, i.e., a determined threshold pressure that is maintained constant despite changes in expiratory airflow.

In a study in 1985, Marini and colleagues [5] showed that spring-loaded PEEP valves produce excessively high expiratory resistances in comparison with systems using a water column or an inflatable diaphragm. In the lung model study, most valves (spring-loaded or magnetic PEEP valves) used in a continuous-flow CPAP system were shown not only to impose high levels of inspiratory work, but also to induce active expiratory work. The high flow resistance of these valves probably explains the induction of a substantial amount of extra work despite the fact that the flow in the CPAP circuit consistently exceeded the flow demands of the model [7]. Some continuous-flow CPAP systems are built with spring-loaded PEEP valves and may induce an excessive effort in patients with acute respiratory failure and high minute ventilation. Moreover, the increase in expiratory resistance may also lead to an increase in the sensation of dyspnea. Because continuous-flow systems do not use valves, the inspired gas enters the patient's lungs directly, and any excess gas delivered to the lung is vented on the expiratory side.

24.2.2 Demand-Valve Systems

Demand-valve CPAP systems are usually built into artificial ventilators. Demand valves are mechanical devices that open when an inspiratory effort is detected. These valves may detect changes in airway pressure, or flow, or both. When a certain threshold level is reached (valve sensitivity), the gas is delivered to the patient's lungs.

The effort required of patients in order to reach a given level of valve sensitivity is variable and depends on the particular characteristics of each valve. In bench studies at least, the performance of pressure-triggered and flow-triggered systems has nowadays become quite similar [8, 9].

When demand-valve and continuous-flow systems are compared the former often exhibits a higher resistance to airflow as PEEP increases, a higher fluctuation between inspiratory and expiratory airway pressures, and also a greater time lag between inspiratory effort and the beginning of inspiratory flow [10].

24.2.3 Continuous-Flow Systems Incorporated in Ventilators

Many modern ventilators incorporate modified continuous-flow mechanisms. These mechanisms significantly reduce the inspiratory effort required to trigger a breath compared with conventional demand valves.

With the aim of improving the demand-valve mechanisms of artificial ventilators, a modified continuous-flow system, called "flow-by", was initially incorporated in the Puritan-Bennett 7200a ventilator [11] and later in other modern microprocessed ventilators. The "flow-by" mechanism consists in a constant and continuous basic flow of gas circulating within the inspiratory and expiratory circuit, with continuous measurement of flow on both the inspiratory and expiratory sides. When the patient is expiring, the total flow measured in the exhalation port becomes higher than the base flow. When inspiration begins, the flow measured in the exhalation port is lower than the base flow. When the difference between the base flow and the measured exhaled flow reaches a certain threshold level, called flow sensitivity, the inspiratory valve opens and delivers a predetermined gas flow to the circuit, in order to maintain the preset airway pressure.

24.3 Effects of the Different Systems on the Work of Breathing

24.3.1 Demand-Valve Versus Continuous-Flow CPAP

In intubated patients recovering from severe acute respiratory failure or from major surgical procedures, demand-valve CPAP systems have been shown to induce a higher work of breathing (WOB) than continuous-flow CPAP systems. This was considered to be related to the high circuit resistances in the former [12].

In a study of a group of intubated patients undergoing weaning from mechanical ventilation, Beydon et al. [13] reported that WOB was significantly lower when the patient was breathing through a continuous flow system than with the demand valves of several ventilators.

The main advantages of conventional demand valves over continuous-flow systems are the considerable gas savings, the possibility of using all the alarm and ventilatory parameter-monitoring capabilities offered by mechanical ventilators, and the availability of back-up ventilation if episodes of apnea ensue.

24.3.2 Effects of "Flow-by"

In COPD patients undergoing weaning from mechanical ventilation, Sassoon et al. [14] evaluated the effects of different CPAP systems on WOB. They found that during CPAP at 0 cmH_2O, there was a significant decrease in WOB (expressed as J/l of ventilation) when comparing CPAP demand-flow with CPAP "flow-by", but when WOB was expressed as J/min they did not detect any differences between the two CPAP systems. During CPAP 8 cm H_2O, WOB, expressed in either J/l or J/min, did not differ significantly between the two CPAP systems. In this study, the WOB during CPAP demand-flow decreased only when a pressure support level of 5 cmH_2O was added. Other authors, however, have reported that during weaning from mechanical ventilation using either CPAP, synchronized intermittent mandatory ventilation, or pressure-support ventilation, the "flow-by" mechanism significantly reduces the WOB and inspiratory effort of these patients, compared with the pressure-triggered demand-valve mechanism [15–19]. The difference, however, is of small magnitude [19]. Aslanian et al. showed, for instance, that no difference was found between the two types of triggering mechanism using assist-control ventilation [19]. The authors presumed this was due to an insufficient peak-flow setting during assist-control, counterbalancing any small difference in the effort to trigger the breath.

24.4 Indications for CPAP

24.4.1 Hypoxemic Respiratory Failure

Pathophysiological Findings
The improvement in oxygenation induced by CPAP presumably results from an increase in functional residual capacity and a decrease in intrapulmonary shunt induced by PEEP. In addition, compared with spontaneous nonassisted breathing, PEEP may improve lung compliance by recruiting alveoli, which decreases the elastic workload that the respiratory muscles must overcome. These effects have been demonstrated by Katz and Marks [20] in intubated patients recovering from acute respiratory failure. These authors found that CPAP increased lung compliance, decreased WOB, and also decreased the alveolar-to-arterial oxygen pressure difference compared with T-piece breathing. In addition, the lung volume increase induced by PEEP may reduce airway resistance, leading to a decrease in resistive WOB. A study by Sassoon et al. [21] of ten patients being weaned from mechanical ventilation showed that lung resistance was decreased during CPAP 5 cmH_2O, compared with T-piece breathing.

In patients with left heart failure, several important pathophysiological abnormalities concern lung function. These patients usually present with orthopnea, which is thought to reflect perivascular, peribronchiolar, and interstitial edema, which compress airways and also may stimulate lung receptors, thus provoking reflex bronchoconstriction (this is the notion of "cardiac asthma"). Interestingly, a recent investigation by Yap et al. indicates that patients with left heart failure have small lung volumes when seated (reduced TLC and similar FRC compared with control subjects) [22]. When subjects lie in the supine posture, those who have heart failure do not exhibit changes in FRC, whereas normals do so. Nevertheless, in supine, patients who have heart failure exhibit significant reductions in vital capacity, whereas this parameter is unchanged in controls. Additionally, the change in posture from seated to supine is associated with major increases in respiratory air flow resistance (Rrs) in patients with left heart failure, whereas normal controls do not exhibit any change in Rrs. The increase in Rrs was not reverted by inhaled ipratropium bromide.

Bradley and colleagues documented the hemodynamic changes that take place in patients with congestive heart failure when they are breathing with CPAP [23]. With CPAP [5], they observed significant increases in cardiac index and stroke volume only in those patients who had elevated pulmonary capillary wedge pressures (PCWP), whereas in patients with low PCWP the cardiac index significantly decreased.

Lenique et al. also studied the effects of CPAP in patients with an acute exacerbation of chronic left heart failure [24]. When comparing spontaneous unassisted breathing with CPAP 10 cmH_2O they observed a significant improvement in lung compliance, significant decreases in both the elastic and the resistive components of WOB, and significant reductions in inspiratory muscle effort. Arterial PO_2 significantly improved and breathing pattern remained essentially unchanged. Additionally, no major changes were seen in cardiac index or stroke volume, although transmural filling pressures decreased with CPAP, which was interpreted as better cardiac performance.

Clinical Findings

There have been numerous cohort studies dealing with the usefulness of CPAP in patients with acute respiratory failure of various etiologies: multiple trauma, ARDS, pneumonia, sepsis, acute pancreatitis, cardiogenic pulmonary edema and pneumonia due to *Pneumocystis carinii* in patients with human immunodeficiency virus infection [4, 25–34]. These investigations have included more than 250 patients and have shown that, in the vast majority of cases, CPAP tended to improve arterial PO_2, with no major changes in arterial PCO_2 and few alterations in cardiac output. A number of patients, however, fail to improve with CPAP for various reasons: no improvement in PaO_2 despite increasing PEEP levels, progressive CO_2 retention, uncooperativeness, fatigue, and other complications associated with the primary disease.

It must be stressed that these studies varied greatly concerning their design: Some authors used face masks and others used CPAP with continuous- or demand-flow systems in intubated patients; the PEEP levels used were not uniform; and etiologies of acute respiratory failure varied. These differences render comparison and interpretation of the studies difficult.

Cardiogenic Pulmonary Edema

The studies mentioned above did not have a controlled and/or randomized design, with the exception of three that were conducted in the setting of cardiogenic pulmonary edema [30, 32, 34].

The studies conducted by Räsänen et al. [32] and Lin et al. [34] had a specific design that essentially allowed evaluation of the effect of CPAP on arterial oxygenation, since:

- The CPAP duration was predetermined (3 h for Räsänen and 6 h for Lin).
- The primary end-point in both studies was treatment failure.

Failure criteria were defined mainly as predetermined level of hypoxemia, rise in arterial carbon dioxide tension, and respiratory rate. For instance, in the study by Räsänen et al. the intubation rate of control patients was very high (60%) and this could have been attributable to the low FiO_2 (28%–30%) used. This is important since the main cause of treatment failure was hypoxemia. In the study by Lin et al., the failure rate over 6 h was 24% (12/50) in the CPAP group and 50% (25/50) in the control group ($p<0.01$), but only 3/12 and 4/25 patients reaching these failure criteria eventually required intubation and mechanical ventilation during their ICU stay (not significant).

Bersten et al. [30] studied 39 patients with cardiogenic pulmonary edema presenting with hypoxemia (mean PaO_2/FiO_2 between 136 and 138 mmHg) and acute hypercapnia (mean $PaCO_2$ between 58 and 64 mmHg), and compared 10 cmH_2O

continuous-flow CPAP with a face mask with conventional therapy with oxygen given by mask. They found a significant improvement in PaO_2 and a significant decrease in $PaCO_2$ in patients treated with CPAP compared with those conventionally treated. Intubation and mechanical ventilation were needed for 35% of patients (7/20) in the conventional treatment group and occurred within 3 h of study entry (CPAP was administered for a total of 9.3±4.9 h). None of the 19 patients treated with CPAP needed intubation. The mortality was similar in both groups. Additionally, a recent study confirmed the benefit of CPAP in patients with severe hypercapnic cardiogenic pulmonary edema [35].

Acute Lung Injury

Delclaux et al. recently investigated whether CPAP delivered by a face mask had physiological benefit and would reduce the need for intubation and mechanical ventilation in patients suffering from permeability pulmonary edema [36]. One hundred and twenty-three patients with acute nonhypercapnic respiratory failure (PaO_2:FiO_2 ratio <300 mmHg) resulting from bilateral pulmonary edema were randomized to receive either oxygen alone (n=61) or oxygen plus CPAP (n=62). Randomization was stratified on the existence of an underlying cardiopathy. In other words, both groups included, in addition to patients with acute lung injury or the acute respiratory distress syndrome, patients with a superimposed noncardiac cause of pulmonary edema in the presence of underlying cardiac disease. After 1 h, both subjective response to treatment (dyspnea) and PaO_2:FiO_2 ratio showed a greater improvement with CPAP than with oxygen alone [203 mmHg (45–431) versus 151 (73–482), p<0.05]. No difference was found in the need for intubation and mechanical ventilation in the CPAP group versus the oxygen group (21/62 versus 24/61, p=0.53), or in in-hospital mortality or length of ICU stay. A higher number of complications occurred in the CPAP group (CPAP: 18 versus oxygen: 6, p=0.03, including four cardiac arrests in the CPAP group observed at the time of intubation or when removing the mask).

Therefore, despite early physiological improvement in oxygenation and in dyspnea obtained with CPAP, these results do not support the use of CPAP in the setting of acute lung injury as a means of avoiding endotracheal intubation. CPAP might thus be reserved for patients in whom distress can be rapidly improved by medications, such as fluid overload. In such patients frank ventilatory failure can be transiently avoided by CPAP, giving time for the medications to act.

24.4.2 Weaning

CPAP has been also proposed for hypoxemic patients being weaned from mechanical ventilation. In these patients, CPAP therapy may improve oxygenation and decrease WOB compared with the classic T-piece trial in patients with restrictive lung disease [21, 37]. Glottic function is suppressed by the presence of the endotracheal tube, and some authors proposed that this may constitute another mechanism to explain why CPAP may be useful during spontaneous breathing through an endotracheal tube [38]. The glottis normally acts as an expiratory brake, facilitates coughing, and helps maintain the intrapulmonary gas volume [37, 39].

Sassoon et al. [21] studied ten patients during weaning from mechanical ventilation and observed that during CPAP with 5 cmH$_2$O PEEP, oxygenation was not better than with a T-piece. However, the pressure-time product of the inspiratory muscles was significantly lower during CPAP than during T-piece breathing. These data were not confirmed in another study conducted by Polese et al. [16] of ten non-COPD patients during weaning. No difference between spontaneous breathing and 5 cmH$_2$O CPAP was detected in terms of work of breathing or the pressure-time product of the inspiratory muscles.

24.4.3 Atelectasis

Postoperative atelectasis has been considered a further indication for CPAP. Andersen et al. [40] have demonstrated radiologic and gas exchange improvements in patients treated after surgery with intermittent CPAP at 15 cmH$_2$O PEEP over 24 h, compared with the conventional treatment. These beneficial effects were attributed to an increase in collateral flow to the obstructed alveolar regions induced by CPAP, and to greater facility in the removal of secretions. However, other investigators [41] were unable to demonstrate that CPAP prevents pulmonary complications, improves gas exchange or vital capacity, or improves chest X-ray findings compared with spontaneous breathing without PEEP in patients undergoing elective abdominal surgery. These findings may be explained partially by the low level of PEEP (5–10 cmH$_2$O) used and the short duration (4 h) of CPAP therapy.

The incidence of postoperative atelectasis may be high [42, 43] after both abdominal (about 20%) and thoracic (about 30%) surgery. The best methods of preventing and treating postoperative atelectasis remain open to debate. Patients with an inspiratory capacity greater than 1 l rarely need additional treatment. In others, any maneuver increasing functional residual capacity and inspiratory capacity may constitute adequate treatment [42, 43].

A study by Stock and co-workers [44], compared the results obtained in a group of 65 postoperative patients (elective abdominal surgery) with incentive spirometry, with deep inspiration and coughing, and with intermittent 7.5 cmH$_2$O CPAP using a face mask and a continuous-flow system. The authors found a lower incidence of atelectasis during CPAP treatment (21%) compared with the other methods (41%). They concluded, however, that although the increment in functional residual capacity was higher and faster with CPAP, all the methods were satisfactory, because the overall incidence of major pulmonary complications in a population considered at high risk was very low in all groups (only two patients developed postoperative pneumonia). In a study [45] performed in 160 patients undergoing cardiac and pulmonary surgery the incidence of postoperative atelectasis was shown to be the same for the three different methods of face-mask physiotherapy: either CPAP, expiratory positive airway pressure (EPAP), or inspiratory resistance with EPAP. All these data suggest that nowadays (an era of better anesthesia and surgical techniques), and at least in postoperative low-risk patients, standard nursing care is as effective in preventing complications as CPAP or other physiotherapeutic techniques [46, 47].

24.5 Contraindications and Complications

When CPAP is delivered via a face mask, the patient's cooperation is important. The presence of fractures or facial anatomical abnormalities and laryngeal, tracheal, or esophageal lesions contraindicate the use of face-mask CPAP.

During face-mask CPAP, patients may complain of facial pain and discomfort and may present with gastric distension with an attendant risk of vomiting and aspiration of the gastric contents. In patients with mild acute respiratory failure, nasal-mask CPAP has been reported to be more comfortable than full face-mask CPAP [48]. In a study of normal subjects, the hemodynamic effects of CPAP were shown to be critically dependent on mouth position [49]. In subjects receiving nasal-mask CPAP (with the mouth closed) or facial-mask CPAP and subjective to progressive increments in PEEP from 0 to 20 cmH$_2$O, a significant decrease in cardiac output and a parallel and significant increase in end-expiratory esophageal pressure were observed. No hemodynamic or esophageal pressure changes were detected when the subjects received nasal-mask CPAP with the mouth open.

24.6 Summary and Recommendations

Hypoxemic patients with acute hypercapnic respiratory failure and low functional residual capacity due to severe cardiogenic pulmonary edema seem to benefit from CPAP treatment, because it usually improves oxygenation and may potentially eliminate the need for intubation and mechanical ventilation in very acute forms of the disease, usually associated with hypercapnia. On the other hand, the benefit of CPAP in noncardiogenic edema has never been clearly demonstrated and its systematic use to prevent intubation in acute lung injury cannot be supported; it can even be hazardous by unnecessarily delaying intubation. Although CPAP may offer some advantages over the T-piece during weaning from mechanical ventilation because it improves gas exchange and decreases the work of breathing, the clinical impact of such a technique has never been demonstrated. Finally, CPAP is also indicated in the treatment of postoperative atelectasis, especially after thoracic and abdominal surgery. However, conventional methods of active respiratory physiotherapy and routine nursing care are also useful in preventing postoperative pulmonary complications. If CPAP is indicated for such patients, the average PEEP levels used are about 10 cmH$_2$O in order to allow significant increments in transpulmonary pressure. It should be stressed, however, that despite the widespread use of CPAP in the ICU, there is a lack of controlled studies to demonstrate its clinical efficacy in most situations.

When the clinical decision to use CPAP is made, it is useful to increase the PEEP levels in serial increments of 5 cmH$_2$O so as to obtain a PEEP value with minimal expiratory air flow resistance. As regards the inspiratory circuit, continuous-flow systems are preferable to demand valves. In continuous-flow systems, it is very important that gas flow within the circuit be at least equal to the patient's spontaneous inspiratory peak flow.

Ideally, the instantaneous gas flow within the circuits should be about 4–5 times the patient's minute ventilation: In this way the WOB done to overcome the impedance of the CPAP system is minimal. A manometer to control the airway pressure may be useful as a help to adjust the PEEP level, and to minimize the fluctuations in airway pressure and the patient's breathing effort.

24.7 References

1. Barach AI, Martini J, Eckman M (1935) Positive pressure respiration and its application to the treatment of acute pulmonary edema. Ann Intern Med 12:754–795
2. Poulton EP, Oxon DM (1936) Left-sided heart failure with pulmonary edema. Lancet 2:981–983
3. Gregory GA, Kitterman JA, Phibbs R, Tooley WH, Hamilton WK, et al (1971) Treatment of the idiopathic respiratory distress syndrome with continuous positive air-way pressure. N Engl J Med 284:1333–1340
4. Civetta JM, Brons R, Gabel JC (1972) A simple and effective method employing spontaneous positive airway pressure ventilation. J Thorac Cardiovasc Surg 63:312–317
5. Marini JJ, Culver BH, Kirk W (1985) Flow resistance of exhalation valves and positive end-expiratory pressure devices used in mechanical ventilation. Am Rev Respir Dis 131:850–854
6. Banner MJ, Downs JB, Kirby RR, Smith RA, Boysen PG, Lampotang S (1988) Effects of expiratory flow resistance on inspiratory work of breathing. Chest 93:795–799
7. Kacmarek RM, Mang E, Barker N, Cycyk-Chapman MC (1994) Effects of disposable or interchangeable positive end-expiratory pressure valves on work of breathing during the application of continuous positive airway pressure. Crit Care Med 22:1219–1226
8. Cox D, Tinloi SF, Farrimond JG (1988) Investigation of the spontaneous modes of breathing of different ventilators. Intensive Care Med 14:532–537
9. Sassoon CSH, Gruer SE (1995) Characteristics of the ventilator pressure- and flow-trigger variables. Intensive Care Med 21:159–168
10. Cox D, Niblett DJ (1984) Studies on continuous positive airway pressure breathing systems. Br J Anaesth 56:905–911
11. Sassoon CSH, Giron AE, Ely EA, Light RW (1989) Inspiratory work of breathing on flow-by and demand-flow continuous positive airway pressure. Crit Care Med 17:1108–1114
12. Viale JP, Annat G, Bertrand O (1985) Additional inspiratory work in intubated patients breathing with continuous positive airway pressure systems. Anesthesiology 63:536–539
13. Beydon L, Chassé M, Harf A, Lemaire F (1988) Inspiratory work of breathing during spontaneous ventilation using demand valves and continuous flow systems. Am Rev Respir Dis 138:300–304
14. Sassoon CSH, Lodia R, Rheeman CH, Kuei HJ, Light RN, Mahutte CK (1992) Inspiratory muscle work of breathing during flow-by, demand-flow, and continuous-flow systems in patients with chronic obstructive pulmonary disease. Am Rev Respir 145:1219–1222
15. Giuliani R, Mascia L, Recchia F, Caracciolo A, Fiore T, Ranieri VM (1995) Patient-ventilator interaction during synchronized intermittent mandatory ventilation. Am J Respir Crit Care Med 151:1–9
16. Polese G, Massara A, Brandolese R, Poggi R, Rossi A (1995) Flow triggering reduces inspiratory effort during weaning from mechanical ventilation. Intensive Care Med 21:682–686
17. Mancebo J, Vallverdú I, Bak E, et al (1993) Effects on the work of breathing (WOB) of different CPAP systems during weaning from mechanical ventilation. Am Rev Respir Dis 147:A876
18. Ranieri VM, Giuliani R, Mascia L, Recchia F, Fiore T (1993) Effects of CPAP on inspiratory muscle effort in COPD patients: flow-by vs. demand flow system. Am Rev Respir Dis 147:A878
19. Aslanian P, El Atrous S, Isabey D, et al (1998) Effects of flow triggering on breathing effort during partial ventilatory support. Am J Respir Crit Care Med 157:135–143
20. Katz JA, Marks JD (1985) Inspiratory work with and without continuous positive airway pressure in patients with acute respiratory failure. Anesthesiology 63:598–607

21. Sassoon CSH, Light RW, Lodia R, Sieck GC, Mahutte CK (1991) Pressure-time product during continuous positive airway pressure, pressure support ventilation and T-piece during weaning from mechanical ventilation. Am Rev Respir Dis 143:459–475

22. Yap J, Moore D, Cleland J, Pride N (2000) Effect of supine posture on respiratory mechanics in chronic left ventricular failure. Am J Respir Crit Care Med 162:1285–1291

23. Bradley TD, Holloway RM, McLaughin PR, Ross BL, Walters J, Liu PL (1992) Cardiac output response to continuous positive airway pressure in congestive heart failure. Am Rev Respir Dis 145:377–382

24. Lenique F, Habis M, Lofaso F, Dubois-Randé JL, Harf A, Brochard L (1997) Ventilatory and hemodynamic effects of continuous positive airway pressure in left heart failure. Am J Respir Crit Care Med 155:500–505

25. Branson RD, Hurst JM, De Haven CB jr (1985) Mask CPAP: state of the art. Respir Care 30:846–857

26. Greenbaum DM, Millen JE, Eroos B, Snyder JV, Grenvik A, Safar P (1976) Continuous positive airway pressure without tracheal intubation in spontaneously breathing patients. Chest 60:615–620

27. Venus B, Jacobs HK, Lim L (1979) Treatment of the adult respiratory distress syndrome with continuous positive airway pressure. Chest 76:257–261

28. Smith RA, Kirby RR, Gooding JM, et al (1980) Continuous positive airway pressure (CPAP) by face mask. Crit Care Med 8:483–485

29. Covelli HD, Weled BJ, Beekman JF (1982) Efficacy of continuous positive airway pressure administered by face mask. Chest 81:147–150

30. Bersten AD, Holt AW, Vedig AE, Skowronski GA, Baggely CJ (1991) Treatment of severe cardiogenic pulmonary edema with continuous positive airway pressure delivered by face mask. N Engl J Med 325:1825–1830

31. Räsänen J, Heikkilä J, Downs J, Nikki P, Vaisänen IT, Viitanen A (1985) Continuous positive airway pressure by face mask in acute cardiogenic pulmonary edema. Am J Cardiol 55:296–300

32. Räsänen J, Vaisanen IT, Heikkilä J, Nikki P (1985) Acute myocardial infarction complicated by left ventricular dysfunction and respiratory failure. Chest 87:158–162

33. Gachot B, Clair B, Wolff M, Régnier B, Vachon F (1992) Continuous positive airway pressure by face mask or mechanical ventilation in patients with human immunodeficiency virus infection and severe Pneumocystis carinii pneumonia. Intensive Care Med 18: 155–159

34. Lin M, Yang YF, Chiang HT, Chang MS, Chiang BN, Cheitlin MD (1995) Reappraisal of continuous positive airway pressure therapy in acute cardiogenic pulmonary edema. Short-term results and long-term follow-up. Chest 107:1379–1386

35. L'Her E, Moriconi M, Texier F, et al (1998) Non-invasive continuous positive airway pressure in acute hypoxaemic respiratory failure – experience of an emergency department. Eur J Emerg Med 5:313–318

36. Delclaux C, L'Her E, Alberti C, et al (2000) Treatment of acute hypoxemic nonhypercapnic respiratory insufficiency with continuous positive airway pressure delivered by face mask. A randomized controlled multicenter study. JAMA 284:2352–2360

37. Annest SL, Gottlieb M, Paloski WH, et al (1980) Detrimental effects of removing end-expiratory pressure prior to endotracheal extubation. Ann Surg 191:539–545

38. Quan SF, Falltrick RT, Schlobohm RM (1981) Extubation from ambient or expiratory positive airway pressure in adults. Anesthesiology 55:53–56

39. Weisman IM, Rinaldo JE (1982) Positive end-expiratory pressure in adult respiratory failure. N Engl J Med 307:1381–1384

40. Andersen JB, Olesen KP, Eikard E, Jansen E, Qvist J (1980) Periodic continuous positive airway pressure. CPAP, by mask in the treatment of atelectasis. Eur J Respir Dis 61:20–25

41. Carlsson C, Sonden B, Thylén U (1981) Can postoperative continuous positive airway pressure (CPAP) prevent pulmonary complications after abdominal surgery? Intensive Care Med 7:225–229

42. O'Donohue WJ (1985) National survey of the usage of lung expansion modalities for the prevention and treatment of postoperative atelectasis following abdominal and thoracic surgery. Chest 87:76–80
43. O'Donohue WJ (1985) Prevention and treatment of postoperative atelectasis. Can it and will it be adequately studied? Chest 87:1–2
44. Stock MC, Downs JB, Gauer PK, Alster JM, Imrey PB (1985) Prevention of postoperative pulmonary complications with CPAP, incentive spirometry, and conservative therapy. Chest 87:151–157
45. Ingwersen UM, Larsen KR, Bertelsen MT, et al (1993) Three different mask physiotherapy regimens for prevention of post-operative pulmonary complications after heart and pulmonary surgery. Intensive Care Med 19:294–298
46. Larsen KR, Ingwersen UM, Thode S, Jakobsen S (1995) Mask physiotherapy in patients after heart surgery: a controlled study. Intensive Care Med 21:469–474
47. Kacmarek RM (1995) Prophylactic bronchial hygiene following cardiac surgery: what is necessary? Intensive Care Med 21:467–468
48. Putensen C, Hörmann C, Baum M, Lingnau W (1993) Comparison of mask and nasal continuous positive airway pressure after extubation and mechanical ventilation. Crit Care Med 21:357–362
49. Montner PK, Greene ER, Murata GH, Stark DM, Timms M, Chick TW (1994) Hemodynamic effects of nasal and face mask continuous positive airway pressure. Am J Respir Crit Care Med 149:1614–1618

25 Closed-Loop Systems for Mechanical Ventilation

L. Brochard and M. Dojat

The consequences of a given form of ventilatory support depend on the work developed by the ventilator, on the opposing forces of the respiratory system, and on the dynamic response of the patient. Therefore, both the passive forces opposing the gas flow into the chest and the active breathing performed by the respiratory muscles of the patient are important for the efficacy of ventilatory assistance. Traditionally, the ventilator did not take this response into account and delivered the same output whatever the response of the system, until the ventilator's limit was reached. More and more now, ventilatory modes tend to adapt to the patient's or the respiratory system's response in order to improve patient-ventilator synchrony, to avoid superimposed work of breathing, and to improve tolerance of assisted ventilation. This important objective is obtained through more or less complex closed-loop systems where the ventilator adapts its output based on the comparison of the result of ventilation with a predefined target.

Simple control-loop systems are aimed at maintaining a preset level of pressure, as in pressure-control or pressure-support ventilation, for instance. In the latter mode, the flow delivered by the ventilator is regulated through a servo-valve in order to obtain airway pressure as close as possible to a predefined value, by comparing the resulting pressure with the actual measured pressure. In the more complex modes, a general strategy can be incorporated into the system, to drive the weaning process for instance.

25.1 Control and Planning: Two Key Points for Automatic Ventilation Management

Modern methods of artificial ventilation partially assist the patient's ventilation by adding to his/her spontaneous activity a variable amount of mechanical support. In this context, because the needs of the patient fluctuate, it is essential to continuously control the ventilatory support to avoid excessive work of breathing and effort, resulting in discomfort and dyspnea on the one hand, or excessive support, hyperinflation, and dysynchrony on the other hand. In parallel to this ideal automatic adaptation, it may be necessary to plan the long-term adaptation of the therapy according to specific medical goals. For instance, there may be an indication for gradually decreasing the level of assistance in order to facilitate the separation from the ventilator or for taking into account large variations of physiological need while the patient is waking up from anesthesia or drug intoxication.

Planning and control are two different tasks that have a common goal: choosing actions over time to influence a process, based on some model of that process (Dean and Wellman 1991). Control is a local task to determine what to do in the next instant. Planning is a strategic task to regulate the process evolution. For control and planning, numerous techniques are available, coming from two disciplines, respectively: control theory and artificial intelligence (AI), which differ mainly in the types of process models used. Control and planning are two complementary and essential tasks that must be combined to design multilevel controllers for the automatic supervision of complex systems such as mechanical ventilation of patients.

25.2 Basic Control Loops in Artificial Ventilation

In the field of mechanical ventilation we can identify three levels of control (Dojat et al. 1997). The complexity and the response time of the levels increase from the lowest to the highest level of control. Each level controls the levels below and is in turn controlled by the levels above.

The first level is a highly reactive basic control loop of the ventilator (response time ~1 ms) that controls essentially the flow or the pressure sent to the patient by driving a servo-valve. This can be used for simple control of pressure, as in pressure-support ventilation, or in much more complex modes such as proportional-assist ventilation (PAV). This level can be characterized as a closed-loop within the breaths.

The second level determines the mode of ventilation and has been used for minute mandatory ventilation (MMV-Hamilton), or for pressure-regulated volume control or volume support, for instance (Servo 300 Siemens). The response time of this level is of approximately one or two cycles (few seconds). Therefore, the closed-loop is used to control breaths based on the preceding ones.

The third level represents the adaptation of the assistance using information about the current state of the patient, its evolution and predefined therapeutic goals. This level of control, relying on specific medical knowledge and therapeutic strategies, is traditionally realized by the clinician in charge. The response time at this level varies from a few seconds in alarming situations to a few minutes in routine patient observation.

The envisaged plan of action can be proposed to the user (*open-loop system*) or performed directly by the computerized system (*closed-loop system*). A minority of medical systems currently work in closed-loop. For scenario recognition and decision-making, knowledge-based systems can rely on an explicit model of the patient or of the medical expertise required to perform a task.

25.3 Importance of the Physiological Reasoning Behind the Rules

Many closed-loop ventilatory systems have been tried in the past and only a very few have proved to be useful in the clinical field. To be efficient, such systems need to incorporate three basic elements. The first of these is the ventilator equipment, which must be fast enough to respond to the changes in drive as soon as needed by the patient and to accurately detect the patient's activity. The second component is the internal capability of the ventilator to use potent processors and function on-line with complex rules. The third one is the physiology beyond the ventilatory mode and the rules. In every new system, however, the theory should be tested in real clinical situations where the complexity of basic respiratory physiology interferes with many nonrespiratory stimuli. A few examples will illustrate the difficulty of designing an adequate system.

25.3.1 Minute Mandatory Ventilation

Minute mandatory ventilation (MMV) was designed to control minute ventilation, either by modifying the number of mandatory breaths in a synchronized intermittent mandatory ventilation (SIMV) type mode or by modifying the level of inspiratory pressure in a pressure-support (PS) mode of ventilation. With both approaches, one major difficulty is for the physician to set the adequate level of minute ventilation. If the level of minute ventilation is set too high with regard to the needs of the patient, the ventilator may do all the ventilatory work and turn assisted ventilation into controlled ventilation. If this level is set too low, the patient may become underassisted and perform all the work of breathing. There is also another drawback that may result in major problems for the patient. Indeed, it has been shown that the breathing pattern, i.e., the distribution between tidal volume and respiratory frequency, and not only the level of minute ventilation, is an essential component of the patient's response to a given workload (Tobin et al. 1986). Therefore, rapid shallow breathing may ensue and still be considered optimal for the ventilator, provided it results in an "adequate" level of minute ventilation. Hazards have also been described with this mode where the pressure-support level was gradually increased up to maximal limits set on the ventilator since the minute ventilation target was never reached. Indeed, increasing volumes were associated with a decrease in spontaneous frequency and no increase in minute ventilation.

25.3.2 Volume-Regulated Pressure-Supported Breaths

Several modes of ventilation propose to assist the patient with pressure-supported breaths, such as pressure-support ventilation, but to target the delivered pressure to a pre-determined tidal volume. This can be done in an assisted or a fully controlled mode of support. Again, major difficulties may arise from the choice of the tidal volume. Because no freedom is left to the patient, the targeted tidal volume may or may not match the patient's own demand. If the patient is actively breathing to get a higher tidal volume than the one delivered, this will automatically decrease the amount of assistance given by the ventilator and the patient may become exhausted because of a lack of ventilator assist.

25.3.3 Frequency-Regulated Pressure-Supported Breaths

Regulation of pressure-support ventilation to reach a pre-set level of respiratory frequency has been proposed as a closed-loop system. There is an inverse relationship between the level of pressure support and the breathing frequency adopted by the patient (Brochard et al. 1987, 1989) . Preliminary evaluation indicated interesting results (Fargier et al. 1987). This mode of ventilation has been shown to adequately ventilate patients with acute respiratory distress syndrome over a short test period (Zakynthinos et al. 1997). The target frequency was the one observed during assist-control ventilation. Controlling pressure support based on frequency makes more sense than controlling based on volume, since thresholds or targets for frequencies may be more universal than for tidal volumes based on body weight (Jubran et al. 1995) . The difficulty with an algorithm of the second level, i.e., regulating on a breath-by-breath basis, may be to find the right time constant to evaluate the patient after a change in the delivered pressure. Indeed, changes in breathing pattern require several cycles to stabilize (Viale et al. 1998). Other more complex systems have adopted a range of breathing frequency within which the patient may be considered to be comfortable (Dojat et al. 1992).

25.3.4 Use of the Occlusion Pressure

Iotti et al. proposed using the occlusion pressure, i.e., the pressure measured in the first 100 ms of an occlusion, to titrate the pressure-support level (Iotti et al. 1996). This index reflects the activation of the respiratory centers and is independent of respiratory mechanics and the patient's conscious response to occlusion (Whitelaw and Derenne 1993). Interestingly, triggering the ventilator is performed through an occlusion, at least with the pressure-triggered systems. In theory, the occlusion pressure could be calculated at each breath. In addition, this simple index has been shown to be well correlated with the patient's work of breathing (Alberti et al. 1995; Mancebo et al. 2000). The level of assistance could thus be controlled by targeting a desired level of $P_{0.1}$. Iotti et al. showed that a closed-loop control pressure support could be designed to control the level of $P_{0.1}$ at around 0.5 cmH$_2$O of the target.

25.3.5 Optimal Alveolar Ventilation

Linton et al. proposed that an optimal level of alveolar ventilation could be calculated and targeted to put the patient in the optimal zone for breathing. The optimal breathing pattern would be determined to optimize work of breathing for a given level of alveolar ventilation, based on classical physiological theories (Laubscher et al. 1994). A study with various groups of patients, using a form of support called "adaptive support or lung ventilation" (ALV) (Amadeus–Hamilton), showed it was an interesting way to decrease the pressure-support level and wean patients from the ventilator (Linton et al. 1994).

25.3.6 Proportional-Assist Ventilation

Proportional-assist ventilation offers the example of a very sophisticated form of closed loop of the first level. It has a very strong physiological background and was designed as a more physiological way to unload the respiratory muscles (Younes 1992, 1994; Younes et al. 1992). It is designed to deliver the appropriate amount of pressure needed at every moment of the inspiratory breathing cycle to counteract both the resistive and the elastic forces opposing gas flow into the lungs. It requires the ventilator to know the resistance and the elastance of the respiratory system measured independently by the clinician. The ventilator measures flow and volume and applies a gain depending on the desired percentage of unloading on both signals, to deliver the appropriate level of resistive and elastic pressure, respectively. The need to measure resistance and elastance is certainly a limitation of this ventilatory mode, since measurements of respiratory mechanics are quite difficult to perform in spontaneously breathing patients under assisted ventilation. In addition, these values may change over time and need to be reassessed frequently. In short-term studies this mode was shown to adapt remarkably well to changes in ventilatory demand (Grasso et al. 2000; Ranieri et al. 1996, 1997). In this mode, there is no pre-set volume, pressure, or time, and the freedom given to the patient is greater than with any other ventilatory mode.

25.4 The Integrated Level

Integration into the controller of an active clinical strategy, represented by production rules (IF conditions, THEN actions), was proposed by Strickland and Hasson (Strickland and Hasson 1991, 1993). Their system used two parameters, tidal volume (Vt) and respiratory frequency (RR), to estimate the patient's current ventilation and modify, if necessary, the machine frequency and the pressure-support level (SIMV+PS mode was used). Oxygen saturation was used as a safety parameter. When ventilation was correct (Vt $\geq$5 ml/kg and 8$\leq$RR$\leq$30 cycles/min), machine frequency and pressure-support level were systematically decreased. The clinical results indicated that the use of the system reduced the time spent with incorrect ventilation and the number of blood gas measurements performed. In this system, the weaning strategy was reactive and fixed and did not take into account temporal evolution of the ventilation, a central point in the clinician's decision-making process. Consequently, only candidates for weaning were ventilated with this system.

The work performed for several years at the LDS Hospital (Salt Lake City, Utah, USA) to elaborate computerized protocols is relevant here (East et al. 1999; Morris 1999; Randolph et al. 1998). The algorithm-oriented approach they have chosen leads to a complicated logic where temporal aspects are intricate. It is largely recognized within the knowledge-acquisition community that the elicitation of the knowledge level (Newell 1982), such as for instance temporal abstractions (Shahar 1997) applied to the context of management of mechanical ventilation, is essential to facilitate reuse, sharing, and maintenance of knowledge-based systems (Musen 1992). Recently, the need to base automatic control on clinical experience rather than on mathematical models of the couple patient-ventilator has led to the introduction of fuzzy logic in working closed-loop (Schaüblin et al. 1996) or open-loop (Nemoto et al. 1999) systems. Fuzzy logic is used to represent the subjective human notions, such as "high", "low", "normal", or "too high", employed in decision-making. Rules, sets, and membership functions, central elements of the fuzzy logic approach, are designed according to medical practice. Promising results were obtained using this type of fuzzy controller for automatic adjustment of the pressure-support level (Nemoto et al. 1999). Here again, the introduction of (fuzzy) temporal reasoning is essential to envisaging the automation of the entire mechanical ventilation with this approach. Indeed, integrating the third level in the system should allow construction of a more comprehensive view of the time course of the patient's state, thereby giving it the ability to manage several ventilation strategies depending on the patient's state. The results we have recently obtained at Henri Mondor Hospital (Créteil, France) demonstrate that this is feasible and that a knowledge-based approach is suitable for modeling a substantial part of the clinician's expertise relevant for the third level.

25.5 A Practical and Successful Experience
Using the NéoGanesh System

The initial objective in designing the knowledge-based system called NéoGanesh was to build a closed-loop system (a) that would be efficient for the automatic control of mechanical support and planning of the weaning process, (b) that could be extended to gradually improve its reasoning and planning capabilities, and (c) that could be tested at the patient's bedside to measure its performance at each step.

25.5.1 A Knowledge-Based System Working in Closed Loop

Instead of computerizing a specific recipe for ventilation management (Randolph et al. 1998; Strickland and Hasson 1993), in designing NéoGanesh we tried to respect the golden rules of knowledge engineering: to make an explicit model of medical tasks and reasoning involved, and to distinguish between the conceptual model (knowledge level) and the representation paradigms (symbolic level) used to implement it (Dojat and Pachet 1995). NéoGanesh is based on current artificial intelligence techniques: knowledge representation mixing objects and rules and temporal abstractions (Dojat and Sayettat 1996) in a distributed architecture (Dojat et al. 1997). It combines a "tactical" component and a strategic component. The "strategic" component relies on the model and representation of the intensivist's decision-making process. The "tactical" component uses three physiological parameters to modify the assistance in pressure-support mode and to maintain the patient within a zone of acceptable ventilation (the zone of respiratory comfort: 15<RR<30 cycles/min, Vt>300 ml or 250 if weight <55 kg, PetCO$_2$<55 mmHg or 65 mmHg if COPD). Therefore, compared with the general architectures of such systems as VENTPLAN (Rutledge et al. 1993) or GUARDIAN (Hayes-Roth et al. 1992; Larsson et al. 1997), the approach is modest. Its originality can be stressed in three points:

The system is based on the modeling of the medical expertise required to perform mechanical ventilation of patients in pressure-support mode. It does not include mathematical equations of a physiological model. There are three reasons for this: (a) In pathological situations, physiological models are uncertain and can require nonavailable data in real-time, the estimation of which is difficult or imprecise. Their validation is still an open problem. (b) Physiological models do not always represent useful information to the clinician in decision-making. For instance, to follow up the recovery of patient after anesthesia, pharmacological equations are imprecise and not used in practice. (c) The decision-making process of clinicians may be less variable than the complex physiology of patients. This is reinforced by the introduction of protocols or guidelines for mechanical ventilation based on such objective measurements as respiratory frequency or the rapid shallow breathing index. In conclusion, it seems simpler to model decision-making based on objective measurements than physiology based on multiple assumptions of the patient's behavior. Therefore, the NéoGanesh system is "decision-driven" as well as "patient-driven", although it indeed uses data coming from the patient.

The introduction of a new mode of ventilation such as PAV (Younes 1992), ALV (Laubscher et al. 1994), or autoregulated inspiratory support (ARIS) (Chambrin et al. 1992) is a long and difficult process. Then, it was decided (a) to ventilate patients with a standard mode of ventilation, pressure support, largely used for weaning, and (b) to add heuristic knowledge to improve its use and facilitate the weaning process.

It is essential to built extensible architectures for patient monitoring and implementation of mechanical ventilation protocols. Most of the recent systems proposed are very ambitious and their validation is possible only through simulators (Larsson et al. 1997). Starting from an extensible architecture Néo-Ganesh integrated modules that are validated in the clinical situation. It is based on a pragmatic bottom-up approach guided by tight collaboration with intensivists and continuous clinical evaluation. The current module is devoted to the control in closed-loop of the mechanical ventilation and decision to extubate. This approach is close to that of the VIE-VENT project in Vienna, Austria (Horn et al. 1997) devoted to the development of a knowledge-based system for artificially ventilated newborn infants to optimize therapy planning and to support neonatologists in their daily routine; a change of the ventilator's settings is evaluated by monitoring the trend of the subsequent changes of the transcutaneous blood gases. A new recommendation is formulated if the short-term trend does not meet present requirements concerning the direction and the amount of the expected change (Miksch et al. 1997). Therapy recommendations, based on transcutaneously and invasively determined blood gas measurements, are formulated in terms of recommended changes of the ventilator settings.

25.5.2 Clinical Results

NéoGanesh has been used in closed-loop and tested in more than 60 ventilated patients at Henri Mondor Hospital. Two types of evaluation have been performed (a) to assess the capacity of the system to control the level of assistance in accordance with the patient's needs (evaluation of the tactical level) and (b) to assess the decision to extubate provided by the system (evaluation of the strategic level).

25.5.3 Evaluation of the Management of Mechanical Ventilation

In a preliminary study, two different groups of patients have been ventilated with the system representing two different steps in the course of mechanical ventilation. The first group ($n=9$) was composed of patients considered candidates for weaning, the second one ($n=10$) of severely ill patients needing to be maintained on mechanical ventilation. The mean time required to reach the zone of respiratory comfort, expressed as the percentage of the total ventilation duration, was 99% for the first group and 90% for the second group (see details in Dojat et al. 1992). In a recent study, ten patients were randomly ventilated over two 24-h periods with and without NéoGanesh (standard PS) (Dojat et al. 2000). In standard PS, the clinician in charge was able to modify the pressure-support level at his or her discretion. The mean PS level was similar with the two modes (17 ± 4 cmH$_2$O and 19 ± 6 cmH$_2$O without and with NéoGanesh, respectively). The percentage of time (over total ventilator time) that patients remained in the zone of respiratory comfort was 66% $\pm24\%$ and 93% $\pm8\%$ without and with NéoGanesh, respectively. These results are shown in Fig. 25.1. The number of PS changes was considerably higher with Néo-Ganesh (56 ±40) than with standard PS (1 ±2). The mean time spent in critical ventilation (RR >35 cycles/min, Vt <300 ml or PetCO$_2$ $\geq$55 mmHg) was 3% with Néo-

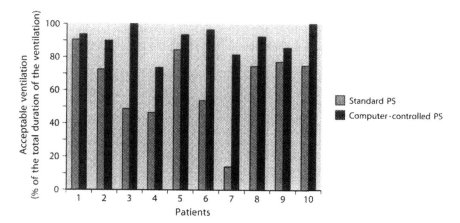

Fig. 25.1. Mean time spent in the zone of respiratory comfort without (*Standard PS*) and with NéoGanesh (*Computer-controlled PS*), expressed as the percentage of the total ventilation duration for ten patients on long-term mechanical ventilation. (From Dojat et al. 2000)

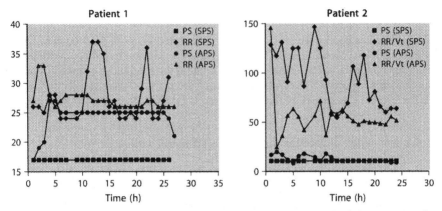

Fig. 25.2. Evolution of pressure-support (*PS*) level and respiratory rate (*RR*) (*patient 1*) or the rapid shallow breathing index (*RR/Vt*) (*patient 2*) without (standard pressure support, or *SPS*) and with NéoGanesh (automated pressure support, or *APS*) over two 24-h periods. Note that the APS prevented excessively high values of the RR or the RR/Vt index by modifying the PS level

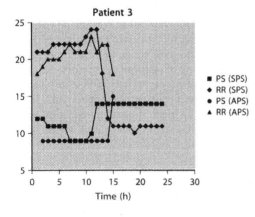

Fig. 25.3. Same legend as in Fig. 25.2 for another patient (patient 3). Note that the mean level of PS was similar for the two periods but that respiratory rate (*RR*) was kept in the normal range only with APS

Ganesh as compared with 23% with standard PS mode. Finally, the time spent at a high level of occlusion pressure ($P_{0.1}$), suggesting a high work of breathing, was significantly reduced with the knowledge-based system.

NéoGanesh tries to automatically decrease the level of assistance. This is illustrated for the patient in Fig. 25.2, where the PS level was modulated depending on the respiratory rate values when NéoGanesh was used, while it was kept constant with the standard PS (Fig. 25.3).

25.5.4 Decision to Extubate

For some patients weaning can be a long and difficult process. Continuous adjustment of mechanical assistance as performed by NéoGanesh may positively influence weaning outcome. The level of pressure support may be a useful guide to determine the optimal time for performing tracheal extubation. This strategy was implemented in NéoGanesh: when the patient was ventilated with a low level of assistance (9 cmH_2O for an endotracheal tube or 5 cmH_2O for a tracheotomy cannula), an observation period was triggered (1 or 2 h, depending on whether the level of pressure support after 1 h of ventilation was <15 or $\geq$15 cmH_2O, respectively) and a decision about extubation was displayed on the computer screen. For 38 patients, we compared the decision given by NéoGanesh with the standard battery of weaning tests (preweaning tests plus 2 h on T-piece plus 48 h follow-up) (Dojat et al. 1996). The negative predictive value was equal in the two cases. However, the positive predictive value was 89% and 77% for NéoGanesh and for the standard PS mode, respectively, and 81% for the rapid shallow breathing index alone (Dojat et al. 1996). NéoGanesh predicted failure of weaning for five patients who tolerated the 2-h T-piece trial but eventually failed to tolerate weaning.

25.6 Conclusion

Modern ventilation needs to be simplified for the user and adapted to the changing needs of the patient. At the same time, the patient might be separated from the ventilator as soon as the risk of separation and subsequent extubation is not deemed superior to the risk of keeping the patient under assisted ventilation. All these actions require a high level of monitoring and frequent reactivity to adapt ventilatory settings. Protocols and guidelines have been designed to help everyone to follow the same rules; clinical practice shows this is extremely difficult to obtain. Closed-loop systems might be of great help in this regard by performing the tasks which are not routinely performed for simple logistic reasons. They do not replace the work performed by the personnel, the therapist, or the physician, but instead perform the necessary tasks which cannot be performed on a 24-h basis. The greatest difficulty in designing such a system is to reliably reproduce the decision-making process of the clinician. It needs to understand both physiology and human reactions.

25.7 References

Alberti A, Gallo F, Fongaro A, Valenti S, Rossi A (1995) $P_{0.1}$ is a useful parameter in setting the level of pressure support ventilation. Intensive Care Med 21:547–553

Brochard L, Pluskwa F, Lemaire F (1987) Improved efficacy of spontaneous breathing with inspiratory pressure support. Am Rev Resp Dis 136:411–415

Brochard L, Harf A, Lorino H, Lemaire F (1989) Inspiratory pressure support prevents diaphragmatic fatigue during weaning from mechanical ventilation. Am Rev Respir Dis 139:513–521

Chambrin M-C, Chopin C, Mangalaboyi KH (1992) Autoregulated inspiratory support system. 14th IEEE-EMBS. Paris, pp 2419–2420

Dean TL, Wellman MP (1991) Planning and control. Morgan Kaufmann, San Mateo, Calif

Dojat M, Pachet F (1995) Effective domain-dependent reuse in medical knowledge bases. Comput Biomed Res 28:403–432

Dojat M, Sayettat C (1996) A realistic model for temporal reasoning in real-time patient monitoring. Applied Artif Intell 10:121–143

Dojat M, Brochard L, Lemaire F, Harf A (1992) A knowledge-based system for assisted ventilation of patients in intensive care units. Int J Clin Monit Comput 9:239–250

Dojat M, Harf A, Touchard D, Laforest M, Lemaire F, Brochard L (1996) Evaluation of a knowledge-based system providing ventilatory management and decision for extubation. Am J Respir Crit Care Med 153:997–1004

Dojat M, Pachet F, Guessoum Z, Touchard D, Harf A, Brochard L (1997) NeoGanesh: a working system for the automated control of assisted ventilation in ICUs. Artif Intell Med 11:97–117

Dojat M, Harf A, Touchard D, Lemaire F, Brochard L (2000) Clinical evaluation of a computer-controlled pressure support mode. Am J Respir Crit Care Med 161:1161–1166

East TD, Bradshaw RL, Lugo A, Sailors M, Ershler L, Wallace CJ, Morris AH, McKinley B, Marquez A, Tonnesen A, Parmley L (1999) Efficacy of computerized decision support for mechanical ventilation: results of a prospective multi-center randomized trial. AMIA'99. AMIA, Washington DC, pp 203–217

Fargier JJ, Robert D, Boyer F, Chagny J, Kopp C, Baulieux J, Meskovtchenko JF, Pouyet M (1987) Positive pressure inspiratory aid VS assisted mechanical ventilation after esophageal surgery. J Crit Care 2:101–108

Grasso S, Puntillo F, Mascia L, Ancona G, Fiore T, Bruno F, Slutsky A, Ranieri M (2000) Compensation for increase in respiratory workload during mechanical ventilation. Pressure-support versus proportional-assist ventilation. Am J Respir Crit Care Med 161:819–826

Hayes-Roth B, Washington R, Ash D, Hewett R, Collinot A, Vina A, Seiver A (1992) Guardian: a prototype intelligent agent for intensive-care monitoring. Artif Intell Med 4:165–185

Horn W, Miksch S, Egghart G, Popow C, Paky F (1997) Effective data validation of high-frequency data: time-point, time-interval, and trend-based methods. Comput Biol Med 27: 389–409

Iotti GA, Brunner JX, Braschi A, Laubscher T, Olivei MC, Palo A, Galbusera C, Comelli A (1996) Closed-loop control of airway occlusion pressure at 0.1 second (P. 01) applied to pressure-support ventilation: algorithm and application in intubated patients. Crit Care Med 24: 771–779

Jubran A, Van de Graaff WB, Tobin MJ (1995) Variability of patient-ventilator interaction with pressure support ventilation in patients with chronic obstructive pulmonary disease. Am J Respir Crit Care Med 152:129–136

Larsson J, Hayes-Roth B, Gaba D, Smith B (1997) Evaluation of a medical diagnosis system using simulator test scenarios. Artif Intell Med 11:119–140

Laubscher TP, Heinrichs W, Weiler N, Hartmann G, Brunner JX (1994) An adaptive lung ventilation controller. IEEE Trans Biol Engin 41:51–58

Linton DM, Potgieter PD, Davis S, Fourie ATJ, Brunner JX, Laubscher TP (1994) Automatic weaning from mechanical ventilation using an adaptative lung ventilation controller. Chest 106:1843–1850

Mancebo J, Albaladejo P, Touchard D, Bak E, Subirana M, Lemaire F, Harf A, Brochard L (2000) Airway occlusion pressure to titrate positive end-expiratory pressure in patients with dynamic hyperinflation. Anesthesiology 93:81–90

Miksch S, Horn W, Popow C, Paky F (1997) Utilizing temporal data abstraction for validation and therapy planning for artificially ventilated newborn infants. Artif Intell Med 8:543–576

Morris A (1999) Computerized protocols and bedside decision support. Crit Care Clin 15:523–545

Musen MA (1992) Dimensions of knowledge sharing and reuse. Comput Biomed Res 25:435–467

Nemoto T, Hatzakis G, Thorpe C, Olivenstein R, Dial S, Bates J (1999) Automatic control of pressure support mechanical ventilation using fuzzy logic. Am J Respir Crit Care Med 160:550–556

Newell A (1982) The knowledge level. Artif Intell 18:87–102

Randolph A, Clemmer T, East T, Kinder A, Orme J, Wallace C, Morris A (1998) Evaluation of compliance with a computerized protocol: weaning from mechanical ventilator support using pressure support. Comput Methods Programs Biomed 57:201–215

Ranieri V, Giuliani R, Mascia L, Grasso S, Petruzzelli V, Puntillo N, Perchiazzi G, Fiore T, Brienza A (1996) Patient-ventilator interaction during acute hypercapnia: pressure support vs. proportional assist ventilation. J Appl Physiol 81:426–436

Ranieri VM, Grasso S, Mascia L, Martino S, Fiore T, Brienza A, Giuliani R (1997) Effects of proportional assist ventilation on inspiratory muscle effort in patients with chronic obstructive pulmonary disease and acute respiratory failure. Anesthesiology 86:79–91

Rutledge GW, Thomsen GE, Farr BR, Tovar MA, Polaschek JX, Beinlich IA, Sheiner LB, Fagan LM (1993) The design and implementation of a ventilator-management advisor. Artif Intell Med 5:67–82

Schaüblin J, Derighetti M, Feigenwinter P, Petersen-Felix S, Zbinden A (1996) Fuzzy control of mechanical ventilation during anesthesia. B J Anaesth 77:636–641

Shahar Y (1997) A framework for knowledge-based temporal abstraction. Artif Intell 90:79–133

Strickland JH, Hasson JH (1991) A computer-controlled ventilator weaning system. Chest 100:1096–1099

Strickland JH, Hasson JH (1993) A computer-controlled ventilator weaning system. Chest 103:1220–1226

Tobin MJ, Perez W, Guenther SM, Semmens BJ, Mader MJ, Allen SJ, Lodato RF, Dantzker D (1986) The pattern of breathing during successful and unsuccessful trials of weaning from mechanical ventilation. Am Rev Respir Dis 134:1111–1118

Viale JP, Duperret S, Mahul P, Delafosse BX, Delpuech C, Weismann D, Annat GJ (1998) Time course evolution of ventilatory responses to inspiratory unloading in patients. Am J Respir Crit Care Med 157:428–434

Whitelaw WA, Derenne JP (1993) Airway occlusion pressure. J Appl Physiol 74:1475–1483

Younes M (1992) Proportional assist ventilation, a new approach to ventilatory support. Am Res Respir Dis 145:114–120

Younes M (1994) Proportional assist ventilation. In: Tobin M (ed) Principles and practice of mechanical ventilation. McGraw-Hill, New-York, pp 349–369

Younes M, Puddy A, Roberts D, Light RB, Quesada A, Taylor K, Oppenheimer L, Cramp H (1992) Proportional assist ventilation. Results of an initial clinical trial. Am Rev Respir Dis 145:121–129

Zakynthinos SG, Vassilakopoulos T, Daniil Z, Zakynthinos E, Koutsoukos E, Katsouyianni K, Roussos C (1997) Pressure support ventilation in adult respiratory distress syndrome: short-term effects of a servocontrolled mode. J Crit Care 12:161–172

26 Tracheostomy in the ICU: Why, When and How?

E. L'Her and L. Brochard

26.1 When to Perform Tracheostomy in the ICU and Why

26.1.1 Reasons for Performing Tracheostomy

Tracheostomy is commonly performed in mechanically ventilated patients with prolonged duration of mechanical ventilation or with difficulties in weaning from the ventilator. This can include patients with chronic respiratory disorders being placed on the ventilator for an acute episode, patients with coma or prolonged inability to protect their airway, trauma patients with major neurological and/or chest injury, patients with upper airway abnormalities, or patients who, for a variety of other reasons, do not seem to tolerate disconnection from the ventilator (Astrachan et al. 1988; Diehl et al. 1994; El Naggar et al. 1976; Plummer and Gracey 1989; Stauffer et al. 1981). Many reasons are often given for the decision to perform tracheostomy in mechanically ventilated patients, very few of then supported by convincing evidence. Tracheostomy also carries a risk of immediate and long-term complications, but new techniques probably allow for fewer immediate complications. Several reasons, however, are often mentioned for the decision to perform tracheostomy on critically ill patients, and these reasons have to be balanced against the risk of the procedure. Tracheostomy is thus frequently performed during weaning from mechanical ventilation without there being strong arguments, substantiated by clinical studies, to support it.

In an international survey of more than 5000 mechanically ventilated patients (Esteban et al. 2001), Esteban et al. found that tracheostomy was performed in 11.5% of all mechanically ventilated patients (for more than 12 h) after a mean of 12.7 ±7.6 days. This percentage varied among countries. For instance, in France, tracheostomy was performed in only 5% of the patients under mechanical ventilation and after a mean of 16.0 ±11.5 days. In a recent survey done in Switzerland, Fischler et al. found a 10% prevalence of tracheostomy for patients requiring ventilation for at least 24 h, with a complication rate of 13%, among which hemorrhage and infections were predominant (Fischler et al. 2000). It is not known whether the absence or presence of financial incentives in different countries might have something to do with these different rates.

26.1.2 Sequels of the Upper Airway

No benefit of tracheostomy, such as a reduction in the risk of laryngeal or tracheal injury or stenosis, has been clearly demonstrated. Retrospective series have suggested that the highest risk of laryngeal or tracheal injury is observed in patients in whom tracheostomy was performed after a prolonged period of translaryngeal intubation, as opposed to early tracheostomy or prolonged intubation alone (Stauffer et al. 1981).Without a controlled study, it is difficult to ascertain that this higher risk is caused by delayed tracheostomy, but this became one of the arguments used against postponing the decision for tracheostomy.

26.1.3 Nosocomial Pneumonia

It is unlikely that tracheostomy changes the colonization rate of the trachea, which is supposed to be one of the major risk factors for subsequent nosocomial pneumonia. In a prospective observational cohort study of children requiring long-term ventilation, Morar et al. assessed the impact of tracheotomy on colonization and infection of the lower airways (Morar et al. 1998). The lower airways were colonized in 71% of children during transtracheal ventilation, whereas post-tracheotomy, this rate reached 95% ($p=0.03$). As in other studies, however, children developed significantly fewer infections following colonization with a micro-organism post-tracheotomy (8/15 pretracheotomy vs 6/21 post-tracheotomy). It is difficult again to relate this lower infection rate to tracheostomy alone. It may simply be that early-onset pneumonia, which may respond to different pathophysiological mechanisms, played a large part in the pneumonia rate occurring before tracheostomy. Although some authors had suggested that tracheostomy might be a risk factor for nosocomial pneumonia, tracheostomy does not seem to increase the risk of pneumonia in critically ill patients. For instance, Blot et al. described the relative safety of tracheotomy in neutropenic mechanically ventilated patients (Blot et al. 1995). In a retrospective study performed on 135 patients requiring tracheotomy for mechanical ventilation (10.6% of the total ICU population), nosocomial pneumonia was found to occur in 26% of the patients (Georges et al. 2000). Nosocomial pneumonia occurred a mean of 8–9 days after tracheotomy. The authors suggested that some episodes of pneumonia, occurring in the 3–5 days after the procedure, could have been caused or favored by the procedure itself. They found that presence of hyperthermia and a high rate of colonization of the trachea were risk factors for these episodes of early pneumonia. Finally, other authors suggested that the use of topical antibiotics on tracheostoma in long-term mechanically ventilated children could prevent exogenous colonization and infection. Clearly, further studies are required on this controversial issue of infection and tracheostomy.

In addition, it has been well-demonstrated that orotracheal intubation carries a lower risk of infectious sinusitis and, likely, of pneumonia than nasotracheal intubation (Holzapfel et al. 1999; Rouby et al. 1994). It makes sense to think that tracheostomy, similar to orotracheal intubation, carries a low risk of infectious sinusitis, and the infectious complications might be compared between orotracheal intubation and tracheostomy.

26.1.4 Comfort and Nursing Care

To date, only one study has prospectively evaluated the effect of tracheotomy in a small group of trauma patients, suggesting a benefit in favor of early tracheotomy as compared with prolonged translaryngeal intubation. Improved patient comfort has been reported, resulting from a facilitation of communication, mobility, oral alimentation, and suctioning of secretions (Astrachan et al. 1988). Comfort and easier nursing care are certainly among the major reasons for performing tracheostomy in mechanically ventilated patients. It is surprising, however, that there has been so little evaluation of this important aspect of patient care.

26.1.5 Weaning and Work of Breathing

Failure of weaning from the ventilator often results from an imbalance between respiratory muscle capacity and the loads imposed on the respiratory system (Lessard and Brochard 1996). Difficult weaning with a prolonged expected duration of mechanical ventilation is often a reason to decide on a tracheostomy. A positive effect of tracheostomy on the work of breathing (WOB) may explain a possible influence on the weaning process, and may therefore help in making individual decisions to perform this invasive procedure. Indeed, both the resistance of the tracheotomy cannula and its internal dead space (volume) may be smaller than those of an endotracheal tube (ETT), and tracheotomy may therefore ease the respiratory workload. On the other hand, the relative influence of the artificial airway in difficult-to-wean patients may be relatively small, and the total effort of breathing may be dictated essentially by the respiratory mechanics of the patient. The study by Diehl et al. was the first to evaluate, in the clinical environment, the effects of tracheotomy on parameters that may have a major influence on the issue of discontinuation of mechanical ventilation (Diehl et al. 1999). Patients were studied just before and right after tracheostomy in the same conditions of ventilation. Pressure-support ventilation was used, since several patients did not tolerate disconnection from the ventilator, and similar levels were used before and after tracheostomy. The study demonstrated mainly a significant reduction in WOB by 55%, as well as in $P_{0.1}$ and in intrinsic PEEP. Interestingly, this reduction was greater than had been predicted or had been calculated in a bench study using new tubes and tracheostomy cannulas. Part of this reduction resulted from substantial extra work imposed by ETTs that had been left in place for prolonged periods. This suggests that part of the imposed work was created by the tube itself and by permanent deposits on the inner wall of the tube (Villafane et al. 1996; Wright et al. 1989) . In this context, changing the tracheotomy cannula in tracheotomized patients is easily performed in a systematic fashion, which can be considered another advantage of this technique.

26.1.6 Impact on Outcome

Tracheostomy is widely performed in intensive care units. Little is known, however, about its effects on weaning from and the duration of mechanical ventilation, or its impact on outcome. Kollef et al. recently described the characteristics and outcome of tracheostomized patients compared with intubated nontracheostomized patients (Kollef et al. 1999). Tracheostomy was performed in 9.8% of 521 mechanically ventilated patients. In a multivariate analysis to identify which patients were selected for tracheostomy, it was found that tracheostomy was significantly associated with nosocomial pneumonia, aerosol therapy, witnessed aspiration, and need for reintubation. Tracheostomy was associated with a longer duration of mechanical ventilation than required for patients with translaryngeal intubation alone: 20 ±16 vs 4 ±5 days (tracheostomy was performed after 9.7 ±6.4 days), a longer length of stay in the intensive care unit or in the hospital (31 vs 13 days), and a lower mortality (13.7%) among medical patients. These interesting results do not help to determine the impact of tracheostomy per se in these patients. Indeed, tracheostomy is performed in patients who have already survived the first 8–10 days of mechanical ventilation and who are expected, by the attending physician, to survive the ICU stay. These two factors favor both a longer duration of ventilation and stay and a lower mortality than the rest of the ICU population, explained by the selection process and not by tracheostomy per se. In order to circumvent these limitations, Esteban et al. recently made use of a large international database of mechanically ventilated patients to perform a matched paired case-control study comparing 373 patients with tracheostomy with the same number of patients without tracheostomy and with endotracheal intubation alone (Esteban et al. 2001). Presented in a preliminary format, the results were quite similar to those of Kollef et al. (Kollef et al. 1999), with prolonged ventilation, a prolonged ICU stay, and a decreased ICU mortality for patients with tracheostomy. By contrast, however, the in-hospital mortality was similar for the two groups due to an increase in non-ICU hospital deaths among tracheostomized patients ("hospital" meaning every institution before home discharge). Therefore, these results seem to indicate that tracheostomy may be a way to discharge patients earlier from the ICU.

26.1.7 Timing of Tracheostomy

This important and much-debated question has no definitive answer. In a review of the literature, Heffner promoted an anticipatory approach in which tracheostomy would be performed after at least 7 days of intubation, when extubation appeared to be distant, and when it was likely to have an important benefit (Heffner 1993). The results of Diehl et al. (Diehl et al. 1999) also indirectly suggest that detecting and/or preventing insidious ETT obstruction may offer an alternative to tracheostomy in some patients.

Maziak and co-workers performed a systematic review of the literature concerning the timing of tracheostomy (Maziak et al. 1998). Five studies were identified, of which three were quasi-randomized and none were blinded. The authors concluded that there was insufficient evidence to support the hypothesis that the timing of tracheostomy alters the duration of mechanical ventilation or the extent of airway injury in critically ill patients.

One group of particular interest may be constituted by patients with central neurological disorders, who have problems both with protecting their airways and with removing secretions. Qureshi et al. assessed the possible prediction and the optimal timing of tracheostomy in patients with infratentorial lesions requiring mechanical ventilatory support (Qureshi et al. 2000). Among 69 patients, 28 (41%) required a surgical procedure. In terms of outcome related to mechanical ventilation, 23 (33%) were successfully extubated, 23 (33%) underwent a tracheostomy (among whom four eventually died), and 23 (33%) died before extubation or tracheostomy was performed. The overall mortality was 39%. Successful extubation (SE) was associated in a multivariate analysis with a Glasgow Coma Scale >7 at admission (odds ratio 4.8) and the absence of deficits at admission (OR 4.3). Reintubation was necessary in 11 patients. This high rate of reintubation was explained by the neurological deficits and the inability of the patients to protect their upper airway or to remove secretions. A high rate of reintubation has already been identified in patients with central neurological disorders (Vallverdu et al. 1998). At day 1, a GCS<7 and the presence of deficits carried a 10% probability of SE, but among the patients with a low probability of SE, many were not going to survive. Indeed, at day 8, the probability of SE for the patients still alive and ventilated had fallen to ~5%, and at day 10 to below 5%. Therefore, at day 8 or 10, among all patients initially predicted to have a low probability of SE, many had died. The patients still alive at day 8 or 10 had an extremely low probability of SE but had survived the first week of ventilation and were likely to survive. These two factors present on admission were therefore strong predictors, for the patients still alive at day 8 or 10, that they were not going to be successfully extubated, and could be used to decide in favor of tracheostomy. Prospective studies in these groups of patients are needed, following these general lines.

26.1.8 Conclusion

Although tracheostomy is a routine procedure in the ICU and there are strong advocates of the technique, it is striking to see how few data exist to help us in determining the best timing of, the best indications for, and the expected benefits of tracheostomy in ICU patients. Prospective controlled trials are needed to provide answers to these important questions.

26.2 How to Perform Tracheostomy

Elective tracheostomy is a widely accepted and commonly performed technique for long-term airway access in critically ill patients. It probably offers several benefits over long-term endotracheal intubation. Different tracheostomy procedures are now established: the conventional open surgical technique (OT), performed worldwide in its actual version for decades (Jackson 1909), and the recently appraised percutaneous tracheostomy techniques (PT), which are more simple to perform at the patient's bedside and are being used increasingly (Ciaglia et al. 1985; Fantoni and Ripamonti 1997; Griggs et al. 1990; Kearney et al. 2000). Data in the literature are now numerous and can help in the choice of practical modalities for tracheostomy. There is convincing evidence that PT, performed at the ICU bedside by an experienced intensivist, can be done safely, with mortality and morbidity at least comparable to those observed for OT, carried out in the operating room by an experienced surgeon (Cheng 2000; Freeman et al. 2000; Friedman et al. 1996; Gysin et al. 1999; Heikkinen and Hannukainen 2000; Holdgaard et al. 1998). In addition, the cost per patient for the procedure is significantly reduced (Cobean et al. 1996; Friedman et al. 1996; Van Natta et al. 1998; Westphal et al. 1999).

26.2.1 Practical Issues

Which Operator and Where?

If the operating room is probably the best location to perform tracheostomy, the low availability of both rooms and staff, combined with risks generated by the transportation of sometimes highly unstable patients (Indeck et al. 1988; Smith and Cernaianu 1990), will make it easier to perform at the ICU bedside. In the literature, peri- and postoperative complication rates do not differ according to the location (Upadhyay et al. 1996; Wease et al. 1996). Every experienced physician, whether surgeon or intensivist, can perform tracheostomy at the ICU bedside under acceptable security conditions (Cobean et al. 1996; Van Natta et al. 1998).

Ease of use, availability of operators and rooms, and low morbidity rates associated with both techniques in experienced hands argue for the performance of tracheostomy by the intensivist at the ICU bedside, thus eliminating the need to transport patients from their optimal ICU environment.

Patient's Installation and Preparation

Installation and preparation are essential issues that may directly influence tracheostomy success. The patient must be sedated and paralyzed, in order to suppress cough and deglutition reflexes. He will then lie supine, with the neck in slight extension (in the absence of any contraindication). The skin is surgically prepared, in association with an oropharyngeal antiseptic toilet. Oxygen concentration is increased to 100% and ventilatory parameters are adapted to the patient's status. Monitoring of the patient will include at least arterial tension, heart rate, and pulse oximetry recordings. End-tidal CO_2 monitoring is interesting to detect hypercarbia related to repeated bronchoscopy. When PT is performed, the endotracheal tube must be placed within or immediately below the vocal cords to avoid puncture of the endotracheal tube cuff. Unlike OT, only one operator is required to perform PT, in association with an experienced intensivist for airway control and endoscopy throughout the procedure.

Anatomical Marks

Whatever technique is chosen, the tracheostomy site should be set between the first and the fourth tracheal ring. Risks of the procedure include subglottic stenosis and irreversible voice changes (Jackson 1921; Kuriloff et al. 1989), venous erosion, and tracheal stenosis that may be cured only by a mediastinal access.

26.2.2 Different Tracheostomy Techniques

Open Surgical Tracheostomy

OT is considered the standard technique for long-term airway access, but many variants do exist: the skin incision may be either vertical or horizontal, large or narrow; the thyroid may be pushed down or sectioned, thus requiring vascular ligation; tracheal access may be a round patch, a U-flap, or a vertical incision. These variants may be responsible for the highly variable complication rate reported in the literature (between 6% and 66%) (Quintel 1999).

Percutaneous Tracheostomy

PT was first described in the early 1960s (Sheldon et al. 1955; Toye 1969) but has gained a worldwide acceptance since the description of the modified technique by Ciaglia and co-workers (Ciaglia et al. 1985). All techniques require the percutaneous placement of a guidewire into the trachea under direct bronchoscopic guidance. Dilation and tracheostomy tube placement are then achieved using the Seldinger catheter over-wire technique. PT may thus result in less tissue dissection and a smaller skin incision. It is also attractive for various logistic reasons: speed of the procedure, elimination of the need to transport the patient to the operating room, and no need to schedule operating room time.

Anterograde PT Techniques

Several steps are common to both anterograde PT techniques, as described by Ciaglia and associates (Ciaglia et al. 1985) and Griggs and colleagues (Griggs et al. 1990) (see Fig. 26.1). The trachea is punctured by a 18-gauge needle with an outer Teflon sheath. When free aspiration of the tracheal air column is confirmed, the Seldinger technique is used to insert a J-guidewire into the tracheal lumen. A short 11-French punch dilator is then inserted after a small skin incision has been made.

Percutaneous Dilational Tracheostomy Using Serial Dilators. This dilational technique was first described by Ciaglia and co-workers in 1985 (Ciaglia et al. 1985). Several commercial kits are now available, with no significant differences between them (Pothmann et al. 1997). After the small dilator is removed, an 8-French clear plastic guiding catheter with a ridge is passed and left in place within the guidewire, to increase its stiffness and facilitate dilator insertion throughout the entire procedure (see Fig. 26.2). Progressive dilation with dilators ranging from 12- to 36-French is then performed over both the guidewire and the guiding catheter. A lubricated tracheostomy tube is introduced into the trachea loaded over an appropriately sized dilator (24-French for an 8-mm ID tracheostomy tube). The endotracheal tube is removed after the tracheostomy tube position has been confirmed under bronchoscopy. Ciaglia's is probably the most popular PT technique. The great majority of published and/or randomized data are derived from this technique.

Percutaneous Dilational Tracheostomy Using a Single Dilator (Blue Rhino Technique). This technique is the newest evolution of the conventional Ciaglia kit. Serial dilation is replaced by one-step progressive dilation, by means of a single curved dilator (see Fig. 26.2). The great simplicity of this device will probably

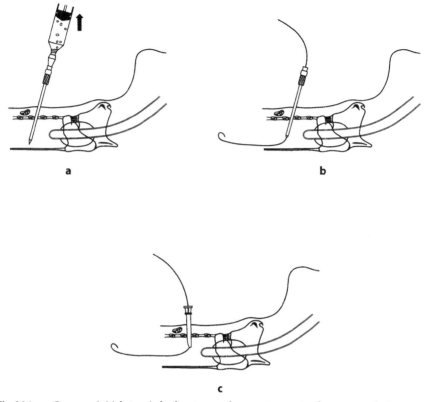

Fig. 26.1a–c. Common initial steps in both anterograde percutaneous tracheostomy techniques, as described by Ciaglia et al. and Griggs et al. The endotracheal tube is withdrawn beneath or immediately below the vocal cords. The trachea is punctured between the first and fourth tracheal ring. Right intratracheal position of the needle is confirmed by free air aspiration and bronchoscopy (**a**). The guidewire is inserted to the carina and the catheter removed (**b**). A first dilation using a small 11-French punch dilator is performed after a 0.5- to 1-cm skin incision has been made (**c**)

make it a widely used technique, even if there are only a few published data at present (Byhahn et al. 2000).

Percutaneous Dilational Tracheostomy Using Forceps (Griggs Technique). Several techniques using forceps have been developed in parallel with dilational techniques (Griggs et al. 1990; Schachner et al. 1989) . The Griggs technique (Portex) is the only available kit to date. A specific and reusable curved forceps is inserted into the trachea in the closed position, guided by a slightly stiffer guidewire. A first dilation is performed by opening the forceps in the pretracheal tissues, and the final dilation is performed by opening the forceps inside the trachea and taking it out in the open position (see Fig. 26.3). A specific tracheostomy tube with a modified obturator is then inserted into the trachea on the guidewire. The Griggs technique is probably the simplest and quickest of the PT techniques.

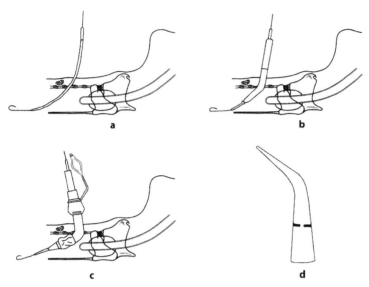

Fig. 26.2a–d. Conventional Ciaglia and Blue Rhino anterograde percutaneous dilational tracheostomy technique. An 8-French specific guiding catheter with a ridge is passed and left in place within the guidewire (**a**). Serial dilation is performed using dilators ranging from 12- to 36-French, over both the guidewire and the guiding catheter (**b**). A conventional tracheostomy tube is introduced into the trachea using an appropriately sized dilator (**c**). The Blue Rhino is the newest evolution of the Ciaglia kit. Serial dilation is replaced by one-step progressive dilation, by means of a single curved dilator (**d**)

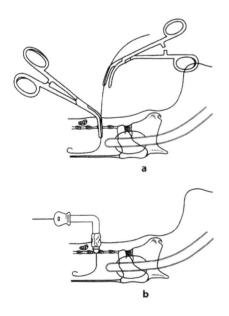

Fig. 26.3a,b. Griggs anterograde percutaneous tracheostomy technique. A specific curved forceps is inserted in the closed position into the trachea over the guidewire. A first dilation is performed opening the forceps in the pretracheal tissues, and the final dilation is performed opening the forceps inside the trachea and taking it out in the open position (**a**). A specific tracheostomy tube with a modified obturator is then inserted into the trachea, loaded over the guidewire (**b**)

Translaryngeal Retrograde PT (Fantoni Technique)

Translaryngeal retrograde PT (TLT) is derived from the percutaneous gastrostomy technique (Fantoni and Ripamonti 1997); i.e., dilation is performed from the inside to the outside, using a specific cone-shaped tube device (see Fig. 26.4). The operator inserts the curved needle into the trachea under bronchoscopic guidance. The metal guide is then inserted in a retrograde fashion, either laterally or inside the endotracheal tube. The cone-shaped tube is connected to the guidewire. The conventional endotracheal tube is withdrawn and replaced by a small 5-mm ID tube with a low-pressure cuff, positioned to the carina. Outward traction of the guidewire begins using the specific grip and the aid of two fingers, exerting a counterpressure to restrict tracheal wall movement. As soon as the metal point of the cone appears, two small incisions are made to favor exiting of the whole cone and part of the tube. The cone is then separated from the tube by sectioning it at the point indicated by the arrows. A special obturator is used to straighten the tube, and after a half rotation on the axis, the cannula is pushed downward.

TLT offers many advantages over anterograde techniques: dilation occurs from the inside to the outside; i.e., tracheal laceration is almost impossible; the bleeding rate is low due to progressive dilation and continuous hemostasis. Aside from these advantages, it seems more complex to learn and requires an initial extubation.

General Issues Concerning PT

Bronchoscopic Guidance. All percutaneous tracheostomy techniques are considered "blind techniques". Bronchoscopic guidance serves several purposes. It has been advocated to avoid injury and ensure correct tracheostomy position (Pothmann et al. 1997; Walz and Schmidt 1999). Perforation risk of the tracheal posterior wall is reduced. The endotracheal tube can be advanced or withdrawn as necessary, and the tracheostomy tube can be seen to enter the tracheal lumen. It may also serve pedagogic goals (Barba et al. 1995), especially during the learning-curve phase. In a prospective study by Berrouschot et al. (Berrouschot et al. 1997) the perioperative complication rates of percutaneous tracheostomy with and without bronchoscopy were similar (6% and 7%). However, the more severe complications occurred in the group that underwent tracheostomy without bronchoscopic guidance.

Contraindications to the Use of PT. Certain contraindications to the use of PT have been identified, such as a neck mass or trauma and inadequate access to the trachea. Although marked obesity has been considered a contraindication by some authors, careful positioning and bronchoscopic guidance may allow the use of PT in such patients (Barba et al. 1995; Mansharamani et al. 2000). In contrast, coagulopathy could be regarded as a specific indication for PT because of the low bleeding rate described with both techniques, especially TLT (McCallum et al. 2000; Westphal et al. 1999), but more experience is needed before recommendations can be made. Emergency situations are also regarded as relative contraindications to PT, but, where an ENT surgeon is unavailable, it could also be lifesaving (Divatia et al. 1999; L'Her et al. 2001).

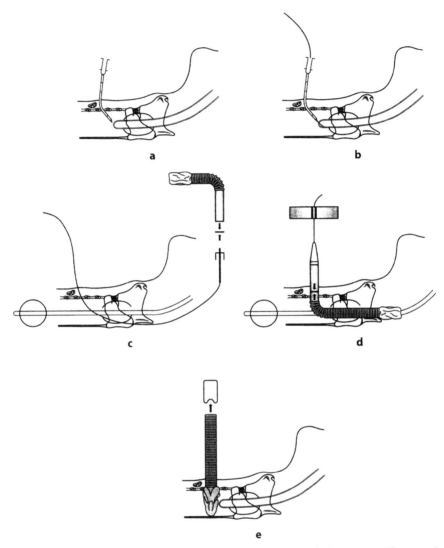

Fig. 26.4a–e. Fantoni retrograde percutaneous tracheostomy technique. A specific curved needle is inserted into the tracheal lumen (**a**). The guidewire is then passed laterally or inside the endotracheal tube, directed to the mouth (**b**). The cone-shaped tube device is loaded over the guidewire. The endotracheal tube is replaced by a small catheter (ID=5 mm) with a low-pressure cuff, positioned to the carina (**c**). Outward traction of the guidewire is performed using the specific grip (**d**). The cone is separated from the tube. A special obturator is used to straighten the tube, and after 180° rotation on the axis the cannula is then pushed downward (**e**)

26.2.3 Comparison Between OT and PT

Specific Disadvantages of PT Techniques

Several common disadvantages need to be addressed. The first is the difficulty of finding the opening stoma into the tracheal lumen during subsequent tracheostomy tube change. This event can be avoided by waiting 5–6 days before the first tube change, in order for the stoma to be fixed. The second is paratracheal-paramedial insertion, which may be limited by using bronchoscopic guidance.

Specific disadvantages such as tracheal ring rupture and tracheal posterior wall laceration can be addressed for the anterograde techniques, even if they seem to be rare and also limited by the use of bronchoscopic guidance. Several main disadvantages to the retrograde technique are the need for endotracheal reintubation with a small-diameter tube and difficulties during the insertion of the tracheostomy tube. Difficult endotracheal intubation can be avoided by using either a specific exchange catheter during endotracheal tube retrieval or a laryngeal mask, which may allow both oxygenation and/or ventilation if the small-diameter tube cannot be inserted.

Comparison Between OT and PT

Both OT and PT are associated with known complications which include local bleeding, stomal infection, and late tracheal stenosis. In the initial otolaryngological reports PT was associated with high complication rates. Wang et al. even recommended that the technique be abandoned (Wang et al. 1992), whereas some large recent open studies did find lower bleeding and stoma infection rates using PT (Kearney et al. 2000). In the first published randomized study, using a serial dilation technique, Hazard observed a significantly decreased postoperative complication rate, especially concerning stomal infection (Hazard et al. 1991). In a similar study by Friedman, no difference was observed between OT and PT, but the authors did question the economic benefits of PT (Friedman et al. 1996). In another randomized study using a dilational technique, Holdgaard also observed a significantly lower stomal infection rate for PT, which could have been related to less subcutaneous tissue dissection and a perfect congruence between the stoma and the cannula (Holdgaard et al. 1998).

Both recent meta-analyses by Freeman (Freeman et al. 2000) and Cheng (Cheng 2000) concluded that OT had a significantly higher complication rate than PT, and that these complications were often more severe. They both concluded that PT was the safer procedure for elective tracheostomy in appropriately selected critically ill patients.

Comparison Between the Different PT Techniques

A number of PT techniques have been established within the past several years. Some, such as the Rapitrach (Schachner et al. 1989) have been abandoned because of a high complication rate. There are only a few studies comparing these techniques. The low number of patients in each study does not allow the definitive choice of one procedure over another, but the main positive prospective studies were published using dilational techniques. Although some data showed very few complications of percutaneous dilational tracheostomy in experienced hands (Escarment et al. 2000; Griggs et al. 1991), there may be a lower risk of bleeding and of posterior tracheal wall laceration with TLT.

26.2.4 Conclusion

Numerous large comparative studies, few randomized studies, and several recent meta-analyses demonstrate that PT has complication rates at least as low or lower than those with OT. It has been shown that PT is significantly quicker to perform than OT, and that it is cost-saving. Both techniques are quite easy to learn, and the associated complications seem to decrease as the operator gains experience. An essential issue with the different percutaneous tracheostomy techniques is adequate puncture of the trachea with the needle. Correct placement will then be confirmed by bronchoscopy.

We believe that PT is the procedure of choice for most critically ill patients who require tracheostomy. Data are still insufficient to guide the choice of one technique over the other. However, a cautionary note is appropriate: The simplicity of the PT procedure should never lead to misuse. A lower risk does not imply a less serious consideration of indications.

26.3 References

Astrachan DI, Kirchner JC, Goodwin WJ jr (1988) Prolonged intubations vs. tracheotomy: complications, practical and psychological considerations. Laryngoscope 98:1165–1169

Barba CA, Angood PB, Kauder DR, Latenser B, Martin K, McGonigal MD, Phillips GR, Rotondo MF, Schwab W (1995) Bronchoscopic guidance makes percutaneous tracheostomy a safe, cost-effective, and easy-to-teach procedure. Surgery 118:879–883

Berrouschot J, Oeken J, Steiniger L, Schneider D (1997) Perioperative complications of percutaneous dilatational tracheostomy. Laryngoscope 107:1538–1544

Blot F, Itemberg G, Guiget M, Casetta M, Antoun S, Pico J, Leclercq B, Escudier B (1995) Safety of tracheotomy in neutropenic patients: a retrospective study of 26 consecutive cases. Intensive Care Med 21:687–790

Byhahn C, Wilke HJ, Halbig S, Lischke V, Westphal K (2000) Percutaneous tracheostomy: Ciaglia Blue Rhino versus the basic Ciaglia technique of percutaneous dilational tracheostomy. Anesth Analg 91:882–886

Cheng E, Fee WE jr (2000) Dilatational versus standard tracheostomy: a meta-analysis. Ann Otol Rhinol Laryngol 109:803–807

Ciaglia P, Firsching R, Syniec C (1985) Elective percutaneous dilatational tracheostomy: a new simple bedside procedure – preliminary report. Chest 87:715–719

Cobean R, Beals M, Moss C, Bredenberg CE (1996) Percutaneous dilatational tracheostomy. A safe and cost-effective bedside procedure. Arch Surg 131:265–271

Diehl JL, Lofaso F, Deleuze P, Similowski T, Lemaire F, Brochard L (1994) Clinically relevant diaphragmatic dysfunction after cardiac operations. J Thoracic Cardiovasc Surg 107:487–498

Diehl JL, El Atrous S, Touchard D, Lemaire F, Brochard L (1999) Changes in the work of breathing induced by tracheotomy of ventilator-dependent patients. Am J Respir Crit Care Med 159:383–388

Divatia JV, Kulkarni AP, Sindhkar S, Upadhye SM (1999) Failed intubation in the intensive care unit managed with laryngeal mask airway and percutaneous tracheostomy. Anaesth Intensive Care 27:409–411

El Naggar M, Sadagopan S, Levine H, Kantor H, Collins VJ (1976) Factors influencing choice between tracheotostomy and prolonged translaryngeal intubation in acute respiratory failure: a prospective study. Anesth Analg 55:195–201

Escarment J, Suppini A, Sallaberry M, Kaiser E, Cantais E, Palmier B, Quinot JF (2000) Percutaneous tracheostomy by forceps dilation: report of 162 cases. Anesthesia 55:125–130

Esteban A, Frutos F, Anzueto A, Alia I, Stewart T, Benito S, Brochard L, Palizas F, Matamis D, Nightingale P, et al (2001) Impact of tracheostomy on outcome of mechanical ventilation. Am J Respir Crit Care Med (In press) A

Fantoni A, Ripamonti D (1997) A non-derivative, non surgical tracheostomy: the translaryngeal method. Intensive Care Med 23:386–392

Fischler L, Erhart S, Kleger G-R, Frutiger A (2000) Prevalence of tracheotomy in ICU patients. A nation-wide survey in Switzerland. Intensive Care Med 26:1428–1433

Freeman BD, Isabella K, Lin N, Buchman TG (2000) A meta-analysis of prospective trials comparing percutaneous and surgical tracheostomy in critically ill patients. Chest 118:1412–1418

Friedman Y, Fildes J, Mizock B, Samuel J, Patel S, Appavu S, Roberts R (1996) Comparison of percutaneous and surgical tracheostomies. Chest 110:480–485

Georges H, Leroy O, Guery B, Alfandari S, Beaucaire G (2000) Predisposing factors for nosocomial pneumonia in patients receiving mechanical ventilation and requiring trachetomy. Chest 118:767–774

Griggs WM, Myburg JA, Worthley LI (1991) A prospective comparison of a percutaneous tracheostomy technique with standard surgical tracheostomy. Intensive Care Med 17:261–263

Griggs WM, Worthley LI, Gilligan JE, Thomas PD, Myburg JA (1990) A simple percutaneous tracheostomy technique. Surgery 170:543–545

Gysin C, Dulguerov P, Guyot JP, Perneger TV, Abajo B, Chevrolet JC (1999) Percutaneous versus surgical tracheostomy. A double-blind randomized trial. Ann Surg 230:708–714

Hazard P, Jones C, Benitone J (1991) Comparative clinical trial of standard operative tracheostomy with percutaneous tracheostomy. Crit Care Med 19:1018–1024

Heffner JE (1993) Timing of tracheotomy in mechanically ventilated patients. Am Rev Respir Dis 147:768–771

Heikkinen M, Aarnio P, Hannukainen J (2000) Percutaneous dilational tracheostomy or conventional surgical tracheostomy? Crit Care Med 28:1399–1402

Holdgaard HO, Pedersen J, Jensen RH, Outzen KE, Midtgaard T, Johansen LV, et al (1998) Percutaneous dilatational tracheostomy versus conventional surgical tracheostomy. Acta Anaesthesiol Scand 42:545–550

Holzapfel L, Chastang C, Demingeon G, Bohe J, Piralla B, Coupry A (1999) A randomized study assessing the systematic search for maxillary sinusitis in nasotracheally mechanically ventilated patients. Am J Respir Crit Care Med 159:695–701

Indeck M, Peterson S, Smith J, Brotman S (1988) Risk, cost, and benefit of transporting ICU patients for special studies. J Trauma 28:1020–1025

Jackson C (1909) Tracheotomy. Laryngoscope 18:285–290

Jackson C (1921) High tracheostomy and other errors: the chief causes of chronic laryngeal stenosis. Surg Gyn Obstet 32:392–398

Kearney PA, Griffen MM, Ochoa JB, Boulanger BR, Tseui BJ, Mentzer RM (2000) A single-center 8-year experience with percutaneous dilational tracheostomy. Ann Surg 231:701–706

Kollef MH, Ahrens TS, Shannon W (1999) Clinical predictors and outcomes for patients requiring tracheostomy in the intensive care unit. Crit Care Med 27:1714–1720

Kuriloff D, Setzen M, Portnoy W, Gadaleta D (1989) Laryngotracheal injury following cricothyroidotomy. Laryngoscope 99:125–130

Lessard MR, Brochard LJ (1996) Weaning from ventilatory support. Clinics Chest Med 17:475–489

L'Her E, Goetghebeur D, Boumediene A, Renault A, Boles JM (2001) Use of the Blue Rhino tracheostomy set for emergency airway management. Intensive Care Med 27:322

Mansharamani NG, Koziel H, Garland R, LoCicero J, Critchlow J, Ernst A (2000) Safety of bedside percutaneous dilatational tracheostomy in obese patients in the ICU. Chest 117:1426–1429

Maziak DE, Meade MO, Todd TR (1998) The timing of tracheotomy: a systematic review. Chest 114:605–609

McCallum PL, Parnes LS, Sharpe MD, Harris C (2000) Comparison of open, percutaneous, and translaryngeal tracheostomies. Otolaryngol Head Neck Surg 122:686–690

Morar P, Singh V, Jones A, Hughes J, van Seene R (1998) Impact of tracheotomy on colonization and infection of lower airways in children requiring long-term ventilation: a prospective observational cohort study. Chest 113:77–85

Plummer AL, Gracey DR (1989) Consensus conference on artificial airways in patients receiving mechanical ventilation. Chest 96:178–180

Pothmann W, Tonner PH, Shulte am Esch J (1997) Percutaneous dilatational tracheostomy: risk and benefits. Intensive Care Med 23:610–612

Quintel M, Roth H (1999) Tracheostomy in the critically ill: clinical impact of new procedures. Intensive Care Med 25:326–328

Qureshi A, Suarez JI, Parekh PD, Bahardwaj A (2000) Prediction and timing of tracheostomy in patients with infratentorial lesions requiring mechanical ventilatory support. Crit Care Med 28:1383–1387

Rouby JJ, Laurent P, Gosnach M, Cambau E, Lamas G, Zouaoui A, Leguillou JL, Bodin L, Do Khac T, Marsault C, et al (1994) Risk factors and clinical relevance of nosocomial maxillary sinusitis in the critically ill. Am J Respir Crit Care Med 150:776–783

Schachner A, Ovil Y, Sidi J, Rogev M, Heilbronn Y, Levy MJ (1989) Percutaneous tracheostomy: a new method. Crit Care Med 17:1052–1056

Sheldon CHPR, Freshwater DB, Crue BL (1955) A new method for tracheostomy. J Neurosurg 12:428–431

Smith I, Fleming S, Cernaianu A (1990) Mishaps during transport from the intensive care unit. Crit Care Med 18:278–281

Stauffer JL, Olson DE, Petty TLE (1981) Complications and consequences of endotracheal intubation and tracheotomy. A prospective study of 150 critically ill adult patients. Am J Med 70:65–76

Toye FJ, Weinstein JD (1969) A percutaneous tracheostomy device. Surgery 65:384–389

Upadhyay A, Maurer J, Turner J, Tiszenkel H, Rosengart T (1996) Elective bedside tracheostomy in the intensive care unit. J Am Coll Surg 182:51–55

Vallverdu I, Calaf N, Subirana M, Net A, Benito S, Mancebo J (1998) Clinical characteristic, respiratory functional parameters and outcome of a 2-hour T-piece trial in patients weaning from mechanical ventilation. Am J Respir Crit Care Med 158:1855–1862

Van Natta TL, Morris JA, Eddy VA, Nunn CR, Rutherford EJ, Neuzil D, et al (1998) Elective bedside surgery in critically injured patient is safe and cost-effective. Ann Surg 227:618–626

Villafane M, Cinnella G, Lofaso F, Isabey D, Harf A, Lemaire F, Brochard L (1996) Gradual reduction of endotracheal tube diameter during mechanical ventilation via different humidification devices. Anesthesiology 85:1341–1349

Walz MK, Schmidt U (1999) Tracheal lesion caused by percutaneous dilatational tracheostomy – a clinico-pathological study. Intensive Care Med 25:102–105

Wang MBG, Ware PH, Calcatera T, Watson D (1992) Early experience with percutaneous tracheostomy. Laryngoscope 102:157–162

Wease GL, Frikker M, Villalba M, Glover J (1996) Bedside tracheostomy in the intensive care unit. Arch Surg 131:552–555

Westphal K, Byhahn C, Wilke HJ, Lischke V (1999) Percutaneous tracheostomy: a clinical comparison of dilatational (Ciaglia) and translaryngeal (Fantoni) techniques. Anesth Analg 89:938–943

Wright PE, Marini JJ, Bernard GR (1989) In vitro versus in vivo comparison of endotracheal tube airflow resistance. Am Rev Respir Dis 140:10–16

Subject Index

Printed in the United States
By Bookmasters